Veterinary Pathology

A Comprehensive Guide

Veterinary Pathology
A Comprehensive Guide

Dr. Shashi Bhushan Sahai

Oxford Book Company
Jaipur • New Delhi

ISBN : 9789355245793

First published in India, 2026

Oxford Book Company
Regd. Off. "Bony Residency", Gate No. 2
Opp. Tilak Public School, Vishweswariya Nagar,
Gopalpura Road, Jaipur - 302018, India
Ph: 0141 - 2761280, Telefax: 2761381
email - oxfordbookjpr@gmail.com
website - oxfordbookcompany.com

Delhi Office: 102, 1st Floor, Satyam House,
4327/3, Ansari Road, Darya Ganj,
New Delhi - 110002, India
Ph: 011-45652440

Distributed By
KEYA INTERNATIONAL PRESS LLP
E-mail: keyainternationalpressllp@gmail.com

Printed and bound in India by Thomson Press Ltd., New Delhi

Contents

Preface

The history of pathology can be traced back to antiquity when people began examining bodies. The examination of bodies led to the dissection of bodies in order to justify the cause of death. During that time, the people already began formulating today what we know as inflammation, tumors, boils, and much more. Pathology began to develop as a subject during the 19th Century through teachers and physicians that studied pathology. They referred to it as "pathological anatomy" or "morbid anatomy." However, pathology as a field of medicine was not recognised until the late 19th and early 20th centuries.

In the 19th century, physicians realised that disease-causing pathogens, germs, created themselves and that symptoms were not the vital characteristics of a disease. Through the new information gathered regarding germ reproduction, physicians began to compare the characteristics of one germ's symptoms as they developed within an affected individual to another germ's characteristics and symptoms. This realisation led to the foundational understanding that diseases are able to create themselves, and that they can affect human beings in unique ways. In order to determine causes of diseases, medical experts used the most common and widely accepted assumptions or symptoms of their times. This is true for those in the past and today. Pathologists are physicians who diagnose and characterize disease in living patients by examining biopsies or bodily fluid. Pathologists may also conduct autopsies to investigate causes of death. Pathology is a core discipline of medical school and many pathologists are also instructors. As managers of medical laboratories, pathologists play an important role in the development of laboratory information systems. Although the medical practice of pathology grew out of the tradition of investigative pathology, most modern pathologists do not perform original research. Pathology is a unique medical speciality in that pathologists typically do not see patients directly, but rather serve as consultants to other physicians (often referred to as "clinicians" within the pathology community). To be licensed, candidates must complete medical training, an approved residency program and be certified by an appropriate body. In the US, certification is by the American Board of Pathology or the American Osteopathic Board of Pathology. The organisation of subspecialities within pathology varies between nations, but usually includes anatomical pathology and clinical pathology.

Many pathologists pursue a broad based training and become certified in both fields. These skills are complementary in many hospital based private practice settings, since the day to day work of many clinical laboratories only intermittently requires the attention of a physician. Thus, pathologists are able to spend much of their time evaluating anatomical pathology cases, while remaining available to cover any special issues which might arise in the clinical laboratories. Pathologists may pursue specialised fellowship training within one or more subspecialities of either anatomical or clinical pathology. Some of these subspecialities permit additional board certification, while others do not.

Hence, this well-knitted; well-researched and well-debated work on this subject is highly academic and research quality will be appreciated and accepted by students; scholars and teachers.

—Dr. Shashi Bhushan Sahai

Chapter 1

Introduction

Pathology

Pathology is the precise study and diagnosis of disease. *Pathologization*, to pathologize, refers to the process of defining a condition or behaviour as pathological, e.g. pathological gambling. Pathologies is synonymous with diseases. The suffix "path" is used to indicate a disease, e.g. psychopath.

Pathology addresses four components of disease: cause/etiology, mechanisms of development (pathogenesis), structural alterations of cells (morphologic changes), and the consequences of changes (clinical manifestations). Pathology is further separated into divisions, based on either the system being studied (e.g. veterinary pathology and animal disease) or the focus of the examination (e.g. forensic pathology and determining the cause of death). General pathology is a broad and complex scientific field which seeks to understand the mechanisms of injury to cells and tissues, as well as the body's means of responding to and repairing injury. Areas of study include cellular adaptation to injury, necrosis, inflammation, wound healing, and neoplasia. It forms the foundation of pathology, the application of this knowledge to diagnose diseases in humans and animals. The term *general pathology* is also used to describe the practice of both anatomical and clinical pathology.

History

The history of pathology can be traced back to antiquity when people began examining bodies. The examination of bodies led to the dissection of bodies in order to justify the cause of death. During that time, the people already began formulating today what we know as inflammation, tumors, boils, and much more. Pathology began to develop as a subject during the 19th Century through teachers and physicians that studied pathology. They referred to it as "pathological anatomy" or "morbid anatomy." However, pathology as a field of medicine was not recognised until the late 19th and early 20th centuries.

In the 19th century, physicians realised that disease-causing pathogens, germs, created themselves and that symptoms were not the vital characteristics of a disease. Through the new information gathered regarding germ reproduction, physicians began to compare the characteristics of one germ's symptoms as they developed within an affected individual to another germ's characteristics and symptoms.

This realisation led to the foundational understanding that diseases are able to create themselves, and that they can affect human beings in unique ways. In order to determine causes of diseases, medical experts used the most common and widely accepted assumptions or symptoms of their times. This is true for those in the past and today.

What set pathology apart from other specialities was the ability to determine a symptom with the naked eye. During the 19th century, Rudolf Virchow gave the biggest contribution to the field by introducing the procedure of analyzing tissue and cells through a microscope to pathologists. This greatly affected the discipline because it was another way to analyze objects, and it led to more advanced technological developments.

By the late 1920s to early 1930s pathology was deemed a medical speciality. During the years following, the decision to split pathology in to sub-specialities arose. Today, anatomical, clinical, molecular, plant, forensic, oral, veterinary, dermato-pathology, hematopathology, and pathology exist as medical specialities. Today, pathologists are discovering new diseases, examining exotic diseases that enter the country, and working on a solution to cure diseases such as AIDS, HIV, Herpes, cancer, and more. Thus the evolution of pathology is evidence of the real value of science, which lies in its ability to continually research and develop new methods while giving credit to those who originally developed the idea.

Anatomical Pathology

Anatomical pathology (*Commonwealth*) or Anatomic pathology (*U.S.*) is a medical speciality that is concerned with the diagnosis of disease based on the gross, microscopic, chemical, immunologic and molecular examination of organs, tissues, and whole bodies (autopsy). Its modern beginner was the Italian scientist Giovan Battista Morgagni from Forlì.

Anatomical pathology is one of two branches of pathology, the other being clinical pathology, the diagnosis of disease through the laboratory analysis of bodily fluids and/or tissues. Often, pathologists practice both anatomical and clinical pathology, a combination known as general pathology.

The distinction between anatomic and clinical pathology is increasingly blurred by the introduction of technologies that require new expertise and the need to provide patients and referring physicians with integrated diagnostic reports. Similar specialities exist in veterinary pathology.

Differences Between Anatomic Pathology and Clinical Pathology

Anatomic pathology relates to the processing of surgical and gynecological specimens. Its subsections usually include surgical pathology, histology and cytology.

Clinical pathology is the division that processes the test requests more familiar to the general public; such as blood cell counts, coagulation studies, urinalysis, blood glucose level determinations and throat cultures. Its subsections include chemistry, hematology, microbiology, immunology, urinalysis and blood bank.

Anatomical pathology is itself divided in subspecialities, the main ones being surgical pathology, cytopathology, and forensic pathology.

In many countries, to be licensed to practice pathology, one has to complete medical school and secure a license to practice medicine. An approved residency program and certification (in the U.S., the American Board of Pathology or the American Osteopathic Board of Pathology) is usually required to obtain employment or hospital privileges.

Skills and Procedures

The procedures used in anatomic pathology include:

- *Gross examination:* the examination of diseased tissues with the naked eye. This is important especially for large tissue fragments, because the disease can often be visually identified. It is also at this step that the pathologist selects areas that will be processed for histopathology. The eye can sometimes be aided with a magnifying glass or a stereo microscope, especially when examining parasitic organisms.
- *Histopathology:* the microscopic examination of stained tissue sections using histological techniques. The standard stains are haematoxylin and eosin, but many others exist. The use of haematoxylin and eosin-stained slides to provide specific diagnoses based on morphology is considered to be the core skill of anatomic pathology. The science of staining tissues sections is called histochemistry.
- *Immunohistochemistry :* the use of antibodies to detect the presence, abundance, and localisation of specific proteins. This technique is critical to distinguishing between disorders with similar morphology, as well as characterizing the molecular properties of certain cancers.
- *In situ hybridization:* Specific DNA and RNA molecules can be identified on sections using this technique. When the probe is labelled with fluorescent dye, the technique is called FISH.
- *Cytopathology:* the examination of loose cells spread and stained on glass slides using cytology techniques.
- *Electron microscopy:* the examination of tissue with an electron microscope, which allows much greater magnification, enabling the visualization of organelles within the cells. Its use has been largely supplanted by immunohistochemistry, but it is still in common use for certain tasks, including the diagnosis of kidney disease and the identification of immotile cilia syndrome among many others.

- *Tissue cytogenetics:* the visualization of chromosomes to identify genetics defects such as chromosomal translocation.
- *Flow immunophenotyping:* the determination of the immunophenotype of cells using flow cytometry techniques. It is very useful to diagnose the different types of leukemia and lymphoma.

Surgical Pathology

Surgical pathology is the most significant and time-consuming area of practice for most anatomical pathologists. Surgical pathology involves the gross and microscopic examination of surgical specimens, as well as biopsies submitted by surgeons and non-surgeons such as general internists, medical subspecialists, dermatologists, and interventional radiologists.

The practice of surgical pathology allows for definitive diagnosis of disease (or lack thereof) in any case where tissue is surgically removed from a patient. This is usually performed by a combination of gross (i.e., macroscopic) and histologic (i.e., microscopic) examination of the tissue, and may involve evaluations of molecular properties of the tissue by immunohistochemistry or other laboratory tests.

Specimens

There are two major types of specimens submitted for surgical pathology analysis: *biopsies* and *surgical resections.* A *biopsy* is a small piece of tissue removed primarily for the purposes of surgical pathology analysis, most often in order to render a definitive diagnosis.

Types of biopsies include *core biopsies*, which are obtained through the use of large-bore needles, sometimes under the guidance of radiological techniques such as ultrasound, CT scan, or magnetic resonance imaging.

Core biopsies, which preserve tissue architecture, should not be confused with fine needle aspiration specimens, which are analyzed using cytopathology techniques. *Incisional biopsies* are obtained through diagnostic surgical procedures that remove part of a suspicious lesion, whereas *excisional biopsies* remove the entire lesion, and are similar to therapeutic *surgical resections.* Excisional biopsies of skin lesions and gastrointestinal polyps are very common. The pathologist's interpretation of a biopsy is critical to establishing the diagnosis of a benign or malignant tumor, and can differentiate between different types and grades of cancer, as well as determining the activity of specific molecular pathways in the tumor. This information is important for estimating the patient's prognosis and for choosing the best treatment to administer. Biopsies are also used to diagnose diseases other than cancer, including inflammatory, infectious, or idiopathic diseases of the skin and gastrointestinal tract, to name only a few.

Surgical resection specimens are obtained by the therapeutic surgical removal of an entire diseased area or organ (and occasionally multiple organs). These procedures are often intended as definitive surgical treatment of a disease in which the diagnosis is already known or strongly suspected. However, pathological analysis of these specimens is critically important in confirming the previous diagnosis, staging the extent of malignant disease, establishing whether or not the entire diseased area was removed (a process called "determination of the surgical margin often using frozen section), identifying the presence of unsuspected concurrent diseases, and providing information for postoperative treatment, such as adjuvant chemotherapy in the case of cancer.

In the determination of surgical margin of a surgical resection, one can use the bread loafing technique, or CCPDMA. A special type of CCPDMA is named after a general surgeon, or the Mohs surgery method.

Surgical Pathology Workflow

- Gross examination
- Frozen section
- Fixation & Embedding
- Histopathologic examination
- Ancillary testing
- The surgical pathology report
- Direct consultation.

Subspecialities

Many pathologists seek fellowship-level training, or otherwise pursue expertise in a focused area of surgical pathology. Subspecialization is particularly prevalent in the academic setting, where pathologists may specialise in an area of diagnostic surgical pathology that is relevant to their research, but is becoming increasingly prevalent in private practice as well. Subspecialization has a number of benefits, such as allowing for increased experience and skill at interpreting challenging cases, as well as development of a closer working relationship between the pathologist and clinicians within a subspeciality area.

Commonly Recognised Subspecialities of Surgical Pathology include the following:

- Bone pathology
- Cardiac pathology
- Cytopathology (A board-certifiable subspeciality in the U.S.)
- Dermatopathology (A board-certifiable subspeciality in the U.S.)
- Endocrine pathology
- Gastrointestinal pathology
- Genitourinary pathology
- Gynecologic pathology
- Head and Neck Pathology
- Hematopathology (A board-certifiable subspeciality in the U.S.)
- Neuropathology (A board-certifiable subspeciality in the U.S. and a recognised speciality in the U.K.)
- Ophthalmic pathology
- Pediatric pathology (A board-certifiable subspeciality in the U.S. and a recognised speciality in the U.K.)
- Pulmonary pathology
- Renal pathology
- Soft tissue pathology.

Cytopathology

Cytopathology "a hollow"; *pathos*, "fate, harm" is a branch of pathology that studies and diagnoses diseases on the cellular level. The discipline was founded by Rudolf Virchow in 1858. A common application of cytopathology is the Pap smear, used as a screening tool, to detect precancerous cervical lesions and prevent cervical cancer.

Cytopathology is also commonly used to investigate thyroid lesions, diseases involving sterile body cavities (peritoneal, pleural, and cerebrospinal), and a wide range of other body sites. It is usually used to aid in the diagnosis of cancer, but also helps in the diagnosis of certain infectious diseases and other inflammatory conditions. Cytopathology is generally used on samples of free cells or tissue fragments, in contrast to histopathology, which studies whole tissues.

Cytopathologic tests are sometimes called smear tests because the samples may be smeared across a glass microscope slide for subsequent staining and microscopic examination. However, cytology samples may be prepared in other ways, including cytocentrifugation. Different types of smear tests may also be used for cancer diagnosis. In this sense, it is termed a *cytologic smear*. Cytopathology is frequently, less precisely, called cytology, which means "the study of cells."

Cell Collection

Two methods of collecting cells for cytopathologic analysis are:

Exfoliative Cytology: In this method, cells are collected after they have been either spontaneously shed by the body ("spontaneous exfoliation") or manually scraped/brushed off of a surface in the body ("mechanical exfoliation").

An example of spontaneous exfoliation is when cells of the pleural cavity or peritoneal cavity are shed into the pleural or peritoneal fluid. This fluid can be collected via various methods for examination. Examples of mechanical exfoliation include Pap smears, where cells are scraped from the cervix with a cervical spatula, or bronchial brushings, where a bronchoscope is inserted into the trachea and used to evaluate a visible lesion by brushing cells from its surface and subjecting them to cytopathologic analysis.

Intervention Cytology: in interventional cytology the pathologist intervenes into the body for sample collection. Nowadays FNAC has become synonymous to interventional cytology.

Fine: Needle Aspiration Cytology *or* Needle aspiration biopsy – *A needle attached to a syringe is used to collect cells from lesions or masses in various body organs by microcoring, often with the application of negative pressure (suction) to increase yield. FNAC can be performed under palpation guidance (i.e., the clinician can feel the lesion) on a mass in superficial regions like the neck, thyroid or breast; FNAC may also be assisted by ultrasound or CAT scan for sampling of deep-seated lesions within the body that cannot be localised via palpation. FNAC is widely used in many countries, but success rate is dependent on the skill of the practitioner. If performed by a pathologist alone, or as team with pathologist-cytotechnologist, the success rate of proper diagnosis is superior than when performed by a non-pathologist. This may be due to the pathologist's ability to immediately evaluate specimens under a microscope and immediately repeat the procedure if sampling was inadequate.*

Fine needles are 23 to 27 gauge. Because needles as small as 27 gauge can almost always yield diagnostic material, FNAC is often the least injurious way to obtain diagnostic tissue from a lesion. Sometime a syringe holder may be used to facilitate using one hand to perform the biopsy while the other hand is immobilizing the mass. Imaging equipment such as a CT scanner or ultrasound may be used to assist in locating the region to be biopsied.

Sediment Cytology: Here, the sample is collected from the fixative that was used for processing the biopsy or autopsy specimen. The fixative is mixed properly and taken into a centrifuge tube and is centrifuged. The sediment is used for smearing. These sediments are the cells that are shed by the autopsy and biopsy specimen during processing.

Parameters

The nucleus of the cell is very important in evaluating the cellular sample. In cancerous cells, altered DNA activity can be seen as a physical change in the nuclear qualities. Since more DNA is unfolded and being expressed, the nucleus will be darker and less uniform, larger than in normal cells, and often show a bright-red nucleolus.

While the cytologist's primary responsibility is to discern whether cancerous or precancerous pathology is present in the cellular sample analysed, other pathologies may be seen such as:

- Microbial infections: parasitic, viral, and/or bacterial
- Reactive changes
- Immune reactions
- Cell aging
- Amyloidosis
- Autoimmune diseases.

Various normal functions of cell growth, metabolism, and division can fail or work in abnormal ways and lead to diseases. Cytopathology is best used as one of three tools, the second and third being the physical exam and medical imaging. Cytology can be used to diagnose a condition and spare a patient from surgery to obtain a larger specimen. An example is thyroid FNA; many benign conditions can be diagnosed with a superficial biopsy and the patient can go back to normal activities right away. If a malignant condition is diagnosed, the patient may be able to start radiation/chemotherapy, or may need to have surgery to remove and/or stage the cancer.

Some tumors may be difficult to biopsy, such as sarcomas. Other rare tumors my be dangerous to biopsy, such as pheochromocytoma. In general, a fine-needle aspiration can be done anywhere it is safe to put a needle, including liver, lung, kidney, and superficial masses.

Many clinicians are not trained to perform fine-needle aspiration biopsies properly and, then when they do not obtain diagnostic material, believe that cytology is not useful. Proper technique takes time to master. Cytotechnologists and cytopathologists can assist clinicians by going to procedures and assisting with collection techniques. A "quick read" is a peek under the microscope and can tell the clinician whether enough diagnostic material was obtained. Cytological specimens must also be properly prepared so that the cells are not damaged.

Sometimes more information about the specimen is helpful. Immunohistochemical stains and molecular testing can be performed, especially if the sample is prepared using liquid based cytology. Often "reflex" testing is performed, such as HPV testing on an abnormal pap test or flow cytometry on a lymphoma specimen.

Body Regions

Cytopathologic techniques are used in the examination of virtually all body organs and tissues:

- *Gynaecologic cytology:* concerning the female reproductive tract.
- *Urinary tract cytology:* concerning the ureters, urinary bladder and urethra.
- *Effusion cytology:* concerning fluids collections, especially within the peritoneum, pleura and pericardium.
- *Breast cytology:* principally concerning the female breast.
- *Thyroid cytology:* concerning the thyroid gland
- *Lymph node cytology:* concerning lymph nodes
- *Respiratory cytology:* concerning the lungs and airways
- *Gastrointestinal cytology:* concerning the alimentary tract
- Soft tissue, bone and skin cytology
- Kidney and adrenal cytology
- Liver and pancreas cytology
- Central nervous system cytology
- Eye cytology
- Salivary gland cytology.

Oral and Maxillofacial Pathology

In the United States, subspeciality-trained doctors of dentistry, rather than medical doctors, can be certified by a professional board to practice Oral and Maxillofacial Pathology.

Molecular Pathology

Molecular pathology is an emerging discipline within pathology which is focused in the study and diagnosis of disease through the examination of molecules within organs, tissues or bodily fluids. Molecular pathology shares some aspects of practice with both anatomic pathology and clinical pathology, molecular biology, biochemistry, proteomics and genetics, and is sometimes considered a "crossover" discipline. It is multi-disciplinary in nature and focuses mainly on the sub-microscopic aspects of disease.

It is a scientific discipline that encompasses the development of molecular and genetic approaches to the diagnosis and classification of human diseases, the design and validation of predictive biomarkers for treatment response and disease progression, the susceptibility of individuals of different genetic constitution to develop disorders.

Forensic Pathology

Forensic pathology is a branch of pathology concerned with determining the cause of death by examination of a corpse. The autopsy is performed by a coroner or medical examiner usually during the investigation of criminal law cases and civil law cases in some jurisdictions. Coroners and medical examiners are also frequently asked to confirm the identity of a corpse. Also see forensic medicine. The word forensics is derived from the Latin *forçnsis* meaning *forum*.

Scope of Forensic Pathology

Forensic pathology is an application of medical jurisprudence. The *forensic pathologist*:

- Is a medical doctor who has completed training in anatomical pathology and who has subsequently sub-specialized in forensic pathology. The requirements for becoming a "fully qualified" forensic pathologist varies from country to country. Some of the different requirements are discussed below.
- Performs autopsies/postmortem examinations to determine the cause of death. The autopsy report contains an opinion about :
  - o The pathologic process, injury, or disease that directly results in or initiates a series of events that lead to a person's death (also called mechanism of death), such as a bullet wound to the head, exsanguination

caused by a stab wound, manual or ligature strangulation, myocardial infarction resulting from coronary artery disease, etc.), and

- o The "manner of death", the circumstances surrounding the cause of death, which in most jurisdictions include:
  - _ Homicide
  - _ Accidental
  - _ Natural
  - _ Suicide
  - _ Undetermined

- The autopsy also provides an opportunity for other issues raised by the death to be addressed, such as the collection of trace evidence or determining the identity of the deceased.
- Examines and documents wounds and injuries, both at autopsy and occasionally in a clinical setting.
- Collects and examines tissue specimens under the microscope (histology) in order to identify the presence or absence of natural disease and other microscopic findings such as asbestos bodies in the lungs or gunpowder particles around a gunshot wound.
- Collects and interprets toxicological analyses on body tissues and fluids to determine the chemical cause of accidental overdoses or deliberate poisonings.
- Forensic pathologists also work closely with the medico-legal authority for the area concerned with the investigation of sudden and unexpected deaths i.e. the coroner (England and Wales), procurator fiscal (Scotland) or coroner or medical examiner (United States).
- Serves as an expert witness in courts of law testifying in civil or criminal law cases.

In an autopsy, he/she is often assisted by an autopsy/mortuary technician (sometimes called a diener in the USA). Forensic physicians, sometimes referred to as 'forensic medical examiners' or 'police surgeons' (in the UK until recently), are medical doctors trained in the examination of, and provision of medical treatment to, living victims of assault (including sexual assault) and those individuals who find themselves in police custody.

Many forensic physicians in the UK practise clinical forensic medicine part-time, whilst they also practise family medicine, or another medical speciality.

In the United Kingdom, Membership of the Royal College of Pathologists is not a prerequisite of appointment as a Coroner's *Medical Expert*, i.e. doctors in the UK that are not forensic pathologists or pathologists are allowed to perform medicolegal autopsies, simply because of the vague wording of 'The Coroners Act', which merely stipulates a 'suitably qualified medical practitioner', i.e. anyone on the GMC Register.

Investigation of Death

Deaths where the known cause and those considered unnatural are investigated. In most jurisdictions this is done by a *"forensic pathologist", coroner, medical examiner*, or hybrid *medical examiner-coroner* offices.

Terminology is not Consistent Across Jurisdictions

In some jurisdictions, the title of "Medical Examiner" is used by a non-physician, elected official involved in medicolegal death investigation. In others, the law requires the medical examiner to be a physician, pathologist, or forensic pathologist. Similarly, the title "coroner" is applied to both physicians and non-physicians. Historically, coroners were not all physicians (most often serving primarily as the town mortician). However, in some jurisdictions the title of "Coroner" is exclusively used by physicians.

Canadian Coroners

In Canada, there is a mix of coroner and medical examiner systems, depending on the province or territory. In Ontario, coroners are licensed physicians, usually but not exclusively family physicians. In Quebec, there is a mix of medical and non-medical coroners, whereas in British Columbia, there is predominantly a non-physican coroner system. Alberta and Nova Scotia are examples of ME systems.

Coroners and Medical Examiners in the United States

In the United States, a coroner is typically an elected public official in a particular geographic jurisdiction who investigates and certifies deaths. The vast majority of coroners lack a Doctor of Medicine degree and the amount of medical training that they have received is highly variable, depending on their profession (e.g. law enforcement, judges, funeral directors, emergency medical technicians, nurses). In contrast, a medical examiner is typically a physician who holds the degree of Doctor of Medicine or Doctor of Osteopathic Medicine. Ideally, a medical examiner has completed both a pathology residency and a fellowship in forensic pathology. In some jurisdictions, a medical examiner must be both a doctor and a lawyer, with additional training in forensic pathology.

History

Forensic pathology was first recognised in the United States by the American Board of Pathology in 1959. In Canada, it was formally recognised in 2003, and a formal training program (a fellowship) is currently being established under the auspices of the Royal College of Physicians and Surgeons of Canada.

Becoming a Forensic Pathologist: Forensic pathology is a subspeciality of anatomical pathology. Training requirements differ from country to country.

Australia

There are currently three paths to qualify as a forensic pathologist in Australia. The first is to train solely in forensic pathology (although a significant amount of anatomical pathology knowledge is still required) and pass two examinations for forensic pathology only. The second is to commence training in anatomical pathology, and complete an initial anatomical pathology examination, which takes a minimum of three years; then go on to train solely in forensic pathology and complete a forensic pathology examination, which takes a minimum of two years. The third is to complete a minimum 5 years' training in anatomical pathology to qualify as a fellow in anatomical pathology, then complete a post-fellowship year in forensic pathology (a minimum twelve months further training plus successful completion of an examination).

Canada

In Canada, anatomical pathology is a five year residency; Then residents who wish to become forensic pathologists must complete a one year fellowship in forensic pathology. Forensic pathology is a subspeciality by the Royal College of Physicians and Surgeons. Currently, the only training program in Canada is in Toronto, with British Columbia, Manitoba, and Alberta possibly offering fellowships in the near future.

India

In India, the speciality is commonly referred to as Forensic Medicine or Legal Medicine. After completion of medical graduation (MBBS), one has to complete three years of study and training including thesis research, which leads to award of degree of MD (Forensic Medicine). One can also alternately pass the board examination conducted by National Board of Examinations, leading to awarding of Diplomate of National Board (DNB).

The majority of the specialists are attached to the Department of Forensic Medicine in various medical colleges. The classification of posts includes Assistant Professor (Lecturer), Associate Professor (Reader) and Professor.

The work profile of the specialists includes conducting autopsies and clinical forensic examinations; apart from teaching the medical students.

They have to regularly appear in the courts as expert witnesses. A typical department in a government institution conducts 100 to 5000 autopsies a year depending upon the jurisdiction. Apart from this the clinical forensic examinations constitute a major part of the work and number of cases can run up to 10000 a year in an average institution.

The largest association of the speciality are the Indian Academy of Forensic Medicine (IAFM), which also publishes its quarterly journal JIAFM regularly. This association has a specialist member strength of more than 800. The another Ntional body is Indian Congress of Forensic Medicine and Toxicology, it is having its official publication as Indian Internet Journal of Forensic Medicine and Toxicology. The most active regional association is the Punjab Academy of Forensic Medicine

& Toxicology (PAFMAT), which also publishes its journal JPAFMAT biannually regularly since 2001. JPAFMAT is also indexed in many listings and also available through HINARI and SafetyLit. PAFMAT has links with many international bodies including WHO.

Indonesia

In Indonesia, forensic medicine, also known as legal medicine (*"kedokteran kehakiman"*), is a 3-year speciality program that can be taken directly after completing medical school. It is separate from anatomical pathology and clinical pathology.

Upon completion of the program, a forensic medicine specialist will obtain the title *Spesialis Forensik*, or *Sp.F.* He or she may be addressed in public as *Dokter Forensik* ("forensic doctor"). Note that there is no pre-medicine program, making the total duration of formal education for one to become a forensic specialist 8 years.

Forensic medicine is also a mandatory round during medical school clerkship. Medical students assist the doctors on autopsies, and they may also be allowed to perform an autopsy under supervision, and to witness in the court.

United Kingdom

In the UK, anatomical pathology is a five year residency. Successful candidates are eligible for inclusion on the specialist register of the General Medical Council (GMC) having obtained Membership of the Royal College of Pathologists (United Kingdom). A specialist training (ST) post is applied for post foundation year to enter a training program in Histopathology.

Imminent changes as a result of the Tooke report may require two years or more to be fulfilled on general rotational placements before the option of histopathology arises, however the Royal College have not issued their response to this matter as of yet. It is then necessary to obtain the MRCPath Part I examination in Histopathology, after which it is then possible to apply to one of few training posts in Forensic Pathology in the UK. Current approved centres include Belfast, Liverpool, Leicester, Cardiff, London, Sheffield, Glasgow and Dundee. Not all the posts are currently actively training. Following 3 years training in Forensic Pathology and completion of the FRCPath Part II slanted to Forensic Pathology you may then obtain CCT (certificate of completion of training) and work as a Consultant Forensic Pathologist.

Another option is to obtain the full FRCPath in general histopathology, followed by another 18–24 months of training in forensic pathology, which will qualify the candidates with either the Diploma of the Royal College of Patholoists in Forensic Pathology (DipRCPath (forensic)), or the Diploma in Medical Jurisprudence (DMJ).

In England & Wales you will also need to be Home Office Accredited, which will require checks of your training portfolio and completion of a security check and the Expert Witness Training Course run by the Forensic Science Service. Foreign graduates and specialists will need to apply to the GMC and the RCPath directly to practise Forensic Pathology in the United Kingdom.

United States

In the United States, forensic pathologists typically complete at least one year of additional training (a fellowship) after completing an anatomical pathology residency and having passed the "board" examination administered by The American Board of Pathology or The American Osteopathic Board of Pathology ("board-certified"). Becoming an anatomic pathologist in the United States requires completing a residency in anatomic pathology, which is on-the-job training one must perform upon completing medical school before one may practice unsupervised. *Anatomic pathology* (as it is called) by itself is a three-year residency. Most U.S. pathologists complete a combined residency in both anatomic and *clinical pathology*, which requires a total of four years.

In the United States, all told, the education after high school is typically 13–15 years in duration (4 years undergraduate training + 4 years medical school + 4–5 years residency [anatomic and clinical pathology combined] + 1-2 year forensic pathology fellowship). Generally, the biggest hurdle is gaining admission to medical school, although the pass rate for anatomic and forensic pathology board examinations (in the U.S.) is approximately 80-90 and 90-100 percent, respectively. The courts do not require American Board of Pathology certification in order for a witness to be qualified as an expert in the field of forensic pathology, and there are several "diploma mills" that give online certificates in the field.

Training and Certification of Anatomical Pathologists

Australia

- (Also New Zealand, Hong Kong, Singapore, Malaysia, and Saudi Arabia)

Anatomical Pathology one of the speciality training programs offered by the Royal College of Pathologists of Australasia (RCPA). The RCPA. To qualify as a Fellow of the RCPA in Anatomical Pathology, the candidate must complete a recognised undergraduate or postgraduate medical qualification, then complete a minimum of 1 year of clinical medical experience (internship) as a prerequisite to selection as a training registrar.

The training program is a minimum of 5 years, served in at least two laboratories, and candidates must pass a Basic Pathological Sciences examination (usually in first year), the Part 1 examination (not before 3rd year) and the Part 2 examination (not before 5th year). Fellows may then continue into subspeciality training.

Canada

Anatomical Pathology (AP) is one of the specialist certificates granted by the Royal College of Physicians and Surgeons of Canada. Other certificates related to pathology include general pathology (GP), forensic pathology, hematopathology, and neuropathology.

Candidates for any of these must have completed four years of medical school and five years of residency training. After becoming certified in either AP or GP, it is common for pathologists to seek further fellowship training in a subspeciality of AP.

USA

Anatomic Pathology (AP) is one of the two primary certifications offered by the American Board of Pathology and one of three primary certifications offered by the American Osteopathic Board of Pathology. The other is Clinical Pathology

(CP). To be certified in anatomic pathology, the trainee must complete four years of medical school followed by three years of residency training. Many U.S. pathologists are certified in both AP and CP, which requires a total of four years of residency. After completing residency, many pathologists enroll in further years of fellowship training to gain expertise in a subspeciality of AP.

Anatomical Pathology Practice Settings

- *Academic anatomical pathology* is practiced at university medical centres by pathologists who are also university faculty. As such, they often have diverse responsibilities that may include training pathology residents, teaching medical students, conducting basic, clinical, or translational research, and/or performing administrative duties, all in addition to the practice of diagnostic anatomical pathology. Pathologists in academic settings often sub-specialize in a particular area of anatomic pathology and may serve as consultants to other pathologists regarding cases in their specific area of expertise.
- *Group practice* is the most traditional private practice model. In this arrangement, a group of senior pathologists will control a partnership that employs junior pathologists and contracts independently with hospitals to provide diagnostic services, as well as attracting referral business from local clinicians who practice in the outpatient setting. The group often owns a laboratory for histology and ancillary testing of tissue, and may hold contracts to run hospital-owned labs. Many pathologists who practice in this setting are trained and certified in both anatomical pathology and clinical pathology, which allows them to supervise blood banks, clinical chemistry laboratories, and medical microbiology laboratories as well.
- Large *corporate providers of anatomical pathology services* have emerged in recent years, the most notable one being *AmeriPath* in the United States. In this model, pathologists are employees, rather than independent partners. This model has been criticized for reducing

physician independence, but defenders claim that the larger size of these practices allows for economies of scale and greater specialization, as well a sufficient volume to support more specialized testing methods.

- *Multispeciality groups*, composed of physicians from clinical specialities as well as radiology and pathology, are another practice model. In some case, these may be large groups controlled by an HMO or other large healthcare organisation. In others, they are in essence clinician group practices that employ pathologists to provide diagnostic services for the group. These groups may own their own laboratories, or, in some cases may make controversial arrangements with "pod labs" that allow clinician groups to lease space, with the clinican groups receiving direct insurance payments for pathology services. Proposed changes to Medicare regulations may essentially eliminate these arrangements in the United States.

Clinical Pathology

Clinical pathology (US, UK, Ireland, Commonwealth, Portugal, Italy), Laboratory Medicine (Germany, Romania, Poland, Eastern Europe), Clinical analysis (Spain) or Clinical/Medical Biology (France, Belgium, Netherlands, Austria, North and West Africa...), is a medical speciality that is concerned with the diagnosis of disease based on the laboratory analysis of bodily fluids, such as blood, urine, and tissues using the tools of chemistry, microbiology, hematology and molecular pathology. This speciality requires a medical residency and should not be confused with Biomedical science, which is not necessarily related to medicine.

Licensing and Subspecialities

The American Board of Pathology certifies clinical pathologists, and recognises the following secondary specialities of clinical pathology:

- Chemical pathology, also called clinical chemistry
- Hematopathology
- Blood banking - Transfusion medicine
- Clinical microbiology

- Cytogenetics
- Molecular genetics pathology.

In some countries other subspecialities fall under certified Clinical Biologists responsibility:

- Assisted reproductive technology, Sperm bank and Semen analysis
- Immunopathology.

Organisation

Clinical pathologists are often medical doctors. In some countries in South-America, Europe, Africa or Asia, this speciality can be practiced by non-physicians, such as Ph.D or Pharm.D after a variable number of years of residency.

In United States of America

Clinical pathologists work in close collaboration with clinical scientists (clinical biochemists, clinical microbiologists, etc.), medical technologists, hospital administrators, and referring physicians to ensure the accuracy and optimal utilisation of laboratory testing. Clinical pathology is one of the two major divisions of pathology, the other being anatomical pathology. Often, pathologists practice both anatomical and clinical pathology, a combination sometimes known as general pathology. Similar specialities exist in veterinary pathology.

Clinical pathology is itself divided in to subspecialities, the main ones being clinical chemistry, clinical hematology/blood banking, hematopathology and clinical microbiology and emerging subspecialities such as molecular diagnostics and proteomics. Many areas of clinical pathology overlap with anatomic pathology. Both can serve as medical directors of CLIA certified laboratories. This overlap includes immunoassays, flow cytometry, microbiology and cytogenetics and any assay done on tissue. Overlap between anatomic and clinical pathology is expanding to molecular diagnostics and proteomics as we move towards making the best use of new technologies for personalized medicine.

In Europe

Recently, EFCCLM has chosen the name of "Laboratory medicine specialist" to define all European Clinical pathologists, regardless of their training (M.D, Ph.D or Pharm.D) . In France,

Clinical Pathology is called Medical Biology ("Biologie médicale") and is practiced by both M.D.s and Pharm.Ds. The residency lasts four years. Specialists in this discipline are called "Clinical Biologist" rather than "Clinical pathologist".

Place of Work

Tools of Clinical Pathology: Microscopes, analysers, strips, centrifugal machines...

Macroscopic Examination: The visual examination of the taken liquid is a first main indication for the pathologist or the physician. The aspect of the liquid, in addition, conditions the analytical assumption of responsibility that follow and the validity of the end-results.

Microscopical Examination

Microscopic analysis is an important activity of the pathologist and the laboratory assistant. They have many different colourings at their disposal (GRAM, MGG, Grocott, Ziehl-Neelsen, ...). Immunofluorescence, cytochemistry, the immunocytochemistry and FISH are also used in order make a correct diagnosis.

This stage allows the pathologist to determine the character of the liquid: "normal", tumoral, inflammatory even infectious. Indeed, microscopic examination can often determine the causal infectious agent, in general a bacterium, a mould, a yeast, or a parasite, more rarely a virus.

Analyzers

The analysers, by the association of robotics and spectrophotometry, allowed these last decades a better reproducibility of the results of proportionings, in particular in medical biochemistry and hematology. The companies of in vitro diagnosis henceforth try to sell chains of automats, i.e. a system allowing the automatic transfer of the tubes towards the various types of automats of the same mark. These systems can include the computer-assisted management of a serum library. These analysers must undergo daily controls to guarantee a result just possible, one speaks about quality control. These analysers must also undergo daily, weekly and monthly maintenances.

Cultures

A big part of the examinations of clinical pathology, primarily in medical microbiology, use culture media. Those allow, for example, the description of one or several infectious agents responsible of the clinical signs.

Dermatopathology

Dermatopathology is a subspeciality of both dermatology and surgical pathology that focuses on the study of cutaneous diseases at a microscopic level. It also encompasses analyses of the potential causes of skin diseases at a cellular level. Dermatopathologists work in close association with dermatologists. In fact, some of them are trained primarily in dermatology themselves. Dermatologists are able to recognise most skin diseases based on their appearances, anatomic distributions, and behaviour. Sometimes, however, those criteria do not allow a conclusive diagnosis to be made, and a skin biopsy is taken to be examined under the microscope. That process reveals the histology of the disease and results in a specific diagnostic interpretation. In some cases, additional specialized testing needs to be performed on biopsies, including immunofluorescence, immunohistochemistry, electron microscopy, flow cytometry, and molecular-pathologic analysis. One of the greatest challenges of dermatopathology is its scope. More than 1500 different disorders of the skin exist, including cutaneous eruptions ("rashes") and neoplasms. Therefore, dermatopathologists must maintain a broad base of knowledge, and be familiar with several other speciality areas in Medicine.

Certification in dermatopathology in the United States requires the completion of a medical degree, followed by residency training of 3 years in dermatology or 4 years in anatomic pathology. Thereafter, an additional 1 or 2 years of post-residency education in dermatopathology is undertaken. For trainees with a primary background in Pathology, the fellowship experience includes the equivalent of 6 months of clinical dermatology, and for those whose training is primarily in Dermatology, 6 months of the fellowship are devoted to anatomic pathology. In the United States, dermatopathologists are first certified by the American Boards of Pathology or Dermatology, or the American Osteopathic Boards of Pathology or Dermatology, and they then obtain subspeciality certification (termed "special competence") in dermatopathology by written examination. Since 2003, the International Board of Dermatopathology (IBDP)— headquartered in Graz, Austria—also has certified candidates from countries around the world. This is done by IBDP review of applicants' professional qualifi-cations, and a formal examination that is given in Europe each year.

Hematopathology

Hematopathology is the branch of pathology which studies diseases of hematopoietic cells. In the United States, hematopathology is a board certified subspeciality (American Board of Pathology) practiced by those physicians who have completed general pathology residency (anatomic, clinical, or combined) and additional fellowship training in hematology. Hematopoietic cells originate from the bone marrow and contribute the cellular components of blood including red blood cells (erythrocytes), white blood cells (leukocytes), and platelets (megakaryocyte-derived bodies). Additionally, leukocytes contribute significantly to the cellular composition of lymph nodes, the spleen, the thymus, and mucosa associated lymphoid tissues, and are present to some degree in all tissues.

Diseases of the hematopoietic system generally manifest as decreases (anemia) or increases (lymphoma/leukemia) in these cell types. Consequently, hematopathologists most frequently evaluate peripheral blood smears, bone marrow aspirates and biopsies, and lymph nodes biopsies to determine the nature of hematopoietic disease. The hematopathologist incorporates traditional microscopy with ancillary techniques including general laboratory values, immunohistochemistry, flow cytometry, and molecular diagnostic tests to make the most accurate diagnosis. The hematopathologist works closely with the hematologist/oncologist speciality doctor who sees the patient and decides on the best treatment based upon the diagnosis made by the hematopathologist.

Diseases of Hematopoietic Cells

Diseases of the hematopoietic system are myriad and include hereditary and congenital disorders as well as acquired disorders. Hereditary and congenital disorders include, in part, bone marrow failure syndromes and primary deficiency syndromes. Acquired disorders may be related to nutritional deficiencies (such as iron, folate, and B12 deficient anemias), infectious processes or neoplastic disorders (cancers). Diagnostic criteria and classification guidelines for the neoplastic diseases are codified in the WHO Classification of Tumours of the Hematopoietic and Lymphoid Tissue, most recently revised in 2008.

The neoplastic diseases of hematopoietic cells fall into two broad categories, myeloid neoplasms and lymphoid neoplasms. Histiocytic and dendritic cell neoplasms are considered separately.

- Myeloid Neoplasms:
  - Myeloproliferative neoplasms
  - Myeloid and lymphoid disorders with eosinophilia
  - Myeloproliferative/myelodysplastic neoplasms
  - Myelodysplastic syndromes
  - Acute myeloid leukemia and related precursor neoplasms
  - Acute leukemia of ambiguous lineage
- Lymphoid Neoplasms
  - Precursor lymphoid neoplasms
  - Mature B-cell neoplasms
  - Mature T-cell neoplasms
  - Hodgkin lymphoma
  - Immunodeficiency associated lymphoproliferative disorders
- Histiocytic and Dendritic Cell Neoplasms

Each category contains several recognised diagnostic entities resulting in nearly 100 different types of hematopoietic cancer, each with defining morphology, pathobiology, treatment, and/or prognostic features. Correct classification, as well as identification of additional factors that may influence prognosis or response to chemotherapy, is essential to allow optimal treatment by the hematologist/oncologist. The hematopathologist is also responsible for additional studies performed after initiation of therapy to monitor for continued remission or disease relapse.

Chapter 2

Veterinary Pathology

Veterinary pathologists are doctors of veterinary medicine who specialize in the diagnosis of diseases through the examination of animal tissue and body fluids. Like medical pathology, veterinary pathology is divided into two branches, anatomical pathology and clinical pathology. Veterinary pathologists are critical participants in the drug development process.

Veterinary Anatomical Pathology

Anatomical pathology (*Commonwealth*) or *Anatomic pathology* (*U.S.*) is concerned with the diagnosis of disease based on the gross, microscopic, and molecular examination of organs, tissues, and whole bodies (necropsy). The Indian, European, Japanese and American Colleges of Veterinary Pathologists certify veterinary pathologists through a certifying exam. The American College of Veterinary Pathologist certification exam consists of four parts - gross pathology, microscopic pathology, veterinary pathology, and general pathology. Only the general pathology section is shared between the anatomic and clinical pathology examinations. Anatomic pathologists are employed in a number of different positions, including diagnostics, teaching, research, and the pharmaceutical industry.

Veterinary Clinical Pathology

Clinical pathology is concerned with the diagnosis of disease based on the laboratory analysis of bodily fluids such as blood and urine, using the tools of chemistry, microbiology, hematology and molecular pathology. The Indian, European, Japanese and American Colleges of Veterinary Pathologists certify veterinary clinical pathologists.

The American College of Veterinary Pathologists certification exam consists of four parts: General Pathology (shared with the Anatomic Pathology certifying examination), Cytology and Surgical Pathology, Hematology, and Clinical Chemistry. The credential, DACVP (Diplomate, American College of Veterinary Pathologists) is usually followed by a parenthetical notation of "(Clinical Pathology)" to distinguish DACVP counterparts certified for anatomic pathology. The European credential is DipECVCP (Diplomate of the European College of Veterinary Clinical Pathology). Clinical pathologists are employed in diagnostic pathology, veterinary and medical teaching, research, and the pharmaceutical industry.

Pathology as a Medical Speciality

Pathologists are physicians who diagnose and characterize disease in living patients by examining biopsies or bodily fluid. Pathologists may also conduct autopsies to investigate causes of death. Pathology is a core discipline of medical school and many pathologists are also instructors. As managers of medical laboratories, pathologists play an important role in the development of laboratory information systems. Although the medical practice of pathology grew out of the tradition of investigative pathology, most modern pathologists do not perform original research.

Pathology is a unique medical speciality in that pathologists typically do not see patients directly, but rather serve as consultants to other physicians (often referred to as "clinicians" within the pathology community). To be licensed, candidates must complete medical training, an approved residency program and be certified by an appropriate body. In the US, certification is by the American Board of Pathology or the American Osteopathic Board of Pathology. The organisation of subspecialities within pathology varies between nations, but usually includes anatomical pathology and clinical pathology.

Training

Pathology in the United States: In the United States, pathologists are physicians (D.O. or M.D.) that have completed a four-year undergraduate program, four years of medical school training, and three to four years of postgraduate training in the form of a pathology residency. Training may be within two primary specialities, as recognised by the American Board of Pathology: anatomical Pathology and clinical Pathology, each of which requires separate board certification. The American Osteopathic Board of Pathology also recognises four primary specialities: anatomic pathology, dermatopathology, forensic pathology, and laboratory medicine.

Many pathologists pursue a broad based training and become certified in both fields. These skills are complementary in many hospital based private practice settings, since the day to day work of many clinical laboratories only intermittently requires the attention of a physician.

Thus, pathologists are able to spend much of their time evaluating anatomical pathology cases, while remaining available to cover any special issues which might arise in the clinical laboratories. Pathologists may pursue specialised fellowship training within one or more subspecialities of either anatomical or clinical pathology. Some of these subspecialities permit additional board certification, while others do not.

Pathology in the United Kingdom

In the United Kingdom, pathologists are medical doctors registered with — and currently licensed by — the UK General Medical Council. The training to become a pathologist is under the oversight of the Royal College of Pathologists.

After four to six years of undergraduate medical study, trainees proceed to a two year foundation programme. Full-time training in Histopathology presently lasts between five to five and a half years. The first year involves structured training and is assessed by an objective structured practical exam (OSPE), which must be passed to progress to year two.

This is followed by further specialist training in surgical pathology, cytopathology, and autopsy pathology. There are two examinations run by the Royal College of Pathologists, termed Part 1 and Part 2. The Part 2 examination is designed to test competence to work as an independent practitioner in pathology and is typically taken after four or five years of specialist training. All postgraduate medical training and education in the UK is overseen by the General Medical Council (GMC). It is possible to take a specialist part 2 examination in forensic pathology, pediatric pathology, or neuropathology. It is also possible to take a Royal College of Pathologists diploma in forensic pathology, dermatopathology, or cytopathology, recognising additional specialist training and expertise.

Pathology in France

In France, Pathology is separate in two distinct specialities, Anatomical pathology and Clinical pathology. Residencies both lasts four years. Residency in anatomical pathology is open to physicians only, while clinical pathology is open to both physicians and pharmacists. Anatomical pathology in France is integrated in the internal medicine speciality track. At the end of the second year of clinical pathology residency, residents can choose between general Clinical pathology and a specialization in one of the disciplines, but they can not practise Anatomical pathology. And conversely, Anatomical pathology residents can not practise Clinical pathology.

Diseases of the Rectum and Anus

Anal Sac Disease

Anal sac disease is the most common disease entity of the anal region in dogs. Small breeds are predisposed; large or giant breeds are rarely affected. In cats, the most common form of anal sac disease is impaction.

Etiology and Pathogenesis: Anal sacs may become impacted, infected, abscessed, or neoplastic. Failure of the sacs to express during defecation, poor muscle tone in obese dogs, and generalized seborrhea (which produces glandular hypersecretion) lead to retention of sac contents. Such retention may predispose to bacterial overgrowth, infection, and inflammation.

Clinical Findings and Lesions: Signs are related to pain and discomfort associated with sitting. Scooting, licking, biting at the anal area, and painful defecation with tenesmus may be noted. Induration, abscesses, and fistulous tracts are common. In impaction, hard masses are palpable in the area of the sacs; the sacs are packed with a thick, pasty, brown secretion, which can be expressed as a thin ribbon only with a large amount of pressure. When the sacs are infected or abscessed, severe pain and often discolouration of the area are present. Fistulous tracts lead from abscessed sacs and rupture through the skin; these must be differentiated from perianal fistulas. Anal sac neoplasms are usually nonpainful and are associated with perineal edema, erythema, induration, or fistula formation. Apocrine gland adenocarcinomas of the anal sac are typically seen in older female dogs.

These dogs are presented for signs secondary to hypercalcemia, such as polyuria and polydipsia, or for problems related to the perineal mass. Diagnosis of impaction, infection, or abscessation is confirmed by digital rectal examination, at which time the sacs can be expressed.

Microscopic examination of the contents from infected sacs reveals large numbers of polymorphonuclear leukocytes and bacteria. A tumor should be suspected (anal sac apocrine adenocarcinoma) in anal sacs that are firm, enlarged, and nonexpressible even with irrigation. In these cases, the diagnosis should be confirmed by biopsy. Regional and systemic metastasis should be evaluated, and serum calcium measured.

Treatment: Impacted anal sacs should be gently manually expressed. A softening or ceruminolytic agent or saline can be infused into the sac if the contents are too dry to express effectively.

Infected sacs should be cleaned with antiseptic, followed by local and systemic antibiotic therapy. Hot compresses, applied every 8-12 hr for 15-20 min each, are beneficial for abscesses. Repeated weekly flushings combined with infusion of a steroid-antibiotic ointment may be needed.

Adding supplemental fibre to the diet may increase fecal bulk, facilitating anal sac compression and emptying. If medical treatment is ineffective, or if neoplasia is present, surgical excision of the sac is indicated.

The closed technique for excision is preferred and has the lowest complication rate. However, fecal incontinence, which is a common complication of anal sac surgery, may result from damage to the caudal rectal branch of the pudendal nerve and may be complete if damage is bilateral. Chronic fistula formation may be seen when sac removal is incomplete or when the sac ruptures. Scar formation in the external anal sphincter may result from surgical trauma and result in tenesmus.

Perianal Fistula

Perianal fistula is characterized by chronic, purulent, malodorous, ulcerating, sinus tracts in the perianal tissues. It is most common in German Shepherds and is also seen in Setters and Retrievers. Dogs >7 yr old are at higher risk.

Etiology and Pathogenesis: The cause is unknown, although many theories have been proposed. Contamination of the hair follicles and glands of the anal area by fecal material and anal sac secretions may result in necrosis, ulceration, and chronic inflammation of the perianal skin and tissues.

Affected animals may be predisposed to generalized skin problems. Hypothyroidism, an immunologic defect, or an immune-mediated component may contribute to susceptibility. The likelihood of contamination is greater in dogs with a broad-based tail; deep anal folds may cause feces to be retained within rectal glands and play a major role.

The draining tracts are lined with chronic inflammatory tissue and often extend to the lumen of the rectum and anus. Infection may spread to deeper structures involving the external anal sphincter and, therefore, should be treated promptly.

Clinical Findings: In dogs, signs include attitude change, tenesmus, dyschezia, anorexia, lethargy, diarrhea, and attempts to bite and lick the anal area. Signs in cats are similar to those in dogs but may include matting of fur and sitting in the litter box.

Treatment: Until recently, management of perianal fistulae was frustrating for both veterinarians and pet owners. Surgical therapy traditionally included anal sacculectomy, in addition to destroying the diseased tissues.

Surgical techniques included excision, debridement, fulguration, and cryosurgery. Amputation of the tail at its base was once advocated alone or adjunctively with other therapy. Surgery is now only recommended for fistulae resistant to medical therapy.

Sequelae of surgery include fecal incontinence, rectal stricture, and recurrence. Cyclosporine has been demonstrated to be an effective treatment; it is usually administered for 16 wk and for an additional 4 wk after all fistulae appear to be healed. Concurrent administration of ketoconazole allows the dosage and cost of cyclosporine therapy to be reduced. Prompt treatment with cyclosporine combined with ketoconazole is recommended early in the course of the disease to reduce the likelihood of recurrence. Other aspects of medical management include the use of stool softeners to reduce dyschezia. Perianal cleansing and antibiotics may reduce inflammation.

Hepatoid Gland Tumors

These common neoplasms arise from modified sebaceous glands that are most abundant in the cutaneous tissues around the anus but may also be present along the ventral midline from the perineum to the base of the skull, the dorsal and ventral tail, and in the skin of the lumbar and sacral regions. Because androgens stimulate the development of hepatoid glands, the incidence of proliferative lesions of hepatoid glands in intact, male dogs is 3 times that in females.

Benign hepatoid gland tumors are divided into hepatoid gland hyperplasias and adenomas; however, as with benign sebaceous gland tumors, there is a continuum from hyperplasia to adenoma. Here, they will be considered as a single entity. Hepatoid gland adenomas are most common in aged dogs. Siberian Huskies, Samoyeds, Pekingese, and Cocker Spaniels are most commonly affected.

Tumors may develop at any site where hepatoid glands are present, but 90% occur in the perianal region. Grossly, they appear as one or (more commonly) multiple intradermal nodules 0.5-10 cm in diametre. Larger lesions commonly ulcerate, and hemorrhagic, keratinaceous material can often be extruded with local pressure.

Large tumors can compress the anal canal and make defecation difficult. Up to 95% of male dogs respond completely to castration; in those that do not, the pituitary-adrenal axis should be evaluated and, if no abnormality is detected, the dog should be reevaluated for the presence of a low-grade hepatoid gland adenocarcinoma. Excision may be used concurrently to remove extremely large or ulcerated tumors that have become secondarily infected. Surgery is the treatment of choice for females with hepatoid gland adenomas but may need to be repeated because recurrence is common. Radiation therapy is also an option and has a 2-yr cure rate of 69% for benign tumors. Cryosurgery is another therapeutic alternative, but because of the complication of fecal incontinence, should be used only when tumors are not amenable to surgical intervention. Diethylstilbestrol has been used in the past as an alternative to castration, but because of severe side effects, including aplastic anemia and cystic prostatic hyperplasia, it should be used with extreme caution, if at all.

Hepatoid gland adenocarcinomas are uncommon canine neoplasms that generally appear as nodular lesions affecting the perianal region. These tumors are found in male dogs 10 times more commonly than in females. Siberian Huskies, Alaskan Malamutes, and Bulldogs are most likely to develop this tumor. Histologic evaluation is the best means of diagnosis; however, there is debate about how to distinguish low-grade malignant tumors from hepatoid adenomas because well-differentiated forms can be confused with adenomas, and anaplastic forms can be confused with apocrine gland adenocarcinomas of anal sac origin. These tumors have metastatic potential and often spread to regional lymph nodes. Treatment consists of wide surgical excision including involved lymph nodes and, possibly, subsequent radiation. These tumors are generally not responsive to castration or to estrogen therapy, and it is unknown whether chemotherapy is of benefit for metastatic disease. The prognosis is guarded.

Perineal Hernia

Perineal hernia is a lateral protrusion of a peritoneally lined hernial sac between the levator ani and either the external anal sphincter muscle or the coccygeus muscle. Incidence in intact 6- to 8-yr-old male dogs is disproportionately high, and Welsh Corgis, Boston Terriers, Boxers, Collies, Kelpies and Kelpie crosses, Dachshunds and Dachshund crosses, Old English Sheepdogs, and Pekingese are at higher risk.

Etiology and Pathogenesis: Many factors are involved, including breed predisposition, hormonal imbalance, prostatic disease, chronic constipation, and weakness of the pelvic diaphragm due to chronic straining. The higher incidence among sexually intact males is evidence that hormonal influences probably play a primary role. Prostatic hypertrophy attributed to sex-hormone imbalance has been strongly implicated. Both estrogens and androgens have been cited as causative agents.

Clinical Findings and Diagnosis: Common signs include constipation and obstipation, tenesmus, and dyschezia. Stranguria and urinary obstruction may develop secondary to retroflexion of the bladder and prostate.

Visceral strangulation may be seen. A perineal swelling ventrolateral to the anus is evident. Herniation may be bilateral, but two-thirds are unilateral and >80% of these are on the right side. The mass is soft and fluctuant and may be reduced digitally. A firm, painful swelling may be compatible with retropulsion of the bladder and prostate.

Determination of contents is often made by rectal examination and perineal centesis (to determine if urine is present). Over 90% of perineal hernias contain a rectal deviation, which is a sacculation of the rectum into the hernial sac, where the layers of the rectal wall remain intact.

Treatment: Perineal hernia is rarely an emergency, except when the bladder has strangulated and the animal is unable to urinate. If catheterization cannot be done, the urine should be removed by cystocentesis and an attempt made to reduce the hernia.

An indwelling urinary catheter may be necessary to ensure urethral patency and prevent recurrence of obstruction. Surgical correction is always indicated, and concurrent castration to reduce recurrence is recommended.

The prognosis is guarded because of the high incidence of recurrence (10-46%) and postoperative complications such as infection, rectocutaneous fistula, anal sac fistula, ischiatic and pudendal nerve entrapment, and rectal prolapse.

Rectal and Anorectal Strictures

Strictures are a narrowing of the lumen due to cicatricial tissue. Injury may result from foreign bodies or trauma (eg, bite wounds, accidents) or as a complication of inflammatory disease.

Neoplasia, enlarged prostate, and scar tissue after perianal fistula or anal sac abscess may all predispose to extraluminal constriction. In small animals, anorectal stricture is more common than rectal strictures, but neither is frequent. Strictures are more common in German Shepherds, Beagles, and Poodles.

Rectal stricture in cattle may result from trauma, neoplasia, or fat necrosis impinging on or within the lumen, or from defects associated with rectal and vaginal strictures. Rectal strictures in pigs are seen secondary to enterocolitis, after repair of rectal prolapse, and as a sequela of ulcerative proctitis induced by salmonellae.

Treatment is Surgical. Rectal Neoplasms

Malignant rectal neoplasms are usually adenocarcinomas in dogs and lymphosarcomas in cats. Adenocarcinomas are slow growing and infiltrative.

Local or systemic metastasis may develop before tenesmus, dyschezia, hematochezia, or diarrhea is seen. Surgery is the treatment of choice for adenocarcinomas, but it may be unrewarding because metastasis has usually occurred before the diagnosis. Cats with rectal lymphosarcoma are treated medically with antineoplastic drugs.

Rectal Polyps

Rectal adenomatous polyps are an infrequent, usually benign disease, primarily of small animals. The larger the polyp, the greater the potential for malignancy. Signs include tenesmus, hematochezia, and diarrhea. The polyp is usually palpable per rectum and bleeds easily with surface ulceration. Periodically, the polyp may prolapse through the anal orifice. Surgical excision is usually followed by rapid clinical recovery and lengthy survival time. New polyps may develop after surgery. A biopsy should always be submitted for histopathologic diagnosis.

Rectal Prolapse

In rectal prolapse, one or more layers of the rectum protrude through the anus due to persistent tenesmus associated with intestinal, anorectal, or urogenital disease. Prolapse may be classified as incomplete, in which only the rectal mucosa is everted, or complete, in which all rectal layers are protruded.

Etiology: Rectal prolapse is common in young animals in association with severe diarrhea and tenesmus. Causal factors include severe enteritis, endoparasitism, disorders of the rectum (eg, foreign bodies, lacerations, diverticula, or sacculation), neoplasia of the rectum or distal colon, urolithiasis, urethral obstruction, cystitis, dystocia, colitis, and prostatic disease. Perineal hernia, or other interruption of normal innervation of the external anal sphincter, may also produce prolapse. Animals of any age, breed, or sex may be affected.

Rectal prolapse is probably the most common GI problem in pigs due to diarrhea or weakness of the rectal support tissue within the pelvis. In cattle, it may be associated with coccidiosis, rabies, or vaginal or uterine prolapse; occasionally, excessive "riding" and associated traumatic injury may be causative in young bulls.

It is common in sheep with short tail docking and especially in feedlot lambs, in which high-concentrate rations may be causative. The use of estrogens as growth promotants, or accidental exposure to estrogenic fungal toxins, may also predispose large animals to rectal prolapse.

Clinical Findings, Lesions, and Diagnosis: An elongated, cylindrical mass protruding through the anal orifice is usually diagnostic. However, it must be differentiated from prolapsed ileocolic intussusception by passing a probe, blunt instrument, or finger between the prolapsed mass and the inner rectal wall.

In rectal prolapse, the instrument cannot be inserted due to the presence of a fornix. Ulceration, inflammation, and congestion of the rectal mucosa is common. Early, there is a short, nonulcerated, inflamed segment; later, the mucosal surface darkens and may become congested and necrotic.

Treatment: In all animals, identifying and eliminating the cause of prolapse is of primary importance. In small animals, treatment includes prompt replacement of viable prolapsed tissue to its proper anatomic location, or amputation if the segment is necrotic.

Small or incomplete prolapses can be manually reduced under anesthesia by using a finger or bougie. Warm saline lavage and lubrication with a water-soluble gel should be applied to the prolapsed tissue prior to reduction. Alternatively, hypertonic sugar solution (50% dextrose or 70% mannitol) applied topically may be used to relieve edematous mucosa. The placement of a loose, anal purse-string suture for 5-7 days is indicated. Straining may be prevented by applying a topical anesthetic (1% dibucaine ointment) or by administering a narcotic epidural injection before or after reduction or correction.

Postoperatively, a moistened diet and a fecal softener (eg, dioctyl sodium sulfosuccinate) are recommended. Diarrhea after surgery may require treatment.

When questionable viability of tissue prohibits manual reduction, rectal resection and anastomosis are required. When rectal tissue is viable but not amenable to manual reduction, celiotomy followed by colopexy is indicated to prevent recurrence. As in medical management, epidural anesthesia may be used to reduce straining.

In large animals, caudal epidural anesthesia is suggested to reduce straining, facilitate repositioning of the prolapse, and permit surgical manipulations. Reduction and retention with a purse-string suture is recommended.

The suture should be loose enough to leave a one-finger opening into the rectum in pigs and sheep, and slightly larger in cattle and horses. Rectal prolapse in mares, if neglected, can lead to prolapse of the small colon.

The blood supply to the small colon is easily disrupted. Replacement of a rectal prolapse with prolapse of the small colon followed by purse-string suture of the anus has a poor prognosis. More aggressive treatment of the prolapse is dictated by the condition of the rectum.

In general, the prolapse may be salvaged by conservative measures, unless obvious deep necrosis or trauma to the tissue exists, or the everted tissue is firm, indurated, and cannot be reduced. Under these circumstances, submucosal resection or amputation should be considered. Amputation of the rectum should be reserved for severe cases. Complete amputation has a higher incidence of rectal stricture formation, especially in swine. A prolapse ring, syringe case, or plastic tubing may be used as an alternative to surgical amputation in pigs and sheep. Postoperatively, the animal should receive antibiotics. Fecal softeners may be used in horses. Usually, it is not economically feasible to repair rectal prolapses in lambs ready for market.

Rectal Tears

A separation, rent, or tear in the rectal or anal mucosa is seen as a result of a laceration inflicted within the lumen. Foreign bodies (eg, sharp bones, needles, and other rough material) have been implicated. Bite wounds and, in large animals, trauma from rectal palpation are common causes. The tear may involve only the superficial layers of the rectum (partial tear) or penetrate all layers (complete tear).

Clinical Findings and Diagnosis: Constipation and reluctance to defecate are usually attributed to pain. Diagnosis is based on tenesmus and hemorrhage, perineal discolouration, and inspection of the rectum and anus; fresh blood found on a glove or on feces after rectal examination is good evidence of a rectal tear. Edema may be present when the injury has persisted. The integrity of the external anal sphincter should be evaluated carefully.

Treatment: In all species, treatment should be initiated immediately. The anorectal area should be cleaned thoroughly and systemic broad-spectrum antibiotics administered. IV fluids and flunixin meglumine may be given to prevent or treat septic and endotoxic shock.

In small animals, lacerations should be debrided and may be sutured through the anal orifice, via laparotomy, or through a combination of both depending on the location and degree of the tear. Antibiotics and fecal softeners should be administered postoperatively.

In cattle and horses, accidental perforation during rectal examination necessitates immediate treatment to reduce the risk of peritonitis and death. Exploration throughout the abdomen should be slow, deliberate, and smooth.

The temptation to use the fingertips excessively or to push the arm through a region of resistance must be avoided. Rectal tears in horses have been classified according to the tissue layers penetrated. Grade I tears involve the mucosa or submucosa. Grade II tears involve rupture of the muscular layers only. Grade III tears involve mucosa, submucosa, and muscular layers, including tears that extend into the mesorectum. Grade IV tears involve perforation of all layers of the rectum and extension into the peritoneal cavity. Grade

I tears may be treated conservatively with broad-spectrum antibiotics and IV fluids. Flunixin meglumine may be given to prevent or treat endotoxic shock.

Mineral oil is given via stomach tube to soften feces, and the diet should consist of pasture grasses or alfalfa. Grade II and III tears require immediate and more extensive surgery. Grade IV tears carry a grave prognosis; they should be repaired only if small and if treatment is instituted before the peritoneal cavity is grossly contaminated.

Chapter 3

Campylobacteriosis: Introduction

Gastrointestinal campylobacteriosis, caused by Campylobacter jejuni or C coli, is associated with diarrhea in various animal hosts, including dogs, cats, calves, sheep, ferrets, mink, several species of laboratory animals, zoo animals, and humans. In humans, it is a leading cause of diarrhea. C jejuni and C coli are also recovered from feces of asymptomatic carriers. Animals, including dogs and cats (especially those recently purchased from shelters), and wild animals maintained in captivity can serve as sources of human infection.

The agents also are isolated frequently from the feces of chickens, turkeys, pigs, and other species. The organism commonly contaminates poultry meat, which serves as one of the major vehicles of spread of C jejuni to humans.

The disease is found worldwide; its prevalence appears to be increasing as proper culture techniques for C jejuni and C coli are refined and updated. Clinical manifestations may be more severe in younger animals.

In studies using monoclonal and polyclonal antibodies, Campylobacter spp (including C jejuni) have been associated with proliferative ileitis in hamsters and proliferative colitis in ferrets. A cause and effect relationship has not been proved experimentally, however. Proliferative bowel disease in these animals is now known to be caused by Lawsonia intracellularis. Etiology:Campylobacter is a gram-negative, microaerophilic, slender, curved, motile bacterium with a polar flagellum. C jejuni is routinely associated with diarrheal disease; however, C coli, distinguished from C jejuni on the basis of hippurate hydrolysis, is occasionally isolated from diarrheic animals and is routinely recovered from asymptomatic pigs. Other intestinal, catalase-negative campylobacters, C upsaliensis and C helveticus, have been isolated from diarrheic dogs and cats as well as asymptomatic dogs and cats.

Campylobacter was once associated with swine dysentery (*Swine Dysentery*), but this is now recognised as being caused by Treponema hyodysenteriae . Most believe that Campylobacter spp do not produce porcine proliferative enteritis (*Porcine Proliferative Enteritis*), even though a new organism, C hyoilei, isolated from swine in Australia, has been associated with porcine proliferative enteritis.

Its role in this disease, however, is not clearly established. C mucosalis and C hyointestinalis have also been isolated from swine but are not considered enteric pathogens. Because of slow growth and microaerobic requirements, standard culture methods require selective media that incorporate various antibiotics to suppress competing fecal microflora.

C jejuni and C coli grow well at 42°C in an atmosphere of 5-10% carbon dioxide and an equal amount of oxygen. Cultures are incubated 48-72 hr; colonies are round, raised, translucent, and sometimes mucoid.

The organism can be identified by a series of biochemical tests readily available in any diagnostic laboratory. Recently, PCR assays have been used to identify Campylobacter spp . Identification is important to distinguish campylobacters from the growing number of novel enterohepatic helicobacters being isolated from a variety of animals.

Transmission and Epidemiology: As with most intestinal pathogens, fecal-oral spread and food- or waterborne transmission appear to be the principal avenues of infection.

One suspected source of infection for pets, as well as mink and ferrets raised for commercial purposes, is ingestion of undercooked poultry and other raw meat products. Asymptomatic carriers can shed the organism in their feces for prolonged periods and contaminate food, water, milk, and fresh processed meats (including pork, beef, and poultry products). The organism can survive in vitro at 41°F (5°C) for 2 mo and can survive in feces, milk, water, and urine. Wild birds also may be important sources of water contamination. Unpasteurized milk has been cited as a principal source of infection in several human outbreaks. Strain identification to study the epizootiology of C jejuni and C coli, in addition to Penner serotyping, is now done using molecular techniques such as restriction fragment length polymorphism and ribotyping.

Clinical Findings: The diarrhea appears to be most severe in young animals. Typical signs in dogs include mucus-laden, watery, and/or bile-streaked diarrhea (with or without blood) that lasts 3-7 days; reduced appetite; and occasional vomiting. Fever and leukocytosis may also be present. In certain cases, intermittent diarrhea may persist >2 wk; in some, it may be present for months. Gnotobiotic puppies inoculated with C jejuni developed malaise, loose feces, and tenesmus within 3 days of inoculation. In calves, signs vary from mild to moderate. The diarrhea is thick and mucoid with occasionally visible blood flecks; body temperature may be normal. Diarrhea with mucus and blood also has been observed in primates, ferrets, mink, and cats. Organisms with ultrastructure similar to that of Campylobacter spp have been seen in hyperplastic ileal epithelial mucosa of hamsters with proliferative ileitis; C jejuni has been isolated from these lesions but has failed to reproduce the syndrome. Organisms with Campylobacter -like morphology also have been associated with proliferative colitis in ferrets and with hyperplastic intestinal lesions in guinea pigs and rats. Campylobacter -like organisms have been described in young rabbits with acute typhlitis. It is now known that these organisms are Lawsonia intracellularis, an organism closely related to Desulfovibrio spp.

Lesions: In 3-day-old chickens infected with C jejuni, the organisms were detected within epithelial cells and mononuclear cells of the lamina propria; the jejunum and ileum were the most severely affected. Congested and edematous colons were found in dogs 43 hr after inoculation; microscopically, epithelial height, brush border, and numbers of goblet cells in the colon and cecum were all reduced. Hyperplastic epithelial glands resulted in a thickened mucosa. Histologic changes in calves primarily involve the jejunum but also can involve the ileum and colon. The lesions vary from mild changes to severe hemorrhagic enteritis. The mesenteric lymph nodes are edematous. Experimentally, some strains of C jejuni produce a hepatitis in mice, and the organism has been isolated from inflamed livers of dogs. A cytotoxin, referred to as cytolethal distending toxin, has been identified in C jejuni ; however, its role in production of intestinal disease is not known. In vitro, the cytotoxin causes distention of cell lines and cell cycle arrest in the G_2M1 phase of the cell cycle.

Diagnosis: The standard method for diagnosis is microaerobic culture of feces at 42°C; a special medium is commercially available. Diagnosis is also possible by using darkfield or phase-contrast microscopy, by which fresh fecal samples are examined for the characteristic darting motility of C jejuni . This method is especially useful during the acute stage of diarrhea when large numbers of organisms are more likely to be shed in the feces. Various techniques can detect serum antibodies to various antigens of Campylobacter spp . Heat-stable or heat-labile antigen schemes are used routinely to serotype various strains. Serial serum samples to demonstrate rising antibody titers are helpful in diagnosis. Intestinal viruses and other intestinal bacterial pathogens must be ruled out as primary or copathogens in animals with Campylobacter - associated diarrhea.

Treatment and Control: Isolation of C jejuni or C coli from diarrheic feces is not, in itself, an indication for antibiotic therapy. Because C jejuni and C coli are not routinely cited as potential intestinal pathogens in animals (except for diarrhea in young cats and dogs and in several species of primates), efficacy of antibiotic therapy has been reported infrequently. In certain cases in which animals are severely affected or are a zoonotic threat, antibiotic treatment may be indicated. In general, C jejuni and C coli isolates from animals are similar to isolates obtained from human populations. Erythromycin, the drug of choice for Campylobacter diarrhea in humans, is also effective in other animals, although erythromycin-resistant strains of Campylobacter spp have been recovered from swine. Gentamicin, furazolidone, and doxycycline also can be used. Ampicillin is relatively inactive against most strains of Campylobacter, and most strains are also resistant to penicillin. Tetracycline and kanamycin resistance in certain C jejuni strains is reported to be plasmid-mediated and transmissible within C jejuni serotypes. Efficacy of sulfadimethoxine and sulfa combinations is variable. Before therapy is instituted, isolation and sensitivity tests should be done. Some animals continue to shed the organism despite antibiotic therapy. Quinolone antibiotics may be useful in eliminating C jejuni and C coli in asymptomatic carriers, but drug resistance may develop.

Intestinal Chlamydial Infections: Introduction

Chlamydiae have been isolated from fecal samples of clinically normal cattle, goats, sheep, and pigs in many parts of the world. Animals with clinically inapparent intestinal infections may shed chlamydiae in the feces for months and possibly years. Accordingly, the GI tract serves as an important reservoir and source for the transmission of these organisms. Chlamydiae, which may cause abortions (*Abortion in Cattle: Overview*) and pneumonia (*Chlamydial Pneumonia: Introduction*), can readily be isolated from feces of normal sheep and cattle.

They have also been recovered from intestinal samples of animals affected with polyarthritis (*Chlamydial Polyarthritis-serositis*), encephalomyelitis (*Sporadic Bovine Encephalomyelitis: Introduction*), and conjunctivitis (*Chlamydial Conjunctivitis: Introduction*). Most fecal isolates from ruminants belong to the species Chlamydia pecorum but some isolates belong to Chlamydophila (Chlamydia) psittaci.

The intestinal infection plays an important role as an initiating event in the pathogenesis of several chlamydia-induced diseases. The intestinal infectious phase also plays an important role in avian chlamydiosis (*Avian Chlamydiosis: Introduction*).

While most of the intestinal chlamydial infections are clinically quiescent, a primary chlamydia-induced enteritis has been seen under field conditions in newborn calves. Such infections may also lead to a change in the number of Escherichia coli in the GI tract, with abnormally high numbers in the abomasum and upper small intestine.

Signs are more severe in colostrum-deprived calves or in those with only a partial transfer of colostral immunity. Affected newborn calves may have a transient watery to mucoid diarrhea with slight fever and nasal discharge. Many veterinary diagnostic laboratories do not routinely check diarrheic feces for chlamydiae; therefore, such an examination must be requested specifically. Treatments of choice are high doses of tetracyclines, administered parenterally or orally, or both.

Salmonellosis: Introduction

Salmonellosis is caused by many species of salmonellae and characterized clinically by one or more of 3 major syndromes —septicemia, acute enteritis, and chronic enteritis. The disease is seen worldwide and in all animals.

The incidence has increased with the intensification of livestock production. Young calves, piglets, lambs, and foals usually develop the septicemic form. Adult cattle, sheep, and horses commonly develop acute enteritis, and chronic enteritis may develop in growing pigs and occasionally in cattle. Pregnant animals may abort.

The clinically normal carrier animal is a serious problem in all host species. Salmonellosis is seen infrequently in dogs and cats and is characterized by acute diarrhea with or without septicemia. The incidence of human salmonellosis has increased in recent years, and animals have been incriminated as the principal reservoir. Transmission to humans occurs via contaminated drinking water, milk, meat, and foods such as cake mixes that use contaminated ingredients; poultry and eggs (*Salmonelloses: Introduction*) are particularly important sources of infection.

Etiology, Epidemiology, and Pathogenesis: While many other Salmonella spp may cause disease, the more common ones in each species are as follows: Cattle— Salmonella serovar typhimurium, Salmonella serovar dublin, and Salmonella serovar newport; Sheep and goats— S typhimurium, S dublin, Salmonella serovar anatum, and Salmonella serovar montevideo; Pigs— S typhimurium and Salmonella serovar choleraesuis ; Horses— S typhimurium, S anatum, S newport, Salmonella serovar enteritidis, and Salmonella serovar IIIa 18:z_4z_{23}.

Although their resulting clinical patterns are not distinct, different species of salmonellae tend to differ in their epidemiology. Plasmid profile and drug-resistance patterns are sometimes useful markers for epidemiologic studies. Feces of infected animals can contaminate feed and water, milk, fresh and processed meats from abattoirs, plant and animal products used as fertilizers or feedstuffs, pasture and rangeland, and many inert materials. The organisms may survive for months in wet, warm areas such as in feeder pig barns or in water dugouts but survive <1 wk in composted cattle manure. Rodents and wild birds also are sources of infection.

Pelleting of feeds reduces the level of contamination by salmonellae. The prevalence of infection varies among species and countries and is much higher than the incidence of clinical disease, which is commonly precipitated by stressful situations such as sudden deprivation of feed, transportation, drought, crowding, parturition, and the administration of some drugs. Salmonellosis is common in hospitalized horses that have been subjected to prolonged surgical procedures.

Use of oral antimicrobial agents is sometimes a risk factor for the disease.The usual route of infection is oral and, after infection, the organism multiplies in the intestine and causes enteritis. Greater susceptibility of the young may be due to high gastric pH, absence of a stable intestinal flora, and limited immunity.

Penetration of bacteria into the lamina propria likely contributes to gut damage and diarrhea. The inflammatory response is marked, and salmonellae are engulfed by phagocytic cells; however, the bacteria can survive and multiply in these cells. Septicemia may follow with subsequent localisation in brain and meninges, pregnant uterus, distal aspects of the limbs, and tips of the ears and tails, which can result, respectively, in meningoencephalitis, abortion, osteitis, and dry gangrene of the feet, tail, or ears.

The organism also frequently localises in the gallbladder and mesenteric lymph nodes, and survivors intermittently shed the organism in the feces. Calves rarely become carriers but virtually all adults do for variable periods—up to 10 wk in sheep and cattle and up to 14 mo in horses. Adult cattle infected with S dublin excrete the organism for years. Infection may persist in lymph nodes or tonsils, with no salmonellae in the feces. Latent carriers may begin shedding the organism or even develop clinical disease under stress. A passive carrier acquires infection from the environment but is not invaded, so that if removed from the environment, it ceases to be a carrier.

Cattle and Sheep: In calves and lambs, the disease is usually endemic on a particular farm, with sporadic explosive outbreaks. Subclinical infection with occasional herd outbreaks may be seen in adult cattle. Stressors that precipitate clinical disease include deprivation of feed and water, minimal levels of nutrition, long transport times, calving, and mixing and crowding in feedlots.

Pigs: Outbreaks of septicemic salmonellosis in pigs are rare and usually can be traced to a purchased, infected pig. Purchase of feeder pigs from salmonellae-free herds and use of the "all-in/all-out" policy in finishing units minimize exposure.

Horses: Many horses may be carriers. In adults, most cases develop after the stress of surgery or transport, especially when horses are moved through sales yards, deprived of feed and water, and then overfed at their destination.

Mares may be inapparent shedders and, despite several negative cultures before foaling, may shed the bacteria at parturition and infect the newborn foal. Salmonellosis in horses hospitalized for other causes is a major problem for equine clinics and stud farms. In these circumstances, carriers are constantly reintroduced, the environment is persistently contaminated, and a large population of vulnerable horses is at risk. Septicemic salmonellosis is also common in foals; it may be endemic on a given premises or there may be outbreaks.

Dogs and Cats: Many dogs and cats are asymptomatic carriers of salmonellae. Clinical disease is uncommon, but when it is seen, it is often associated with hospitalization, another infection or debilitating condition in adults, or exposure to large numbers of the bacteria in puppies and kittens.

Clinical Findings: *Septicemia* is the usual syndrome in newborn calves, lambs, foals, and piglets, and outbreaks may occur in pigs up to 6 mo old. Illness is acute, depression is marked, fever (105-107°F [40.5-41.5°C]) is usual, and death occurs in 24-48 hr. In pigs, a dark red to purple discolouration of the skin is common, especially of the ears and ventral abdomen. Nervous signs may be seen in calves and pigs; these animals may also suffer from pneumonia. Mortality may reach 100%. Acute enteritis is the common form in adults as well as in calves that are usually ≥1 wk old. Initially, there is fever

(105-107°F [40.5-41.5°C]), followed by severe watery diarrhea, sometimes dysentery, and often tenesmus. In a herd outbreak, several hours may lapse before the onset of diarrhea, at which time the fever may disappear.

The feces, which vary considerably, may have a putrid odor and contain mucus, fibrinous casts, shreds of mucous membrane, and in some cases, large blood clots. Rectal examination causes severe discomfort, tenesmus, and commonly dysentery. Milk production often declines precipitously in dairy cows. Abdominal pain is common and severe in horses.

Affected horses are severely dehydrated and may die within 24 hr of the onset of diarrhea; mortality may reach 100%. A marked leukopenia and neutropenia are characteristic of the acute disease in horses.

In dogs and cats, clinical disease takes the form of acute diarrhea with septicemia and is seen occasionally in puppies and kittens or in adults stressed by concurrent disease. Pneumonia may be evident. Abortion is likely to occur in pregnant bitches or queens.

Conjunctivitis is sometimes seen in affected cats. Subacute enteritis may develop in adult horses and sheep on farms where the disease is endemic. The signs include mild fever (103-104°F [39-40°C]), soft feces, inappetence, and some dehydration. There may be a high incidence of abortion in cows and ewes, some deaths in ewes after abortion, and a high mortality rate due to enteritis in lambs younger than a few weeks of age.

In cattle, the first signs may be fever and abortion, followed several days later by diarrhea. Chronic enteritis is a common form in pigs and adult cattle. There is persistent diarrhea, severe emaciation, intermittent fever, and poor response to treatment. The feces are scant and may be normal or contain mucus, casts, or blood. In growing pigs, rectal stricture may be a sequela if the terminal part of the rectum is involved. Affected pigs are anorectic and lose weight; the abdomen becomes grossly distended. The stricture is obvious on digital palpation and necropsy. A number of Salmonella spp are found in foxes, especially kits, and produce a peracute enteritis. Fur-bearing and zoo carnivores may be affected. Contaminated feed is often the source of infection. Several rodents (eg, guinea pigs, hamsters, rats, and mice) and rabbits are susceptible. Rodents commonly act as a source of infection on farms where the disease is endemic. Pet turtles were once a common source of infection in humans that has been virtually eliminated by the curtailment of commercial trafficking in turtles.

Diagnosis: This depends on the clinical signs and on the laboratory examination of feces, tissues from affected animals, feed (including all mineral supplements used), water supplies, and feces from wild rodents and birds that may inhabit the premises.

The clinical syndromes usually are characteristic but must be differentiated from several similar diseases in each species as follows: Cattle—diarrhea due to enterotoxigenic Escherichia coli, dysentery due to verotoxigenic E coli, coccidiosis, cryptosporidiosis, the alimentary tract form of infectious bovine rhinotracheitis, bovine viral diarrhea, hemorrhagic enteritis due to Clostridium perfringens types B and C, arsenic poisoning, secondary copper deficiency (molybdenosis), winter dysentery, paratuberculosis, ostertagiasis, and dietetic diarrhea; Sheep—enteric colibacillosis, septicemia due to Haemophilus sp or pasteurellae, and coccidiosis; Pigs—enteric colibacillosis of newborn pigs and weanlings, swine dysentery, campylobacteriosis, and the septicemias of growing pigs (which include erysipelas, classical swine fever, and pasteurellosis); Horses—septicemia (due to E coli, Actinobacillus equuli, or streptococci) and colitis-X.

The lesions are those of a septicemia or a necrotizing fibrinous enteritis, or both. Lesions are most severe in the lower ileum and the large intestine and vary from shortening of villi with loss of the epithelium to complete loss of intestinal architecture.

There is a neutrophilic reaction in the lamina propria, and thrombi may be seen in blood vessels in this region. Hemorrhage and fibrin strands are usually seen. Culture techniques that involve suppression of fecal E coli are usually necessary, and several daily fecal cultures may be necessary to isolate the organism. Blood cultures in septicemic animals may be rewarding but are costly. Serologic testing is difficult to interpret.

Treatment: Early treatment is essential for septicemic salmonellosis, but there is controversy regarding the use of antimicrobial agents for intestinal salmonellosis. Oral antibiotics may deleteriously alter the intestinal microflora, interfere with competitive antagonism, and prolong shedding of the organism. There is also concern that antibiotic-resistant strains of salmonellae selected by oral antibiotics may subsequently infect humans.

Broad-spectrum antibiotics are used parenterally to treat the septicemia. Initial antimicrobial therapy should be based on knowledge of the drug resistance pattern found in the area. Nosocomial infections often involve highly drug-resistant organisms. Trimethoprim-sulfonamide combinations are often effective. Alternatives are ampicillin, fluoroquinolones, or third-generation cephalosporins.

Treatment should be continued daily for up to 6 days. Oral medication should be given in drinking water because affected animals are thirsty due to dehydration, and their appetite is generally poor. Fluid therapy to correct acid-base imbalance and dehydration is necessary.

Calves, adult cattle, and horses need large quantities of fluids. Antibiotics such as ampicillin or cephalosporins lead to lysis of the bacteria with release of endotoxin. NSAID may be used to reduce the effects of endotoxemia. Horses with acute intestinal salmonellosis are severely acidotic and hyponatremic and may need to be treated initially with 5% sodium bicarbonate, IV, at 5-8 L/450 kg body wt.

This is followed by balanced electrolytes containing potassium to correct the hypokalemia that may follow correction of the acidosis. In horses, flunixin meglumine is recommended for its antiendotoxic properties. Corticosteroids are not recommended because of their immunosuppressive effects and their potential to exacerbate laminitis. IV administration of plasma with a high titer of Salmonella lipopolysaccharide core antibodies may be beneficial in horses. Plasma with serotype-specific antibodies is even more beneficial. Septicemic salmonellosis in pigs usually responds favourably if treated early. However, the intestinal form is difficult to treat effectively in all species. Although clinical cure may be achieved, bacteriologic cure is difficult, particularly in adult animals, because the organisms become established in the biliary system and are intermittently shed into the intestinal lumen, which causes chronic relapsing enteritis and contamination of the environment.

Control and Prevention: These are major problems because of carrier animals and contaminated feedstuffs. Drain swabs or milk filters may be cultured to monitor the salmonellae status of a herd. The principles of control include prevention of introduction and limitation of spread within a herd.

Prevention of Introduction: Every effort must be made to prevent introduction of a carrier; animals should be purchased directly only from farms known to be free of the disease and should be isolated for ≥1 wk while their health status is monitored. Ensuring that feed supplies are free of salmonellae depends on the integrity of the source.

Limitation of Spread Within a Herd: In an outbreak, the following procedures should be implemented: 1) Carrier animals should be identified and either culled or isolated and treated vigorously. Treated animals must be rechecked several times before there can be confidence that they are not carriers. 2) The prophylactic use of antibiotics in feed or water supplies may be considered (but the hazards have been mentioned above). 3) Movement of animals around the farm should be restricted to limit infection to the smallest group. Random mixing of animals should be avoided. 4) Feed and water supplies must be protected from fecal contamination. 5) Contaminated buildings must be vigorously cleaned and disinfected. 6) Contaminated material must be disposed of carefully. 7) All persons should be aware of the hazards of working with infected animals and the importance of personal hygiene. 8) Use of a vaccine should be considered, particularly in an outbreak involving pregnant cattle in which a vaccine has been shown to confer some protection in adults and calves. Commercial killed bacterins or autogenous bacterins may be used. Live attenuated vaccines show considerable promise, but they are not available commercially. 9) Stresses should be minimized. 10) Fetal membranes of mares should be placed in a plastic bag until the mare eliminates them, and the foal should be fed colostrum before contact with the mare.

Salmonella Vaccines: Salmonellae are intracellular parasites, and a live vaccine is therefore expected to be necessary for optimal immune protection against disease. Several studies with live attenuated Salmonella vaccines in pigs, cattle, and chickens have shown them to be effective in stimulating a strong cell-mediated immune response and protecting animals against disease.

A live attenuated S choleraesuis vaccine that has been licensed for use in swine appears to be effective in reducing colonization of tissues and protecting pigs from disease following challenge with virulent organisms. This vaccine has also been reported to reduce the prevalence of Salmonella infections in pigs under field conditions.

This vaccine also protected calves against experimental challenge with S Dublin following intranasal or subcutaneous administration of the vaccine. The administration of the S choleraesuis vaccine to pregnant dairy cows reduced the frequency of shedding of serogroup C1 salmonellae during the peripartum period.

Live S enteritidis has been effective in significantly reducing the infection of laying hens challenged with S enteritidis. The commercial vaccines available for use in cattle are bacterins and appear to induce a modest level of protection. When given to pregnant cows, they induce antibodies in colostrum, which provide an important measure of protection to calves, which are most susceptible in the first week of life.

Salmonellosis in Veterinary Teaching Hospitals: The risk of equine salmonellosis epidemics is particularly high in veterinary teaching hospitals.

A high case load, the presence of animals with severe illnesses, and the stresses of transportation contribute to this risk. The serotype most commonly implicated is S typhimurium but other serotypes that have been identified include Salmonella serovar heidelberg, Salmonella serovar krefeld, Salmonella serovar infantis, and S anatum .

They are frequently resistant to multiple drugs. Contamination of the hospital environment often begins with the introduction of the organisms by a carrier animal. Animals in the hospital (which are often highly susceptible) readily develop diarrhea and contribute to further contamination of the hospital. Infection rates as high as 18% have been reported. Nosocomial infection can be identified by development of salmonellosis ≤3 days after hospitalization and by isolation of hospital-associated Salmonella from cases. The identification of hospital-associated Salmonella involves determination of serotype, drug resistance patterns, and possibly other strain markers such as pulsed field gel electrophoresis patterns, ribotype, and plasmid profiles.

Many hospitals have developed protocols designed to minimize the occurrence of these epidemics, including isolating horses with diarrhea, controlling animal traffic patterns, routinely disinfecting the hospital with an agent of known effectiveness, controlling rodents, using footbaths, limiting access to the hospital area, regularly monitoring drains and other areas of the hospital for salmonellae, routinely repeatedly monitoring horses admitted to the hospital to determine whether they are shedding Salmonella, wearing barrier clothing when attending animals at high risk, and educating personnel. Renovations to the hospital may be required to facilitate thorough cleaning. Closing the hospital for a period of time is often necessary to thoroughly clean and disinfect the premises and to break the cycle of transmission. Outbreaks of salmonellosis have been reported among dogs in veterinary teaching hospitals, but these occurrences are uncommon; antibacterial therapy is a predisposing factor.

Tyzzer's Disease: IntroductionTyzzer's disease is an acute bacterial infection of a wide range of animals that is seen worldwide. Sporadic fatal infection of foals is common, and acute fatal epidemics occur in laboratory animals. The disease is rare in dogs, cats, and calves. It primarily affects young, stressed animals; however, some species appear resistant unless stressed or immunosuppressed, while others are susceptible without immunosuppression. Immunosuppressive drugs and some antibacterials, especially sulfonamides, predispose animals to the disease.

Etiology and Pathogenesis: The cause is Clostridium piliforme (previously Bacillus piliformis), a motile, filamentous, gram-negative, sporeforming, obligate, intracellular bacterium. It does not grow in cell-free media but can be cultured in the yolk sac of chick embryos or tissue culture cells. The vegetative phase is very labile; spores may survive in soiled bedding at room temperature for 1 yr and can also survive at ~133°F (60°C) for 1 hr.The pathogenesis is poorly understood. Infection most likely results from oral exposure.

Possible sources include infective spores from the environment, contact with carrier animals, and in foals, ingestion of horse feces. The primary site of infection is the lower intestinal tract with subsequent dissemination via the blood or lymphatics. The bacterium has an affinity for the intestine (epithelial and smooth muscle cells), hepatocytes, and cardiac myocytes. Stress factors such as capture, overcrowding, shipping, and poor sanitation appear to be predisposing.

Sulfonamide administration predisposes rabbits to the disease. Mortality is highest at weaning age except in foals, in which the disease is seen between 1 and 6 wk of age, with most cases between 1 and 2 wk. In some species, the disease has been identified concurrently with other diseases, eg, feline infectious peritonitis in cats, distemper and mycotic pneumonia in dogs, and cryptosporidial and coronaviral enteritis in calves. The disease most often affects well-nourished animals during periods of stress. Under laboratory conditions, stress is created by immunosuppressive drugs or other factors that can be easily identified. With many experiments, stress may be involved as part of the protocol, and when the disease develops, it is devastating.

Clinical Findings: After experimental infection, the incubation period in foals is 3-7 days; under natural conditions, the period is unknown. Most foals are found in a coma or dead. Clinical signs, if seen, are of short duration (a few hours to 2 days). Signs are variable, but may include depression, anorexia, pyrexia, jaundice, diarrhea, and recumbency. Terminally, there are convulsions and coma. Signs vary slightly between species. Laboratory animals may show depression, ruffled coat, and varying degrees of watery diarrhea; at the start of an outbreak, they often are found dead. Clinicopathologic tests are of little value in laboratory animals because they die so rapidly. In foals, the serum enzymes sorbitol dehydrogenase, AST, alkaline phosphatase, lactate dehydrogenase, and ã-glutamyltransferase are increased. There is also hyperbilirubinemia, leukopenia, hemoconcentration, and terminally profound hypoglycemia.

Lesions: Characteristic lesions are seen in the liver, myocardium, and intestinal tract. In the liver, white, gray, or yellowish foci of necrosis, 2 mm in diametre, are few to disseminated. The hepatic necrosis is most marked and disseminated in foals in which the multiple necrotic foci with slightly depressed hemorrhagic centres appear to infect almost every hepatic lobule.

In addition, there is marked hepatomegaly, and the hepatic lymph nodes are hyperplastic. In rabbits, severe lesions develop in the intestines and heart. The terminal ileum, cecum, and proximal colon are diffusely reddened.

Diffuse ("paint-brush") hemorrhage is frequently seen on the serosa of the cecum. Patchy areas of mucosal necrosis are present in the cecum and colon, together with marked edema of the wall of the cecum. Mesenteric lymph nodes may be enlarged and edematous.

White streaks in the myocardium may be present, especially near the apex. Intestinal and heart lesions are generally milder or absent in other animals. Microscopically, randomly distributed and coalescing foci of necrosis in the liver are associated with scant to moderate infiltration of neutrophils and macrophages.

The causative bacteria are found in a crisscross pattern in viable hepatocytes at the periphery of the necrotic foci. In the cecum and colon of rabbits, patchy areas of necrosis extend as deep as the muscularis externa with associated mucosal and submucosal infiltrates of neutrophils. Organisms may be found in the epithelium, muscularis mucosa, and muscularis externa of the affected intestine. When cardiac lesions are present, they consist of foci of fibre fragmentation, vacuolation, loss of cross-striations, and minimal inflammatory cell infiltration.

Diagnosis: Treatment and Control: Little is known about the effectiveness of antibiotics for treatment; some antibiotics are known to aggravate the disease. C piliforme is sensitive to tetracycline and partially sensitive to streptomycin, erythromycin, penicillin, and chlortetracycline; it is resistant to sulfonamides and chloramphenicol. In foals, the disease seems to be nearly 100% fatal, although it is likely that some foals survive. A definitive clinical diagnosis is not possible due to the lack of a definitive diagnostic test. Once the disease is present on a farm, it may be seen sporadically year after year. Animals suspected of being infected may be treated IV initially with 50% dextrose, followed by 10% dextrose (slowly), other fluid therapy, and antibiotics. Most foals respond dramatically to the dextrose therapy but relapse into a coma and die in a few hours. Rarely, an occasional foal appears to survive the disease after prolonged treatment with dextrose given slowly IV with antibiotics.

Because the disease in foals is sporadic and not highly contagious, specific preventive measures are usually not indicated. Reducing factors that cause stress and immunosuppression lessens the incidence. When the disease is seen in a colony, treatment is not recommended because it prolongs the disease and possibly produces carrier animals. It is best to destroy all animals in the colony and attempt to restock with disease-free animals.

Amebiasis: Introduction (Amebiosis) Amebiasis is an acute or chronic colitis, characterized by persistent diarrhea or dysentery, that is prevalent in tropical and subtropical areas worldwide. Its prevalence has declined in the USA over the past several decades, but the disease is still important in many tropical areas, particularly in times of disasters.

It is common in people and nonhuman primates, sometimes seen in dogs and cats, and rare in other mammals. Several species of amebae are found in mammals, but the only known pathogen is Entamoeba histolytica. Humans are the natural host for this species and the usual source of infection for domestic animals. Mammals become infected by ingesting food or water contaminated with feces containing infective cysts. E dispar is a noninvasive, nonpathogenic amoeba that is molecularly distinct but morphologically indistinguishable from the pathogenic species E histolytica. E invadens of reptiles is also morphologically identical to E histolytica, but it is not transmissible to mammals.

Clinical Findings: E histolytica is a pathogen with variable virulence. It lives in the lumen of the large intestine and cecum and may produce no obvious clinical signs or invade the intestinal mucosa and produce mild to severe, ulcerative, hemorrhagic colitis. In acute disease, fulminating dysentery may develop, which may be fatal, progress to chronicity, or resolve spontaneously. Chronic cases may show weight loss, anorexia, tenesmus, and chronic diarrhea or dysentery, which may be continuous or intermittent. In addition to the colon and cecum, amebae may invade perianal skin, genitalia, liver, brain, lungs, kidneys, and other organs. Signs may resemble those of other colonic diseases (eg, trichuriasis, balantidiasis). Invasive amebiasis is exacerbated by immunosuppression.

Diagnosis: Definitive diagnosis depends on finding E histolytica trophozoites or cysts in feces. Trophozoites are best seen in direct saline smears or in stained sections of affected colonic tissue. These parasites are difficult to find because many animals with extraintestinal amebiasis have no concurrent intestinal infection.

Colonoscopy with scraping or biopsy of ulcerations is more effective than fecal examination in diagnosing amebic colitis. In intestinal infections, repeated examinations may be necessary because parasites may be passed periodically in the feces. Trophozoites range in size from 10-60 μm but usually are >20 μm in diametre, have a single vesicular nucleus, (usually with a central karyosome), are motile, and may contain ingested RBC. Feces should be examined promptly because the trophozoites die quickly once outside the body.

Fecal leukocytes may be mistaken for amebae, so fixed and stained fecal smears (iodine, trichrome, iron, hematoxylin, or periodic acid-Schiff reaction) may be necessary for identification. Cysts range from 10-20 μm in diametre; the usual size is 12-15 μm. Mature cysts have 4 nuclei, while immature cysts may have 1 or 2. In primates, the cysts may be recovered and identified on zinc sulfate flotations or in fixed and stained preparations (iodine, trichrome, or iron hematoxylin); however, E histolytica cysts are seldom if ever excreted by dogs or cats. An ELISA-based antigen test, available for diagnosis in humans, may also aid diagnosis in other mammals. Immunostaining may also be useful.

Treatment: Scant information on treatment in animals is available. Metronidazole (10-25 mg/kg, PO, bid for 1 wk) or furazolidone (2-4 mg/kg, PO, tid for 1 wk) has been suggested. Dogs may continue to shed trophozoites after therapy.

Coccidiosis: Introduction

Coccidiosis is a usually acute invasion and destruction of intestinal mucosa by protozoa of the genera Eimeria or Isospora . Infection is characterized by diarrhea, fever, inappetence, weight loss, emaciation, and sometimes death. Coccidiosis is a serious disease in cattle, sheep, goats, pigs, poultry (*Coccidiosis: Introduction*), and also rabbits, in which the liver as well as the intestine can be affected (*Coccidiosis*). In dogs, cats, and horses, it is less often diagnosed but can result in clinical illness. Other genera, of both hosts and protozoa, can be involved.

Etiology and Epidemiology: Eimeria and Isospora typically require only one host in which to complete their life cycles. Some species of Isospora have facultative intermediate (paratenic or transfer) hosts. A new genus name, Cystoisospora, has been proposed but has not gained wide acceptance. Coccidia are host-specific, and there is no cross-immunity between species of coccidia.

Coccidiosis is seen universally, most commonly in animals housed or confined in small areas contaminated with oocysts. Coccidia are opportunistic pathogens; if pathogenic, their virulence may be influenced by various stressors.

Therefore, clinical coccidiosis is most prevalent under conditions of poor nutrition, poor sanitation, or overcrowding, or after the stresses of weaning, shipping, sudden changes of feed, or severe weather. In general, for most species of farm animals, the infection rate is high and rate of clinical disease is low (5-10%), although up to 80% of animals in a high-risk group may show signs. Most animals acquire Eimeria or Isospora infections of varying severity when between 1 mo and 1 yr old. Older animals usually are resistant to clinical disease but may have sporadic inapparent infections. Such clinically healthy, mature animals usually can be sources of infection to young, susceptible animals.

Pathogenesis: Infection results from ingestion of infective oocysts. Oocysts enter the environment in the feces of an infected host, but oocysts of Eimeria and Isospora are unsporulated and therefore not infective. Under favourable conditions of oxygen, humidity, and temperature, oocysts sporulate and become infective in several days. During sporulation, the amorphous protoplasm develops into small bodies (sporozoites) within secondary cysts (sporocysts) in the oocyst. In Eimeria spp, the sporulated oocyst has 4 sporocysts, each containing 2 sporozoites; in Isospora spp, the sporulated oocyst has 2 sporocysts, each containing 4 sporozoites. When the sporulated oocyst is ingested by a susceptible animal, the sporozoites escape from the oocyst, invade the intestinal mucosa or epithelial cells in other locations, and develop intracellularly into multinucleate schizonts (also called meronts). Each nucleus develops into an infective body called a merozoite; merozoites enter new cells and repeat the process. After a variable number of asexual generations, merozoites develop into either macrogametocytes (females) or microgametocytes (males). These produce a single macrogamete or a number of microgametes in a host cell. After being fertilized by a microgamete, the macrogamete develops into an oocyst. The oocysts have resistant walls and are discharged unsporulated in the feces. Oocysts do not survive well at temperatures below -30°C or above 40°C; within this range, they may survive up to 1 yr or more. Of the numerous species of Eimeria or Isospora that can infect a particular host, not all are pathogenic. Concurrent infections with 2 or more species, some of which may not normally be considered pathogenic, also influence clinical disease. Within pathogenic species, strains may vary in virulence.

Clinical Findings: Clinical signs of coccidiosis are due to destruction of the intestinal epithelium and, frequently, the underlying connective tissue of the mucosa. This may be accompanied by hemorrhage into the lumen of the intestine, catarrhal inflammation, and diarrhea. Signs may include discharge of blood or tissue, tenesmus, and dehydration. Serum protein and electrolyte levels may be appreciably altered, but changes in Hgb or PCV are seen only in severely affected animals.

Diagnosis: Oocysts can be identified in feces by salt or sugar flotation methods. Finding appreciable numbers of oocysts of pathogenic species in the feces is diagnostic, but because diarrhea may precede the heavy output of oocysts by 1-2 days and may continue after the oocyst discharge has returned to low levels, it is not always possible to find oocysts in a single fecal sample; multiple examinations may be required. The number of oocysts present in feces is influenced by the genetically determined reproductive potential of the species, the number of infective oocysts ingested, stage of the infection, age and immune status of the animal, prior exposure, consistency of the fecal sample, and method of examination. Therefore, the results of fecal examinations must be related to clinical signs and intestinal lesions (gross and microscopic). Furthermore, the species must be determined to be pathogenic in that host. The finding of numerous oocysts of a nonpathogenic species concurrent with diarrhea does not constitute a diagnosis of clinical coccidiosis.

Treatment: The life cycles of Eimeria and Isospora are self-limiting and end spontaneously within a few weeks unless reinfection occurs. Prompt medication may slow or inhibit development of stages resulting from reinfection and, thus, can shorten the length of illness, reduce discharge of oocysts, alleviate hemorrhage and diarrhea, and lessen the likelihood of secondary infections and death.

Sick animals should be isolated and treated individually whenever possible to ensure delivery of therapeutic drug levels and to prevent exposure of other animals. Sulfonamides may be used.

Sulfaquinoxaline has been reported to give excellent clinical results in beef and dairy calves, sheep, dogs, and cats. Because the soluble sulfonamides may be given PO or parenterally, they are more effective than intestinal sulfonamides. Amprolium has been reported to be effective during outbreaks in calves, sheep, and goats. In outbreaks in feedlots or on lush pastures, preventive treatment of healthy exposed animals as a safeguard against additional morbidity should be considered.

Prevention: Prevention is based on limiting the intake of sporulated oocysts by young animals so that an infection is established to induce immunity but not clinical signs. Good feeding practices and good management, including sanitation, contribute to this goal.

Neonates should receive colostrum. Young susceptible animals should be kept in clean and dry quarters. Feeding and watering devices should be clean and protected from fecal contamination. Stresses (eg, weaning, sudden changes in feed, and shipping) should be minimized. Preventive administration of coccidiostats is recommended when animals under various management regimens can be predictably expected to develop coccidiosis.

In virtually all cases, Eimeria spp are implicated. Decoquinate, amprolium, and ionophorous antibiotics are effective in cattle. Continuous low-level feeding of amprolium, decoquinate, lasalocid, or monensin during the first month of feedlot confinement has been reported to have preventive value. Both amprolium and ionophorous antibiotics have been reported to be effective in goat kids, as have sulfas and amprolium in pigs.

Coccidiosis of Cattle

E zuernii, E bovis, and E auburnensis are the species most often associated with clinical disease in cattle. Experimentally, other species have been shown to be mildly or moderately pathogenic. Coccidiosis is commonly a disease of young cattle (1-2 mo to 1 yr) and usually is sporadic during the wet seasons of the year. "Summer coccidiosis" and "winter coccidiosis" in range cattle probably result from severe weather stress and crowding around a limited water source, which concentrates the hosts and parasites within a restricted area.

Although particularly severe epidemics have been reported in feedlot cattle during extremely cold weather, cattle confined to feedlots are susceptible to coccidiosis throughout the year. Outbreaks usually occur within the first month of confinement. The incubation period is 17-21 days. The most typical syndrome is chronic or subclinical disease in groups of growing animals. Calves may appear unthrifty and have fecal-stained perineal areas. In light infections, cattle appear healthy and oocysts are present in normally formed feces, but feed efficiency is reduced.

The most characteristic sign of clinical coccidiosis is watery feces, with little or no blood, and the animal shows only slight discomfort for a few days. Severe infections are rare. Severely affected cattle develop thin, bloody diarrhea that may continue for >1 wk, or thin feces with streaks or clots of blood, shreds of epithelium, and mucus. They may develop a fever; become anorectic, depressed, and dehydrated; and lose weight. Tenesmus is common. During the acute period, some cattle die; others die later from secondary complications (eg, pneumonia).

Cattle that survive severe illness can lose significant weight that is not quickly regained or can remain permanently stunted. Calves with concurrent infections (eg, coronavirus) may be more severely affected than calves with coccidia infections alone.

In addition, management factors, such as weather, housing, feeding practices, and how animals are grouped, are important in determining the expression of clinical coccidiosis in cattle. The pathogenic coccidia of cattle can damage the mucosa of the lower small intestine, cecum, and colon. The first-generation schizonts of E bovis appear as white macroscopic bodies in the villi of the small intestine.

Nervous signs (eg, muscular tremors, hyperesthesia, clonic-tonic convulsions with ventro flexion of the head and neck, nystagmus) and a high mortality rate (80-90%) are seen in calves with acute clinical coccidiosis. Outbreaks of this "nervous form" have occurred in which 30-50% of all susceptible calves are affected.

It has been seen most commonly during, or following, severely cold weather in midwinter in Canada and the northern USA. Affected calves may die <24 hr after the onset of dysentery and nervous signs, or they may live for several days, commonly in a laterally recumbent position with a mild degree of opisthotonos. In spite of intensive supportive therapy, the mortality rate is high.

Nervous signs have not been reported in experimental clinical coccidiosis in calves, which suggests that the nervous signs may be unrelated to the dysentery or, indeed, even to coccidiosis.

Diagnosis is by finding oocysts on fecal flotation or direct smear or by the McMaster's technique. Differential diagnoses include salmonellosis, bovine virus diarrhea, malnutrition, toxins, or other intestinal parasites. Coccidiosis is a self-limiting disease, and spontaneous recovery without specific treatment is common when the multiplication stage of the coccidia has passed. The chemotherapeutic agents in common use for clinical coccidiosis are unlikely to have any effect on the late stages of the coccidia. Most of the coccidiostats have a depressant effect on the early, first-stage schizonts and are used for control. Drugs that can be used for therapy of clinically affected animals include amprolium (10 mg/kg/day for 5 days) and sulfaquinoxaline (6 mg/lb/day for 3-5 days). Sulfaquinoxaline is particularly useful for feedlot cattle that develop bloody diarrhea after arrival. For prevention, amprolium (5 mg/kg/day for 21 days), decoquinate (22.7 mg/45 kg/day for 28 days) and lasalocid (1 mg/kg/day to a maximum of 360 mg/head/day), or monensin (100-360 mg/head/day) can be used.

The major benefits of the coccidiostats are through improved feed efficiency and rate of gain. In an outbreak, the clinically affected animals should be isolated and given supportive oral and parenteral fluid therapy as necessary. The population density of the affected pens should be reduced. All feed and water supplies should be high enough off the ground to avoid fecal contamination.

Mass medication of the feed and water supplies may be indicated in an attempt to prevent new cases and to minimize the effects of an epidemic. Cattle with coccidiosis and nervous signs should be brought indoors, kept well-bedded and warm, and given fluid therapy orally and parenterally. However, the case fatality rate is high despite intensive supportive therapy.

Parenteral sulfonamide therapy may be indicated to control the development of secondary bacterial enteritis or pneumonia, which may develop in calves with coccidiosis during very cold weather. Corticosteroids are contraindicated. Coccidiosis has been difficult to control reliably.

Overcrowding of animals should be avoided while they develop an immunity to the coccidial species in the environment. Calving grounds should be well drained and kept as dry as possible.

All measures that minimize fecal contamination of hair coats and fleece should be practiced regularly. Feed and water troughs should be high enough to avoid heavy fecal contamination. Control of coccidiosis in feeder calves brought into a crowded feedlot depends on management of population density, or use of chemotherapeutics, to control the numbers of oocysts ingested by the animals while effective immunity develops. Coccidiostats are used for the control of naturally occurring coccidiosis. The ideal coccidiostat suppresses the full development of the life cycle of the coccidia, allows immunity to develop, and does not interfere with production performance. Sulfonamides in the feed at 25-35 mg/kg for ≥15 days are effective for the control of coccidiosis in calves. Monensin is an effective coccidiostat and growth promotant in calves. Withdrawal of monensin may be followed by development of fatal coccidiosis in some animals, presumably because the drug suppressed the development of immunity.

Postweaning coccidiosis in beef calves has been controlled using monensin administered via intraluminal continuous release devices. Lasalocid is related to monensin and is also an effective coccidiostat for ruminants. Mixing lasalocid in the milk replacer of calves beginning at 2-4 days of age is an effective method of controlling coccidiosis.

Lasalocid is also effective as a coccidiostat when fed free-choice in salt at a level of 0.75% of the total salt mixture. A level of 1 mg/kg is the most effective and rapid, and is recommended when outbreaks of coccidiosis are imminent. Decoquinate in the feed at 0.5-1.0 mg/kg suppressed oocyst production in experimentally induced coccidiosis of calves. It is most effective in preventing coccidial infections when fed continuously in dry feed at 0.5 mg/kg.

Monensin, lasalocid, and decoquinate at the manufacturer's recommended levels are equally effective. Toltrazuril administered at 20 mg/kg as a single dose, 10 days after animals are turned out to pasture, almost completely prevents coccidiosis. Control of infection should include changes in management factors that contribute to the development of clinical disease. Inadequate housing and ventilation should be corrected, feeding practices adopted that avoid fecal contamination of feed, calves grouped by size, and an "all-in/all-out" method of calf movement from pen to pen adopted.

Coccidiosis of Sheep

Infection with Eimeria is one of the most economically important diseases of sheep. Historically, some Eimeria spp were thought to be infectious and transmissible between sheep and goats, but the parasites are now considered host-specific. The names of some species of goat coccidia are still erroneously applied to species of similar appearance found in sheep. E ahsata and E ovinoidalis (ninakohlyakimovae) are pathogens of lambs, usually 1-6 mo old; E ovina appears to be somewhat less pathogenic. Older sheep serve as sources of infection for the young.

All other Eimeria of sheep are essentially nonpathogenic, even when large numbers of oocysts are present in feces. Signs include diarrhea (sometimes containing blood or mucus), dehydration, fever, inappetence, weight loss, anemia, wool breaking, and death. The ileum, cecum, and upper colon are usually most affected and may be thickened, edematous, and inflamed; sometimes, there is mucosal hemorrhage. Thick, white, opaque patches containing large numbers of E ovina oocysts may develop in the small intestine.

Because oocysts are prevalent in feces of sheep of all ages, coccidiosis cannot be diagnosed based solely on finding oocysts. Peak oocyst counts of >100,000/g of feces have been reported in 8- to 12-wk-old lambs that appeared healthy. However, diarrhea with oocyst counts of a pathogenic species of >20,000/g is characteristic of coccidiosis in sheep.

Immune complex glomerulonephritis has also been attributed to coccidiosis. Fly strike and secondary bacterial enteric infections may accompany coccidiosis. Lambs 1-6 mo old in lambing pens, intensive grazing areas, and feedlots are at greatest risk as a result of shipping, ration change, crowding stress, severe weather, and contamination of the environment with oocysts from ewes or other lambs.

Because occurrence of coccidiosis under these management systems often becomes so predictable, coccidiostats should be administered prophylactically for 28 consecutive days beginning a few days after lambs are introduced into the environment. A concentrated ration containing monensin at 15 g/tonne can be fed to ewes from 4 wk before lambing until weaning, and to lambs from 4-20 wk of age.

The toxic level of monensin for lambs is 4 mg/kg. Lasalocid (15-70 mg/head/day, depending on body wt) may be effective. A combination of monensin and lasalocid at 22 and 100 mg/kg of diet, respectively, is an effective prophylactic against naturally occurring coccidiosis in early weaned lambs under feedlot conditions. Treatment of affected sheep once coccidiosis has been diagnosed is not effective, but severity can be reduced if treatment is begun early. A single treatment of toltrazuril (20 mg/kg) can significantly reduce the oocyst output in naturally infected lambs for ~3 wk after administration. Sulfaquinoxaline in drinking water at 0.015% concentration for 3-5 days may be used for treatment of affected lambs.

In groups of lambs at pasture, the frequent rotation of pastures for parasite control will also help control coccidial infection. However, when lambs are exposed to infection early in life as a result of infection from the ewe and a contaminated lambing ground, a solid immunity usually develops and only when the stocking density is extremely high will a problem develop.

Coccidiosis of Goats

Numerous species of Eimeria are found in goats in North America. The Eimeria spp are host-specific and are not transmitted from sheep to goats. E arloingi, E christenseni, and E ovinoidalis are highly pathogenic in kids.

Clinical signs include diarrhea with or without mucus or blood, dehydration, emaciation, weakness, anorexia, and death. Some goats are actually constipated and die acutely without diarrhea. Usually, stages and lesions are confined to the small intestine, which may appear congested, hemorrhagic, or ulcerated, and have scattered pale, yellow to white macroscopic plaques in the mucosa.

Histologically, villous epithelium is sloughed, and inflammatory cells are seen in the lamina propria and submucosa. In addition, there have been several reports of hepatobiliary coccidiosis with liver failure in dairy goats.

Diagnosis of intestinal coccidiosis is based on finding oocysts of the pathogenic species in diarrheal feces, usually at tens of thousands to millions per gram of feces. It is not unusual to find oocyst counts as high as 70,000 in kids without overt disease, but weight gain may be affected. Angora and dairy goats, raised under different management practices, may have similar patterns of exposure of kids. Just after parturition, nursery pens and surrounding areas may be heavily contaminated with oocysts from does. Resistance to infection is decreased just after shipping, changing rations, introducing new animals, or mixing young with older animals. Coccidiostats can be administered to a herd immediately after diagnosis or as a preventive in predictable situations such as those mentioned above. Diagnosis and treatment are similar to those for cattle and sheep. Sulfadimidine at 55 g/tonne is also effective for the control of coccidiosis in goats. In nonlactating goats, adding monensin to the feed at 18 g/tonne is preventive.

Coccidiosis of Pigs

Eight species of Eimeria and 1 of Isospora infect pigs in the USA. Piglets 5-15 days old are characteristically infected with only I suis, which produces enteritis and diarrhea. These agents must be differentiated from viruses, bacteria, and helminths that also cause scours in neonatal pigs. I suis is prevalent in neonatal pigs.

Infection is characterized by a watery or greasy diarrhea, usually yellowish to white and foul smelling. Piglets may appear weak, dehydrated, and undersized; weight gains are depressed, and sometimes piglets die. A contributing factor to mortality is that piglets become covered with diarrheic feces and stay damp. Oocysts are usually shed in the feces and can be identified by their size, shape, and sporulation characteristics; however, in peracute infections, diagnosis must be based on finding stages of the parasite in impression smears or histologic sections of the small intestine because pigs can die before oocysts are formed.

In severely affected piglets, histologic lesions confined to the jejunum and ileum are characterized by villous atrophy, blunting of villi, focal ulceration, and fibrinonecrotic enteritis with parasite stages in epithelial cells.

Preventive control by feeding anticoccidials to sows from 2 wk before farrowing through lactation or to neonatal pigs from birth to weaning has been reported; however, effectiveness of the latter has not been confirmed. Although the sow is a logical source of infection for piglets, this has not been well documented. Thorough removal of feces and disinfection of farrowing facilities between litters greatly decreases infection. Piglets that recover from infection are highly resistant to reinfection. Although less commonly associated with clinical coccidiosis, E debliecki, E neodebliecki, E scabra, and E spinosa have been found in pigs ~1-3 mo old with diarrhea. Illness may last 7-10 days, with pigs remaining unthrifty. Treatment may include sulfamethazine in drinking water. The control of coccidiosis in newborn piglets infected with I suis has been unreliable. The use of coccidiostats in the feed of the sow for several days or a few weeks prior to, and following, farrowing has been recommended and used in the field, but the results are variable.

Amprolium and monensin are ineffective for the prevention of experimental coccidiosis in piglets. A control program designed to decrease the number of oocysts has been recommended and consists of proper cleaning, disinfection, and steam cleaning of the farrowing housing.

Amprolium (25% feed grade) at the rate of 10 kg/tonne of sows' feed started 1 wk before farrowing and continued until the piglets are 3 wk of age has been recommended, but the results are unsatisfactory. A single oral dose of 1.0 mL of toltrazuril given to piglets 3-6 days old reduced the occurrence of coccidiosis from 71% to 22%, and the number of days that oocysts were excreted in the feces was reduced from 4.9 to 2.5.

Coccidiosis of Cats and Dogs

Many species of coccidia infect the intestinal tract of cats and dogs. All species appear to be host-specific. Cats have species of Isospora, Besnoitia, Toxoplasma, Hammondia, and Sarcocystis. Dogs have species of Isospora, Hammondia, and Sarcocystis. Neither dogs nor cats have Eimeria .Hammondia has an obligatory 2-host life cycle with cats or dogs as final hosts and rodents or ruminants as intermediate hosts, respectively. Hammondia oocysts are indistinguishable from those of Toxoplasma and Besnoitia but are nonpathogenic in either host. The most common coccidia of cats and dogs are Isospora. Some Isospora spp of cats and dogs can facultatively infect other mammals and produce in various organs an encysted form that is infective for the cat or dog.

Two Species Infect Cats: I felis and I rivolta ; both can be identified easily by oocyst size and shape. Almost every cat eventually becomes infected with I felis . Four species infect dogs: I canis, I ohioensis, I burrowsi, and I neorivolta . In dogs, only I canis can be identified by the oocyst structure; the other

3 Isospora overlap in dimensions and can be differentiated only by endogenous developmental characteristics. Clinical coccidiosis, although not common, has been reported in kittens and puppies. In kittens, it is seen primarily during weaning stress. The most common clinical signs in severe cases are diarrhea (sometimes bloody), weight loss, and dehydration. Usually, coccidiosis is associated with other infectious agents, immunosuppression, or stress.

Treatment may be unnecessary in cats because they usually spontaneously eliminate the infection. In clinically affected cats, trimethoprim-sulfa (30-60 mg/kg/day for 6 days) can be used. In kennel conditions when the need for prophylaxis might be predicted, amprolium is said to be effective, although it is not approved for use in dogs.

In severe cases, in addition to supportive fluid therapy, sulfonamides such as sulfadimethoxine (50 mg/kg the first day and 25 mg/kg/day for 2-3 wk thereafter) can be used. Sanitation is important, especially in catteries and kennels, or where large numbers of animals are housed. Feces should be removed frequently. Fecal contamination of feed and water should be prevented. Runs, cages, and utensils should be disinfected daily. Raw meat should not be fed. Insect control should be established.

Cryptosporidiosis

Cryptosporidiosis is recognised worldwide, primarily in neonatal calves but also in lambs, kids, foals, and piglets. It is considered a cause of varying degrees of naturally occurring diarrhea in neonatal farm animals. The parasites commonly act in concert with other enteropathogens to produce intestinal injury and diarrhea.

Etiology and Epidemiology: Cryptosporidium parvum infection is common in young ruminants and is found in many species of mammals, including humans. Infection is common in calves. Cryptosporidia have been detected in 70% of 1- to 3-wk-old dairy calves. Infection can be detected as early as 5 days of age, with the greatest proportion of calves excreting organisms between days 9 and 14. Many reports associate infection in calves with diarrhea occurring at 5-15 days of age. C parvum is also a common enteric infection in young lambs and goats. Diarrhea can result from a monoinfection, but more commonly is associated with mixed infections. Infection can be associated with severe outbreaks of diarrhea, with high case fatality rates in lambs 4-10 days of age and in goat kids 5-21 days of age. Cryptosporidial infection in pigs is seen over a wider age range than in ruminants and has been observed in pigs from 1 wk of age through market age.

The majority of infections are asymptomatic, and the organism does not appear to be an important enteric pathogen in pigs, although it may contribute to postweaning malabsorptive diarrhea. Cryptosporidial infection in foals appears less prevalent and is seen at a later age than in ruminants, with excretion rates peaking at 5-8 wk of age.

Infection is not usually detected in yearlings or adults. Most studies indicate that cryptosporidiosis is not a common disease in foals; infections in immunocompetent foals are usually subclinical. Persistent clinical infections are seen in Arabian foals with inherited combined immunodeficiency. Cryptosporidiosis is also recorded in young deer and can be a cause of diarrhea in artificially reared orphans.

Transmission: The source of infection is oocysts that are fully sporulated and infective when excreted in the feces. Large numbers are excreted during the patent period, resulting in heavy environmental contamination.

Transmission may occur directly from calf to calf, indirectly via fomite or human transmission, from contamination in the environment, or by fecal contamination of the feed or water supply. A periparturient rise in the excretion of oocysts may occur in ewes.

C parvum is not host-specific, and infection from other species (eg, rodents, farm cats) via contamination of feed is also possible. Oocysts are resistant to most disinfectants and can survive for several months in cool and moist conditions.

Oocyst infectivity can be destroyed by ammonia, formalin, freeze-drying, and exposure to temperatures <32°F (0°C) or >149°F (65°C). Ammonium hydroxide, hydrogen peroxide, chlorine dioxide, 10% formol saline, and 5% ammonia are effective in destroying oocyst infectivity. Infectivity in calf feces is reduced after 1-4 days of drying. Concurrent infections with other enteric pathogens, especially rotavirus and coronavirus, are common, and epidemiologic studies suggest that diarrhea is more severe in mixed infections. Immunocompromised animals are more susceptible to clinical disease than immunocompetent animals, but the relationship between disease and failure of passive transfer of colostral immuno-globulins is not clear.

Age-related resistance, unrelated to prior exposure, is observed in lambs but not calves. Infection results in the production of parasite-specific antibody, but both cell-mediated and humoral antibody are important in protection, as well as local antibody in the gut of the neonate. Case fatality rates in cryptosporidiosis are generally low unless complicated by other factors (eg, concurrent infections, energy deficits from inadequate intake of colostrum and milk, chilling from adverse weather conditions).

Pathogenesis: The life cycle of Cryptosporidium consists of 6 major developmental events. Following ingestion of the oocyst there is excystation (release of infective sporozoites), merogony (asexual multiplication), gametogony (gamete formation), fertilization, oocyst wall formation, and sporogony (sporozoite formation).

Oocysts of Cryptosporidium spp can sporulate within host cells and are infective when passed in the feces. Infection persists until the host's immune response eliminates the parasite. In natural and experimentally produced cases in calves, cryptosporidia are most numerous in the lower part of the small intestine and less common in the cecum and colon. Prepatent periods are 2-7 days in calves and 2-5 days in lambs. Oocysts are usually passed in the feces of calves for 3-12 days.

Clinical Findings: Calves usually have a mild to moderate diarrhea that persists for several days regardless of treatment. The age at onset is later, and the duration of diarrhea tends to be a few days longer than are seen in the diarrheas caused by rotavirus, coronavirus, or enterotoxigenic Escherichia coli . Feces are yellow or pale, watery, and contain mucus. The persistent diarrhea may result in marked weight loss and emaciation. In most cases, the diarrhea is self-limiting after several days. Varying degrees of apathy, anorexia, and dehydration are present. Only rarely do severe dehydration, weakness, and collapse occur, in contrast to other causes of acute diarrhea in neonatal calves. Case fatality rates can be high in herds with cryptosporidiosis when the calf feeder withholds milk and feeds only electrolyte solutions during the episode of diarrhea. The persistent nature of the diarrhea leads to a marked energy deficit in these circumstances, and the calves die of inanition at 3-4 wk of age.

Lesions: Calves with persistent diarrhea have villous atrophy in the small intestine. Histologically, large numbers of the parasite are embedded in the microvilli of the absorptive enterocytes. In low-grade infections, only a few parasites are present, with no apparent histologic changes in the intestine. The villi are shorter than normal, with crypt hyperplasia and a mixed inflammatory cell infiltrate.

Diagnosis: Diagnosis is based on detection of oocysts by examination of fecal smears with Ziehl-Neelson stains, by fecal flotation, or by immunologically assisted methods. It has been suggested that if the diarrhea is caused by cryptosporidia, there should be 10^5 -10^7 oocysts/mL of feces. The oocysts are small (5-6 mm in diametre) and relatively nonrefractile. They are difficult to detect by normal light microscopy but are readily detected by phase-contrast microscopy.

Treatment: There are no currently licensed therapeutics available in the USA for C parvum infection in food animals. Anecdotal reports of success with extra-label use of various compounds have not been replicated in controlled trials. Experimental treatments have for the most part been toxic or ineffective.

Halofuginone is reported to markedly reduce oocyst output in experimentally infected lambs and naturally and experimentally infected calves; therapy was also reported to prevent diarrhea.

Paromomycin sulfate (100 mg/kg, PO, sid for 11 days from the second day of age) proved successful in preventing natural disease in a controlled clinical field trial in goat kids. Affected calves should be supported with fluids and electrolytes, both orally and parenterally, as necessary until recovery occurs. Cows' whole milk should be given in small quantities several times daily (to the full level of requirement) to optimize digestion and to minimize weight loss. Several days of intensive care and feeding may be required before recovery is apparent. Parenteral nutrition may be considered for valuable calves.

Control: The disease is difficult to control. Reducing the number of oocysts ingested may reduce the severity of infection and allow immunity to develop. Calves should be born in a clean environment, and adequate amounts of colostrum should be fed at an early age.

Calves should be kept separate without calf-to-calf contact for at least the first 2 wk of life, with strict hygiene at feeding. Diarrheic calves should be isolated from healthy calves during the course of the diarrhea and for several days after recovery. Great care must be taken to avoid mechanical transmission of infection. Calf-rearing houses should be vacated and cleaned out on a regular basis; an "all-in/all-out" management system, with thorough cleaning and several weeks of drying between batches of calves, should be used.

Rats, mice, and flies should be controlled when possible, and rodents and pets should not have access to calf grain and milk feed storage areas.

Hyperimmune bovine colostrum can reduce the severity of diarrhea and the period of oocyst excretion in experimentally infected calves. Protection is not related to circulating levels of specific antibody but requires a high titer of C parvum antibody in the gut lumen for prolonged periods. Vaccination with lyophylized C parvum given orally shortly after birth gave partial protection to calves challenged experimentally at 1 wk of age. It was not effective in protecting against natural challenge in a field trial, presumably because natural infection occurred too early to allow development of immunity. In the same trial, lactic acid-producing probiotics had no protective effect.

Zoonotic Risk: Infections in domestic animals may be a reservoir for infection of susceptible humans. Cryptosporidium is considered to be a relatively common nonviral cause of self-limiting diarrhea in immunocompetent persons, particularly children. In immunocompromised persons, clinical disease may be severe. The infection is transmitted predominantly from person to person, but direct infection from animals and waterborne infection from contamination of surface water and drinking water by domestic or wild animal feces can also be important. Animal handlers on a calf farm can be at high risk of diarrhea due to cryptosporidiosis transmitted from infected calves. Immunocompromised people should be restricted from access to young animals and possibly from access to farms.

Diseases of the Mouth in Large Animals: IntroductionLip Lacerations

Wounds of the lips and cheeks are most common in horses. They may be caused by a fall, a kick, or the use of inappropriate bits or restraint devices or, more commonly, from the horse having its lips and sometimes mandible caught as it "plays" in its stall. Lip lacerations may be accompanied by mandibular or incisive bone and dental fractures and avulsions in some cases (eg, if the horse panics). Because of the vascularity of the region, healing is usually rapid. However, once the wound has penetrated into the mouth, careful management is needed to avoid formation of a fistula. First-stage healing is best achieved by the construction of intraoral mucosal flaps to achieve an oral seal. Subsequent skin or mucosal grafts may be necessary to correct large defects or fistulae.

Glossoplegia (Paralysis of the Tongue): This may be seen in newborns as a result of the placement of obstetric snares. Such neonates need to be managed carefully to ensure that they are able to eat; ingestion of colostrum is particularly important. Fluid therapy (IV) and anti-inflammatory treatments are required. If the condition persists for >10 days after birth, the likelihood of regaining normal function is slight. Inflammatory diseases and trauma may also result in transient glossoplegia. Glossoplegia of central origin may accompany or follow such conditions as strangles, upper respiratory infections, meningitis, botulism, encephalomyelitis, leukoencephalomalacia, or cerebral abscessation in horses. In cattle, glossoplegia may accompany severe actinobacillosis (*Actinobacillosis: Introduction*). There may be complete paralysis of the tongue accompanied by necrosis of the tip. Such conditions are occasionally seen in outbreaks in feedlot cattle and may follow an initiating viral stomatitis.

Neoplasia: Neoplasia of the mouth and lips other than viral papillomas are uncommon in younger animals. In gray horses, melanomas may develop and infiltrate the commissures of the mouth and cause hard, thickened, tumorous plaques that may not be detected until well advanced. Treatment of oral and lip melanomas in the horse is unrewarding, although prolonged cimetidine therapy may be palliative. Both verrucose and fibrous forms of equine sarcoid around the mouth should be treated as early as possible to maintain lip function.

Slaframine Toxicosis: The causes are ingestion of forages, particularly clovers, infected with the fungus Rhizoctonia leguminicola, which produces the toxic alkaloid slaframine. The only clinical signs that may be diagnostic are profuse salivation; no lesions have been described within the mouth. Usually, there is complete recovery. Differential diagnoses in large animals, particularly in ruminants, include bluetongue, vesicular stomatitis, vesicular exanthema, and foot-and-mouth disease. Removal of infected forages results in rapid recovery.

Stomatitis: Inflammation of the mouth is a clinical sign of many diseases in large animals. Oral trauma or contact with chemical irritants (eg, horses that lick at their legs after having been blistered) may result in transient stomatitis. Traumatic injury from the ingestion of the awns of barley, foxtail, porcupine grass, and spear grass, as well as feeding on plants infested with hairy caterpillars, also will result in severe stomatitis in horses and cattle.

Frothy salivation and reluctance to eat or resistance to oral examination are the clinical signs of acute active stomatitis. The animal should be sedated, and the mouth examined carefully with a speculum.

Any ulcers should be curetted to expose embedded foreign material, eg, grass awns, etc. If the etiology is ingestion of foreign material, changing the quality and quantity of the hay may effect recovery. Differential diagnoses include actinobacillosis, foot-and-mouth disease, malignant catarrhal fever, and bovine viral diarrhea. Epidemic diseases such as bluetongue in ruminants, swine vesicular disease, and vesicular stomatitis in horses must be differentiated from other forms of acute noninfectious or contagious stomatitis.

Papillar Stomatitis: Viral papillomas are found around the lips and mouths of all young animals, particularly in cattle from 1 mo to 2 yr old. In some instances, the rate of occurrence may be 100%. The lesions are characteristic and usually resolve spontaneously. However, in some cases, the lesions may coalesce to form cosmetically unacceptable masses around the muzzles of young horses, and owners may request therapy. Application of cryogenetics (liquid nitrogen), use of autologous vaccines, or combinations of such therapies may be effective.

Esophageal Obstruction (Choke): Overview

Esophageal obstruction or choke, in which the esophagus is obstructed by food masses or foreign objects, is by far the most common esophageal disease in large animals. Horses most frequently obstruct on greedily eaten dried grains or hay. Cattle more usually obstruct on a single solid object, eg, apples, beets, potatoes, turnips, corn stalks, or ears of corn.

Clinical Findings: In horses, the classic clinical findings associated with esophageal obstruction are overflow of esophageal food and regurgitation of that food through the nostrils. Nasal discharge of saliva and food material, which usually also spills from the pharynx into the airway, induces coughing.

The horse is anxious and may stretch and arch its neck but may still attempt to continue to either eat or drink. In cattle, acute and complete esophageal obstruction is an emergency because it prohibits the eructation of ruminal gases, and free-gas bloat develops.

This in turn may result in asphyxia as the expanding rumen puts pressure on the diaphragm and reduces return of blood to the heart. The cow may be bloated and in distress or recumbent, or there may be protrusion of the tongue, extension of the head, and grinding of the teeth with excess salivation.

Diagnosis: The clinical signs are extremely suggestive. Objects lodged in the cervical esophagus may be located via palpation. Endoscopic evaluation and the inability to pass a stomach or nasogastric tube in horses or cattle can also confirm the diagnosis.

Each case should be carefully evaluated independently because, in many instances, the complications of esophageal disease (eg, aspiration pneumonia) may prohibit or limit the effectiveness of treatment. In such cases, thoracic radiography, hematology, and biochemical serum analyses are indicated.

Treatment: In horses, many cases of obstruction caused by greedily eaten grain or hay may resolve spontaneously. The horse should be held off feed and water, and mild sedation and smooth muscle relaxants may be effective. (Compounds such as acepromazine have some effect in these cases, even though the esophagus has striated muscle, ie, special visceral muscle.) Oxytocin may be useful to facilitate relaxation and esophageal movement.

Horses should be monitored because spontaneous resolution may take from a few hours to several days. However, the longer the horse is obstructed, the greater the danger of pressure necrosis or esophagitis and complications of aspiration pneumonia. If the obstruction does not resolve spontaneously and the horse resists attempts at passage of a nasogastric tube and subsequent irrigation, then irrigation of the esophagus under general anesthesia is recommended.

A nasogastric tube should be placed before general anesthesia is induced; a cuffed endotracheal tube must be used to protect the airway. Repeated pumping and siphoning of warm water usually loosens the impacted food material. Oral food should be introduced gradually. The horse should receive parenteral antibiotics and analgesics, and the esophagus should be examined endoscopically to monitor the healing of mucosal ulcers. In cattle, esophageal obstruction accompanied by ruminal tympany is an emergency, and if clinical signs of distress indicate, the bloat (*Bloat*) must be relieved by trocarization through the left sublumbar fossa. Once the tympany has been relieved, then solid objects (eg, potatoes) may often be massaged free or spontaneously dislodge as their outer surfaces are softened by saliva. Caution should be used if any attempt is made to push an offending object down the esophagus using a probang; esophageal rupture and fatal septic mediastinitis may result. In both horses and cattle, elective esophagotomy may be used in some cases to relieve cervical choke.

Complications of Esophageal Obstruction

In both horses and cattle, inhalation pneumonia and resultant fulminating septic pleural pneumonia may be complications of esophageal obstruction. Longterm obstruction may be associated with pressure necrosis of the esophageal mucosa due to prolonged contact with the foreign body. A 360° mucosal slough may result in development of a postobstruction esophageal stricture. When large animals gulp food material and become obstructed, the etiology may be esophageal spasm; therefore, if the animal's respiratory system is healthy, conservative management should be practiced in most cases before any attempts to irrigate, siphon, or use a probang to loosen the object. Intrathoracic esophageal rupture is a fatal event. Cervical esophageal rupture can be managed in horses by local drainage, wound hygiene, and nasogastric feeding. If secondary healing does not occur, delayed surgical repair may be effective.

Esophageal Obstruction Secondary to Extraesophageal Disease

Cervical and prethoracic trauma may result in scar formation that may lead to constriction of the esophagus. Such cases may be diagnosed from a history of recurrent choke or recurrent obstruction. The use of radiography and contrast material may delineate the site of the obstruction within the esophagus. If the lesion is extrathoracic, it may be explored and relieved surgically.

Esophageal Strictures

Idiopathic esophageal strictures are seen in foals. Initial diagnosis based on clinical signs may be difficult in that horses may be presented because they are thought to have either cleft palates or pharyngeal cysts. The diagnosis is confirmed by endoscopic evaluation of the esophagus. Treatment is based on either dilation (bougienage) or surgical relief of the lesion. Critical cases should be referred to advanced surgical centres, and esophagomyotomy or esophageal resection and anastomosis may be attempted.

Esophageal Neoplasia

In ruminants, bovine viral papillomas (ie, warts) occasionally develop in the cranial esophagus and pharynx and, in the presence of other agents, may result in development of esophageal carcinoma. In some areas of the world (eg, Scotland and South America), such disease may follow ingestion of natural bracken fern toxins. There is also a causal relationship between such bracken fern tumors and bladder cancers in cattle.

Gastrointestinal Ulcers in Large Animals: Introduction

Gastric Ulcers in Horses: Mild gastric ulcers are seen in ~50% of foals. In most cases, these ulcers heal without treatment or clinical signs. The prevalence of clinical signs from ulcers in foals is not known. In adult horses, ~30% have mild gastric erosions, and the prevalence and severity of ulcers increase as the intensity of work increases—90% of race horses have gastric lesions, and in 50% the lesions are moderate to severe. Prevalence also varies by location of ulcers within the stomach and tends to be highest in the nonglandular squamous mucosa. Within the glandular mucosa, prevalence differs between the mucosa of the corpus (<10%) and that of the antrum and pylorus (>50%). Duodenal ulceration in foals has been considered part of the ulcer syndrome and hence a peptic (acid-induced) disorder. Duodenitis appears, instead, to be an enteritis syndrome. Duodenal ulceration, perforation, and stricture can occur, and it is not known whether these problems develop solely as a result of enteritis (duodenitis) or whether peptic factors have a role.

Etiology: Causes of gastric ulcers vary and can differ for nonglandular squamous mucosa and glandular mucosa. Horses' stomachs secrete hydrochloric acid continuously, and gastric acidity of a horse or foal is very high between periods of eating or nursing. Ulcers in the squamous mucosa result from increased exposure to hydrochloric acid, which can be secondary to prolonged periods of not eating or nursing, intensive exercise, or delayed gastric emptying. The effects of different feeds on gastric acidity and ulcerogenesis have not been thoroughly studied, although one report indicated that alfalfa hay was associated with reduced ulcer severity in research horses. The causes of most ulcers in the glandular mucosa of the stomach are not known. Excessive doses of NSAID are known to induce ulceration, but most horses with ulcers in this part of the stomach have had no recent exposure to NSAID. Recent research suggests that horses may be infected with a species of Helicobacter, but a role for this organism in equine gastric ulcers has not been shown.

Clinical Findings: Most foals with gastric ulcers do not exhibit clinical signs. Clinical signs become apparent when the ulceration is widespread or severe. The classic clinical signs for gastric ulcers in foals include diarrhea, bruxism, poor nursing, dorsal recumbency, and ptyalism. None of these signs is specific for gastric ulcers. In fact, ptyalism is a sign of esophagitis, which in most foals is secondary to gastric outflow obstruction and gastroesophageal reflux. Other causes, including esophageal obstruction and Candida infection, should be considered. Importantly, when a foal exhibits clinical signs, the ulcers are severe and should be diagnosed and treated immediately. Sudden gastric perforation without prior signs occurs sporadically in foals. Adult horses with ulcers display nonspecific signs that can include abdominal discomfort (colic), poor appetite, mild weight loss, poor body condition, and attitude changes. Complications related to gastric ulcers are most frequent and severe in foals and include perforation, delayed gastric emptying, gastroesophageal reflux and esophagitis, and megaesophagus secondary to chronic gastroesophageal reflux. Ulcers in the proximal duodenum or at the pylorus can cause fibrosis and stricture. The latter complication is seen in both foals and adult horses. In rare cases, severe gastric ulceration causes fibrosis and contracture of the stomach.

Diagnosis: Neither clinical signs nor laboratory tests are specific for gastric ulcers, and an abnormality in a laboratory test does not preclude the possibility that another disorder may be present. Gastric ulcers can develop secondary to problems in many organ systems. Endoscopy is the only reliable method of diagnosis.

Treatment: Suppression of gastric acidity is the primary treatment objective. This can be accomplished with over-the-counter antacids, with the histamine type-2 receptor antagonists (cimetidine and ranitidine), and with the proton pump inhibitor omeprazole. Of these, omeprazole is the most effective, and antacids are the least effective. Ranitidine (6.6 mg/kg, PO) is effective in healing and preventing gastric ulcers, but recent evidence suggests that cimetidine is not effective. Omeprazole is the only medication approved by the FDA for treatment of gastric ulcers in horses. It is effective for treatment and prevention of ulcers in race horses and other types of horses. Sucralfate binds to the gastric glandular mucosa and may promote healing there, although no efficacy data is available to support its use in horses.

Gastric Ulcers in Pigs

Ulcers affect the pars esophagea in pigs and cause sporadic cases of acute gastric hemorrhage resulting in death or slow growth due to chronic ulceration.

Etiology: The specific causes are unknown. Ulcers are seen in pigs of all ages but are most common in growing pigs (100-200 lb [45-90 kg]) fed pelleted feed or finely ground rations, and also in pigs fed large quantities of skimmed milk or whey. It is thought that promotants of hyperacidity may contribute to ulcer development. A combination of finely ground feeds, transportation, hot weather, deprivation of feed and water, and mixing with unfamiliar pigs results in a significant increase in the incidence of gastric ulcers in rapidly growing pigs. Variability in daily feed intake secondary to a systemic illness, particularly pneumonias, also result in an increased incidence of ulcers. This condition is particularly significant in pigs gathered for slaughter at abattoirs, especially those transported long distances.

Clinical Findings: In the peracute form, the pig dies quickly; it is found dead with paleness as the only sign. In the acute form, hemorrhage results in anorexia, weakness, anemia, and black, tarry feces; death can occur in hours or days. In the chronic form, unthriftiness, anemia, and black, tarry feces are characteristic; the pig may survive for several weeks. Pigs with the subclinical form may not reach maturity at the expected time; in these pigs, the ulcer usually heals and a scar remains. In some herds, up to 90% of pigs may be affected; in other herds, the incidence is sporadic. In findings at abattoirs, the incidence of ulcers may be quite high in pigs that have grown normally, although the lesion may have developed in some during transport. Clinical disease apparently develops only after hemorrhage of the ulcer.

Lesions: The typical terminal lesion is found in the gastric mucosa near the esophageal opening in a rectangular area of white, glistening, nonglandular, squamous epithelium. It is common to find a crater ≥ 2.5-5 cm in diametre encompassing the entrance of the esophagus. The crater appears as a cream or gray, punched-out area and may contain blood clots or debris. In acute hemorrhage, the stomach and upper small intestine contain dark blood. Earlier lesions are characterized by hyperkeratosis and parakeratosis of the squamous epithelium in the area of the esophageal opening into the stomach. Later, the proliferative lesion erodes to form the ulcer. The healed ulcer appears as a stellate scar.

Diagnosis and Treatment: Appearance in a pen of 1 or 2 listless, anorectic pigs that show weight loss, anemia, dark feces, and sometimes dyspnea is suggestive of gastric ulceration, as is the sudden death of an apparently healthy pig.

No economically feasible treatments are currently available. Palliative care—removing the affected pig from the pen and feeding a coarse and fibrous diet—can be attempted. Early marketing of affected pigs should be considered. Controlling chronic respiratory disease is important.

Feeding meal rather than pellets with a recommended particle size ^{3}600-700 µm in diametre is of value but may have a negative effect on feed conversion. Strategic use of such diets during stages of production that are at higher risk is useful.

Diseases of the Ruminant Forestomach

Simple Indigestion (Mild Dietary Indigestion)

Simple indigestion is a minor disturbance in ruminant GI function that is seen in cattle and rarely in sheep. It is usually related to a change in the quality or quantity of the diet.

Etiology: Almost any dietary factor that can alter the ruminal environment can cause simple indigestion. The disease is common in hand-fed dairy and beef cattle because of variability in the quality and quantity of their feed.

Dairy cattle may suddenly eat excessive quantities of highly palatable feeds such as corn or grass silage; beef cattle may eat excessive quantities of relatively indigestible, poor-quality roughage during winter.

During drought, cattle and sheep may be forced to eat large quantities of poor-quality straw, bedding, or scrub. Simple indigestion can result from suddenly changing the feed, using spoiled or frozen feeds, introducing urea to a ration, turning cattle onto a lush cereal grain pasture, or introducing feedlot cattle to a high-level grain ration. It can also result from ingestion of placentas by postparturient cows. Simple indigestion, which is primarily ruminal atony, may follow a sudden change in the pH of the ruminal contents caused by excessive fermentation or putrefaction of ingested feed. The simple accumulation of excessive quantities of relatively indigestible feed may physically impair rumen function for 24-48 hr.

Clinical Findings: The signs depend on the type of animal affected and cause of the disorder. Silage overfeeding causes anorexia and a moderate drop in production in dairy cattle. The rumen is usually full, firm, and doughy; primary contractions are absent, but secondary contractions may be present. Temperature, pulse, and respiration are normal. The feces are normal to firm in consistency but reduced in amount. Recovery usually is spontaneous within 24-48 hr. Simple indigestion due to excessive feeding of grain results in anorexia and ruminal stasis. The rumen is not necessarily full and may contain excessive fluid. The feces are usually soft and foul smelling. The affected animal is bright and alert and usually begins to eat within 24 hr. A more severe upset from the same cause is described as grain overload.

Diagnosis: This is based largely on elimination of other possibilities and a history of a change in the nature or amount of the diet. The systemic reaction and painful responses to deep palpation of the xiphoid in traumatic reticuloperitonitis are not seen. The history and the absence of ketonuria help eliminate ketosis from consideration. The possibility of displaced abomasum usually can be eliminated by auscultation. Vagal indigestion and abomasal torsions become more readily detectable as they progress because they have a longer course, but initial differentiation may be difficult. Grain overload is distinguishable by its greater severity and the pronounced fall in the pH of the rumen contents. Phytobezoars cause partial or complete anorexia and scant feces; on rectal examination, distended loops of intestine and the firm phytobezoar masses are palpable.

Treatment: Treatment is aimed at correcting the suspected dietary factors. Spontaneous recovery is usual. Administration of 20-40 L of warm water or saline via a stomach tube, followed by vigorous kneading of the rumen, may help restore rumen function. Magnesium hydroxide PO seems to be useful when excessive amounts of high-energy feeds have been ingested. If too much urea or protein has been ingested, acetic acid or vinegar may be administered PO. If the activity of the ruminal microbes is reduced, administration of 4-8 L of ruminal fluid from a healthy cow will help.

Grain Overload (Lactic Acidosis, Carbohydrate Engorgement, Rumen Impaction)

Grain overload is an acute disease of ruminants that is characterized by indigestion, rumen stasis, dehydration, acidosis, toxemia, incoordination, collapse, and frequently death.

Etiology and Pathogenesis: The disease is most common in cattle that accidentally gain access to large quantities of readily digestible carbohydrates, particularly grain. It also is common in feedlot cattle when they are introduced to heavy grain diets too quickly.

Wheat, barley, and corn are the most readily digestible and oats less digestible. Less common causes include engorgement with apples, grapes, bread, batter's dough, sugar beets, mangels, or sour wet brewer's grain that was incompletely fermented in the brewery.

The amount of a feed required to produce acute illness depends on the kind of grain, previous experience of the animal with that grain, the nutritional status and condition of the animal, and the nature of the microflora. Cattle accustomed to heavy grain diets may consume 30-45 lb (15-20 kg) of grain and develop only moderate illness, while others may become acutely ill and die after eating 20 lb (10 kg) of grain.

Ingestion of toxic amounts of highly fermentable carbohydrates is followed within 2-6 hr by a change in the microbial population in the rumen. The number of gram-positive bacteria (Streptococcus bovis) increases markedly, which results in the production of large quantities of lactic acid. The rumen pH falls to d”5, which destroys protozoa, cellulolytic organisms, and lactate-utilising organisms, and impairs rumen motility. The low pH allows the lactobacilli to utilise the carbohydrate and to produce excessive quantities of lactic acid. The superimposition of lactic acid and its salt, lactate, on the existing solutes in the rumen liquid causes osmotic pressure to rise substantially, which results in the movement of excessive quantities of fluid into the rumen, causing dehydration. The lactic acid causes a chemical rumenitis, and its absorption results in lactic acidosis. In addition to acidosis and dehydration, the pathophysiologic consequences are hemoconcentration, cardiovascular collapse, renal failure, muscular weakness, shock, and death. Animals that survive may develop mycotic rumenitis in several days, hepatic necrobacillosis several weeks or months later, or chronic laminitis, as well as evidence of ruminal scars at slaughter.

Clinical Findings: Carbohydrate engorgement results in conditions ranging from simple indigestion (*Simple Indigestion*) to a rapidly fatal acidosis. The interval between overeating and onset of signs is shorter with ground feed than with whole grain, and severity increases with the amount eaten.

A few hours after engorgement, the only detectable abnormality may be an enlarged rumen and possibly some abdominal pain (manifest by belly kicking). In the mild form, the rumen movements are reduced but not entirely absent, the cattle are anorectic but bright and alert, and diarrhea is common. The animals usually begin eating again 3-4 days later without any specific treatment.

Within 24-48 hr of the onset of severe overload, some animals will be recumbent, some will be staggering, and others will be standing quietly; all will be completely off feed. Immediately after consuming large quantities of dry grain, cattle may engorge themselves on water, but once ill they usually do not drink at all.

Body temperature is usually below normal, 98-101°F (36.5-38.5°C); however, in animals exposed to the sun in hot weather, it may be increased to 106°F (41°C). Respirations tend to be shallow and rapid, up to 60-90/min. The heart rate usually is increased in accordance with severity of the acidosis; prognosis is poor for cattle with rates of 120-140/min. Diarrhea is common and usually profuse. The feces are soft to liquid, yellow or tan, and have an obvious sweet-sour odor. The feces frequently contain undigested kernels of the feed that has induced the overload. In mild cases, dehydration equals 4-6% body wt; in severe cases, up to 10-12%. In severe overload, the primary contractions of the rumen are completely absent, although the gurgling sounds of gas rising through the large quantity of fluid are usually audible on auscultation. Ballottement and auscultation of the left flank may elicit fluid-splashing sounds in the rumen. The contents of the rumen, as palpated through the left paralumbar fossa, may feel firm and doughy in cattle that were previously on a roughage diet and have consumed a large amount of grain.

In cattle that have become ill on smaller amounts of grain, the rumen will feel not necessarily full, but rather resilient because of the excessive fluid. Severely affected animals stagger and may bump into objects; their palpebral reflex is sluggish or absent, and the pupillary light reflex is usually present but slower than normal.

They commonly lie quietly, often with the head turned into the flank, and their response to any stimulus is much decreased so that they resemble cases of parturient paresis (*Parturient Paresis in Cows*). Acute laminitis may be present and is most common in those animals that are not severely affected; chronic laminitis may develop weeks or months later.

Anuria is a common finding in acute cases, and diuresis after fluid therapy is a good prognostic sign. Death may occur in 24-72 hr, and rapid development of acute signs, particularly recumbency, indicates an urgent need for radical treatment. A reduction in heart rate, rise in temperature, return of ruminal movement, and passage of large amounts of soft feces are more favourable signs. However, some animals appear to improve temporarily but become severely ill again 3-4 days later, probably because of severe fungal rumenitis; death from acute diffuse peritonitis usually follows in 2-3 days. In pregnant cattle that survive the severe form of the disease, abortion may occur 10-14 days later.

Diagnosis: The diagnosis is usually obvious if the history is available. It may be confirmed by the clinical findings, a low ruminal pH (<5), and examining the microflora of the rumen for the presence of live protozoa. When only one animal is involved and there is no history of engorgement, the diagnosis is less obvious, but the clinical signs—a static rumen with gurgling fluid sounds, diarrhea, ataxia, and a normal temperature—are characteristic. Although parturient paresis (*Parturient Paresis in Cows*) may resemble rumen overload, diarrhea and dehydration are not typical, the intensity of heart sounds is reduced, and the response to calcium injection is usually dramatic. Peracute coliform mastitis and acute diffuse peritonitis may also resemble overload, but usually a careful examination will reveal the cause of the toxemia. To avoid an increase in pH on exposure to air, rumen fluid obtained by stomach tube or paracentesis should be checked promptly. Normally, the pH in cattle on roughage is 6-7; in those on a grain diet, 5.5-6.

Values below those ranges are strongly suggestive of overload, and a pH <5 indicates severe acidosis. Wide-range (2-11) pH indicator paper is suitable for field use. Ruminal fluid may be examined microscopically; 5-7 protozoa are normally seen under low power.

In acidosis, the protozoa are virtually absent. A Gram's stain of the fluid will reveal a change from predominantly gram-negative bacteria (normal) to predominantly gram-positive bacteria in acidosis. Increased blood lactate and inorganic phosphate levels, mild hypocalcemia, and reduced urinary pH are also seen, but it is seldom necessary to check such values to make a firm diagnosis.

The diagnostic problem is to properly assess which animals require vigorous therapy (or slaughter), which require supportive therapy, which have only a mild indigestion that will correct itself if water and grain intake are restricted and hay and exercise are provided, and which need nothing beyond their routine care and ration.

In an outbreak of overload involving several animals, it is necessary to identify those animals that need the most intensive therapy and those that will recover with minimal medical therapy. If the cattle are found while still eating, it is possible that some of the group will fall into each category, and close monitoring is necessary to minimize losses.

Cattle found while engorging or shortly thereafter should be allowed no more concentrate or water, but plenty of good hay for up to 24 hr, and forced to exercise periodically. Cattle that appear normal at the end of the first day are probably in good health, although if even one is ill, all should be monitored closely for 48 hr. Most of those that have eaten enough concentrate to be affected seriously show signs within 6-8 hr.

Treatment: For all cattle suspected of having eaten large quantities of concentrate, it is important to restrict water intake for the first 18-24 hr. If overload is serious, slaughter for salvage should be considered; in feeders nearing the end of their feeding period, it may well be the most economical choice. Mortality is high in severely affected animals unless vigorous therapeutic measures are initiated early.

In such animals, removal of rumen contents and replacement with ingesta taken from healthy animals is necessary. In animals that are still standing, rumen lavage may be accomplished with a large stomach tube if sufficient water is available. A large-bore tube (2.5 cm inside diametre, 3 m long) should be used, and enough water added to distend the left paralumbar fossa; gravity flow is then allowed to empty out what it will.

Repeating this 15-20 times achieves the same results (and requires about as much time) as using rumenotomy to empty and wash out the rumen with a siphon. Emptying the rumen should be followed by rumen inoculation (*Drugs for Specific Purposes*) and, if not accomplished before signs of severe toxicosis are evident, by rigorous fluid therapy to correct the acidosis and dehydration and to restore renal function.

Initially, over a period of ~30 min, 5% sodium bicarbonate solution should be given IV (5 L/450 kg). During the next 6-12 hr, a balanced electrolyte solution, or a 1.3% solution of sodium bicarbonate in saline, may be given IV, up to as much as 60 L/450 kg body wt.

Urination should resume during this period. Usually, it is unnecessary and even undesirable to also administer antacids PO (or intraruminally). In less severe cases, emptying the rumen is unnecessary.

In these, magnesium hydroxide (500 g/450 kg body wt) should be added to warm water, pumped into the rumen, and mixed therein via kneading the flank. This may be all that is necessary if the rumen pH is >5, and the animal is still standing and reasonably alert several hours after the engorgement. A heart rate of 70-85 bpm, weak ruminal contractions, normal body temperature, and especially willingness to eat are additional reassurances that this therapy will suffice. If any question remains, additional fluids should be given. During the convalescent period, which may last 2-4 days, good-quality hay and no grain should be given, and the grain then reintroduced gradually. If good appetite returns within 3 days, the prognosis is good. However, if treatment was not started early enough to prevent acidification of the ruminal contents, and mycotic infection of the rumen wall ensues, relapse is likely within 3-5 days, and the prognosis is grave.

Prevention: Accidental access to concentrates for which the cattle have developed an appetite, in quantities to which they are unaccustomed, should be avoided. Feedlot cattle should be introduced gradually to concentrate rations over a period of ~3 wk, beginning with a mixture of d”50% concentrate in the milled feed containing roughage.

Subacute Ruminal Acidosis (Chronic Ruminal Acidosis, Subclinical Ruminal Acidosis)

Ruminant animals are adapted to digest and metabolize predominantly forage diets; however, growth rates and milk production are increased substantially when they consume high-grain diets. One consequence of feeding excessive amounts of rapidly fermentable carbohydrates in conjunction with inadequate fibre to ruminants is subacute ruminal acidosis, characterized by periods of low ruminal pH, depressed feed intake, and subsequent health problems.

Chronic disease conditions secondary to subacute ruminal acidosis can negate the production gains accomplished by high grain feeding. Dairy cattle, feedlot cattle, and feedlot sheep are all at high risk for developing this condition. Although dairy cattle are typically fed diets that are higher in forage and fibre compared with feedlot animals, this advantage is offset by their much higher dry-matter intakes. Field observations suggest that periparturient cows are at risk of subacute ruminal acidosis because of the time required for the rumen microflora and papillae to adapt to increased intakes of concentrates immediately before parturition and during early lactation when feed intake increases rapidly to meet the energy needs of high-producing dairy cows. The adaptation of the ruminal microflora and papillae from a system appropriate for forage to a system capable of utilising high-energy lactation rations requires a gradual change over a period of 3-5 wk.

Etiology: Ruminal pH drops below ~5.5 (the normal physiologic nadir) when ruminants consume excessive amounts of rapidly fermentable carbohydrates. Any additional intake puts the ruminant at risk of subacute ruminal acidosis because it results in the fermentation of carbohydrates into volatile fatty acids (VFA). Ruminal pH typically drops 0.5-1.0 pH units after the major meal of the day.

The ability of the rumen to rapidly absorb organic acids contributes greatly to the stability of ruminal pH. It is rarely difficult for peripheral tissues to utilise VFA already absorbed from the rumen; however, absorption of these VFA from the rumen can be an important bottleneck.

VFA from the rumen are absorbed passively across the rumen wall. This passive absorption is enhanced by finger-like papillae, which project away from the rumen wall. Ruminal papillae increase in length when cattle are fed higher-grain diets; this presumably increases ruminal surface area and absorptive capacity, which protects the animal from acid accumulation in the rumen.

If the absorptive capacity of these cells is impaired (eg, chronic rumenitis with fibrosis), it becomes much more difficult for the animal to maintain a stable ruminal pH following a meal. Intake depression is the ruminant's last resort for regulating ruminal pH.

Depressed dry-matter intake becomes especially evident if ruminal pH falls to <~5.5. Intake depression may be mediated by pH receptors and/or osmolality receptors in the rumen. Inflammation of the ruminal epithelium (rumenitis) could cause pain and contribute to intake depression during subacute ruminal acidosis.

Unfortunately, lactate production at low ruminal pH can offset gains from VFA absorption. As pH drops, lactate-synthesizing bacteria such as Streptococcus bovis begin to ferment glucose to lactate instead of VFA. This is a dangerous situation, since lactate has a much lower pK_a than VFA (3.9 vs 4.8) and lactate is 5.2 times less dissociated than VFA at pH 5.0. As a result, lactate stays in the rumen longer and contributes to the downward spiral in ruminal pH. Additional adaptive responses are invoked if lactate production begins.

Lactate-utilising bacteria, such as Megasphaera elsdenii and Selenomonas ruminantium, begin to proliferate. These beneficial bacteria convert lactate to other VFA, which are then easily protonated and absorbed.

However, the turnover time of lactate utilisers is much slower than that of lactate synthesizers. Thus, this mechanism may not be invoked quickly enough to fully stabilize ruminal pH. Periods of very high ruminal pH, as during feed deprivation, may inhibit populations of lactate utilisers (which are sensitive to higher ruminal pH) and leave them more susceptible to severe ruminal acidosis.

Besides disrupting microbial balance, feed deprivation causes cattle to overeat when feed is reintroduced. This creates a double effect in lowering ruminal pH. Cycles of feed deprivation and refeeding are critical risk factors for subacute ruminal acidosis.

Low ruminal pH during subacute ruminal acidosis also reduces the number of species of bacteria in the rumen, although the metabolic activity of the bacteria that remain is very high. Protozoal populations are limited as ruminal pH approaches 5.0. When fewer species of bacteria and protozoa are present, the ruminal microflora are less stable and less able to maintain normal ruminal pH during periods of sudden dietary change. Thus, pre-existing subacute ruminal acidosis increases the risk of acute ruminal acidosis in the event of accidental ingestion of excessive amounts of grain.

Pathogenesis: Ruminal epithelial cells are not protected by mucus, so they are vulnerable to chemical damage by acids. Low ruminal pH leads to rumenitis, erosion, and ulceration of the ruminal epithelium. Once the ruminal epithelium is inflamed, bacteria may colonize the papillae and leak into the portal circulation. These bacteria may cause liver abscesses, which may eventually lead to peritonitis around the site of the abscess. If the ruminal bacteria clear the liver (or if bacteria from liver infections are released into circulation), they may colonize the lungs, heart valves, kidneys, or joints. The resulting pneumonia, endocarditis, pyelonephritis, and arthritis are often difficult to diagnose antemortem. Postmortem evaluation of these conditions in animals that are slaughtered, culled, or that died on the farm can be very beneficial. Caudal vena cava syndrome can cause hemoptysis and peracute deaths due to massive pulmonary hemorrhage in affected cows. In these cases, septic emboli from liver abscesses can lead to lung infections, which ultimately invade pulmonary vessels and cause them to rupture.

Subacute ruminal acidosis has also been associated with laminitis and subsequent hoof overgrowth, sole abscesses, and sole ulcers. The severity of laminitis depends on the duration and frequency of metabolic insult. These foot problems generally do not appear until weeks or months after the initiating event. The mechanism by which subacute ruminal acidosis increases the risk of laminitis has not been fully characterized.

Clinical Findings: The major clinical manifestation is reduced or cyclic feed intake, or both. Other associated signs include decreased efficiency of milk production, reduced fat test, poor body condition score despite adequate energy intake, unexplained diarrhea, and episodes of laminitis. High rates of culling or unexplained deaths may be noted in the herd. Sporadic nosebleeds due to caudal vena cava syndrome may also be observed.

The clinical signs are delayed and insidious. Actual episodes of low ruminal pH are not identified; in fact, by the time an animal is observed to be off-feed, its ruminal pH has probably been restored to normal. Diarrhea may follow periods of low ruminal pH; however, this finding is subtle and difficult to evaluate.

Diagnosis: Subacute ruminal acidosis is diagnosed on a group rather than individual basis. Measurement of pH in the ruminal fluid of a representative portion of apparently healthy animals in a group has been used to assist in making the diagnosis of subacute ruminal acidosis in dairy herds.

Animal selection should be from high-risk groups, eg, in the first 60 days of lactation. Ruminal fluid is collected by rumenocentesis or stomach tube and can be measured in the field using wide-range pH (2-12) indicator paper, although a pH metre yields more accurate results. Twelve or more animals are typically sampled at ~2-4 hr after a grain feeding (in component-fed herds) or 6-10 hr after the first daily total mixed ration feeding. If >25% of the animals tested have a ruminal pH <5.5, then the group is considered to be at high risk of subacute ruminal acidosis. This type of diagnostic tool should be used in conjunction with other factors such as ration evaluation, evaluation of management practices, and identification of health problems on a herd basis. Milk fat depression is a poor and insensitive indicator of subacute ruminal acidosis in dairy herds. Cows and herds with severe subacute ruminal acidosis may have normal milk fat tests. Thus, it is vitally important not to exclude the diagnosis in a dairy herd that has a normal milk-fat test.

Treatment: Because subacute ruminal acidosis is not detected at the time of depressed ruminal pH, there is no specific treatment for it. Secondary conditions may be treated as needed.

Prevention: The key to prevention is reducing the amount of readily fermentable carbohydrate consumed at each meal. This requires both good diet formulation (proper balance of fibre and nonfibre carbohydrates) and excellent feed bunk management. Animals consuming well-formulated diets remain at high risk for this condition if they tend to eat large meals because of excessive competition for bunk space or following periods of feed deprivation.

Field recommendations for feeding component-fed concentrates to dairy cattle during the first 3 wk of lactation are usually excessive. Feeding excessive quantities of concentrate and insufficient forage results in a fibre-deficient ration likely to cause subacute ruminal acidosis.

The same situation may be seen during the last few days before parturition if the ration is fed in separate components; as dry-matter intake drops before calving, dry cows preferentially consume concentrate over fibre and develop acidosis.

Subacute ruminal acidosis may also be caused by errors in delivery of the rations or by formulation of rations that contain excessive amounts of rapidly fermentable carbohydrates or a deficiency of fibre. Recommendations for the fibre content of dairy rations are available in the National Research Council report, *Nutrient Requirements of Dairy Cattle*. Dry-matter content errors in total mixed rations are commonly related to a lack of adjustment for changes in moisture content of forages. Including long-fibre particles in the diet reduces the risk of subacute ruminal acidosis by encouraging saliva production during chewing and by increasing rumination after feeding. However, long-fibre particles should not be easily sorted away from the rest of the diet; this could delay their consumption until later in the day or cause them to be refused completely. Ruminant diets should also be formulated to provide adequate buffering.

This can be accomplished by feedstuff selection and/or by the addition of dietary buffers such as sodium bicarbonate or potassium carbonate. Dietary anion-cation difference is used to quantify the buffering capacity of a diet.

Supplementing the diet with direct-fed microbials that enhance lactate utilisers in the rumen may reduce the risk of subacute ruminal acidosis. Yeasts, propionobacteria, lactobacilli, and enterococci have been used for this purpose. Ionophore (eg, monensin sodium) supplementation may also reduce the risk by selectively inhibiting ruminal lactate producers; however, ionophores are not currently approved for use in lactating dairy cows in North America.

Bloat (Ruminal Tympany)

Bloat is an overdistention of the rumenoreticulum with the gases of fermentation, either in the form of a persistent foam mixed with the ruminal contents—called primary or frothy bloat, or in the form of free gas separated from the ingesta—called secondary or free-gas bloat.

It is predominantly a disorder of cattle but may also be seen in sheep. The susceptibility of individual cattle to bloat varies and is genetically determined.

Etiology and Pathogenesis: In primary ruminal tympany, or frothy bloat, the cause is entrapment of the normal gases of fermentation in a stable foam. Coalescence of the small gas bubbles is inhibited, and intraruminal pressure increases because eructation cannot occur. Several factors, both animal and plant, influence the formation of a stable foam. Soluble leaf proteins, saponins, and hemicelluloses are believed to be the primary foaming agents and to form a monomolecular layer around gas rumen bubbles that has its greatest stability at about pH 6.0. Salivary mucin is antifoaming, but saliva production is reduced with succulent forages. Bloat-producing pastures are more rapidly digested and may release a greater amount of small chloroplast particles that trap gas bubbles and prevent their coalescence.

The immediate effect of feeding is probably to supply nutrients for a burst of microbial fermentation. However, the major factor that determines if bloat will occur is the nature of the ruminal contents. Protein content and rates of digestion and ruminal passage reflect the forage's potential for causing bloat. Over a 24-hr period, the bloat-causing forage and unknown animal factors combine to maintain an increased concentration of small feed particles and enhance the susceptibility to bloat. Bloat is most common in animals grazing legume or legume-dominant pastures, particularly alfalfa, ladino, and red and white clovers, but also is seen with grazing of young green cereal crops, rape, kale, turnips, and legume vegetable crops.

Legume forages such as alfalfa and clover have a higher percentage of protein and are digested more quickly. Other legumes, such as sainfoin, crown vetch, milk vetch, and birdsfoot trefoil, are high in protein but do not cause bloat, probably because they contain condensed tannins, which precipitate protein and are digested more slowly than alfalfa or clover. Leguminous bloat is most common when cattle are placed on lush pastures, particularly those dominated by rapidly growing leguminous plants in the vegetative and early bud stages, but can also be seen when high-quality hay is fed.

Frothy bloat also is seen in feedlot cattle, and less commonly in dairy cattle, on high-grain diets. The cause of the foam in feedlot bloat is uncertain but is thought to be either the production of insoluble slime by certain species of rumen bacteria in cattle fed high-carbohydrate diets or the entrapment of the gases of fermentation by the fine particle size of ground feed.

Fine particulate matter, such as in finely ground grain, can markedly affect foam stability as can a low roughage intake. Feedlot bloat is most common in cattle that have been on a grain diet for 1-2 mo. This timing may be due to the increase in the level of grain feeding or to the time it takes for the slime-producing rumen bacteria to proliferate to large enough numbers. In secondary ruminal tympany, or free-gas bloat, physical obstruction of eructation is caused by esophageal obstruction due to a foreign body (eg, potatoes, apples, turnips, kiwifruit), stenosis, or pressure from enlargement outside the esophagus (as from lymphadenopathy). Interference with esophageal groove function in vagal indigestion and diaphragmatic hernia may cause chronic ruminal tympany. This also occurs in tetanus.

Tumors and other lesions of the esophageal groove or the reticular wall are less common causes of obstructive bloat. There also may be interference with the nerve pathways involved in the eructation reflex. Lesions of the wall of the reticulum (which contains tension receptors and receptors that discriminate between gas, foam, and liquid) may interrupt the normal reflex that is essential for escape of gas from the rumen.

Ruminal tympany also can be secondary to the acute onset of ruminal atony that occurs in anaphylaxis and in grain overload; this causes a reduction in rumen pH and possibly an esophagitis and rumenitis that can interfere with eructation. Ruminal tympany also develops with hypocalcemia.

Chronic ruminal tympany is relatively frequent in calves up to 6 mo old without apparent cause; this form usually resolves spontaneously. Unusual postures, particularly lateral recumbency, are commonly associated with secondary tympany. Ruminants may die of bloat if they become accidentally cast in dorsal recumbency or other restrictive positions in handling facilities, crowded transportation vehicles, or irrigation ditches.

Clinical Findings: Bloat is a common cause of sudden death. Cattle not observed closely, such as pastured and feedlot cattle and dry dairy cattle, usually are found dead. In lactating dairy cattle, which are observed regularly, bloat commonly begins within 1 hr after being turned onto a bloat-producing pasture. Bloat may develop on the first day after being placed on the pasture but more commonly develops on the second or third day. In primary pasture bloat, the rumen becomes obviously distended suddenly, and the left flank may be so distended that the contour of the paralumbar fossa protrudes above the vertebral column; the entire abdomen is enlarged. As the bloat progresses, the skin over the left flank becomes progressively more taut and, in severe cases, cannot be "tented." Dyspnea and grunting are marked and are accompanied by mouth breathing, protrusion of the tongue, extension of the head, and frequent urination. Occasionally, vomiting occurs. Rumen motility does not decrease until bloat is severe. If the tympany continues to worsen, the animal will collapse and die. Death may occur within 1 hr after grazing began but is more common ~3-4 hr after onset of clinical signs.

In a group of affected cattle, there are usually several with clinical bloat and some with mild to moderate abdominal distention. Death rates as high as 20% are recorded in cattle grazing bloat-prone pasture, and in pastoral areas, the annual mortality rate from bloat in dairy cows may approach 1%. There is also economic loss from depressed milk production in nonfatal cases and from suboptimal use of bloat-prone pastures.

Bloat can be a significant cause of mortality in feedlot cattle. In secondary bloat, the excess gas is usually free on top of the solid and fluid ruminal contents, although frothy bloat may be seen in vagal indigestion when there is increased ruminal activity.

Secondary bloat is seen sporadically. There is tympanic resonance over the dorsal abdomen left of the midline. Free gas produces a higher pitched ping on percussion than frothy bloat. The distension of the rumen can be detected on rectal examination. In free-gas bloat, the passage of a stomach tube or trocarization releases large quantities of gas and alleviates distention.

Lesions: Necropsy findings are characteristic. Congestion and hemorrhage of the lymph nodes of the head and neck, epicardium, and upper respiratory tract are marked. The lungs are compressed, and intrabronchial hemorrhage may be present. The cervical esophagus is congested and hemorrhagic, but the thoracic portion of the esophagus is pale and blanched—the demarcation known as the "bloat lin" of the esophagus. The rumen is distended, but the contents usually are much less frothy than before death. The liver is pale due to expulsion of blood from the organ.

Diagnosis: Usually, the clinical diagnosis of frothy bloat is obvious. The causes of secondary bloat must be ascertained by clinical examination to determine the cause of the failure of eructation.

Treatment: Bloat (Ruminal tympany) Etiology and Pathogenesis Clinical Findings Lesions Diagnosis Treatment Control and Prevention Bloat is an overdistention of the rumenoreticulum with the gases of fermentation, either in the form of a persistent foam mixed with the ruminal contents—called primary or frothy bloat, or in the form of free gas separated from the ingesta—called secondary or free-gas bloat. It is predominantly a disorder of cattle but may also be seen in sheep. The susceptibility of individual cattle to bloat varies and is genetically determined.

Etiology and Pathogenesis: In primary ruminal tympany, or frothy bloat, the cause is entrapment of the normal gases of fermentation in a stable foam. Coalescence of the small gas bubbles is inhibited, and intraruminal pressure increases because eructation cannot occur.

Several factors, both animal and plant, influence the formation of a stable foam. Soluble leaf proteins, saponins, and hemicelluloses are believed to be the primary foaming agents and to form a monomolecular layer around gas rumen bubbles that has its greatest stability at about pH 6.0. Salivary mucin is antifoaming, but saliva production is reduced with succulent forages.

Bloat-producing pastures are more rapidly digested and may release a greater amount of small chloroplast particles that trap gas bubbles and prevent their coalescence. The immediate effect of feeding is probably to supply nutrients for a burst of microbial fermentation.

However, the major factor that determines if bloat will occur is the nature of the ruminal contents. Protein content and rates of digestion and ruminal passage reflect the forage's potential for causing bloat.

Over a 24-hr period, the bloat-causing forage and unknown animal factors combine to maintain an increased concentration of small feed particles and enhance the susceptibility to bloat. Bloat is most common in animals grazing legume or legume-dominant pastures, particularly alfalfa, ladino, and red and white clovers, but also is seen with grazing of young green cereal crops, rape, kale, turnips, and legume vegetable crops. Legume forages such as alfalfa and clover have a higher percentage of protein and are digested more quickly. Other legumes, such as sainfoin, crown vetch, milk vetch, and birdsfoot trefoil, are high in protein but do not cause bloat, probably because they contain condensed tannins, which precipitate protein and are digested more slowly than alfalfa or clover. Leguminous bloat is most common when cattle are placed on lush pastures, particularly those dominated by rapidly growing leguminous plants in the vegetative and early bud stages, but can also be seen when high-quality hay is fed.

Frothy bloat also is seen in feedlot cattle, and less commonly in dairy cattle, on high-grain diets. The cause of the foam in feedlot bloat is uncertain but is thought to be either the production of insoluble slime by certain species of rumen bacteria in cattle fed high-carbohydrate diets or the entrapment of the gases of fermentation by the fine particle size of ground feed. Fine particulate matter, such as in finely ground grain, can markedly affect foam stability as can a low roughage intake. Feedlot bloat is most common in cattle that have been on a grain diet for 1-2 mo.

This timing may be due to the increase in the level of grain feeding or to the time it takes for the slime-producing rumen bacteria to proliferate to large enough numbers. In secondary ruminal tympany, or free-gas bloat, physical obstruction of eructation is caused by esophageal obstruction due to a foreign body (eg, potatoes, apples, turnips, kiwifruit), stenosis, or pressure from enlargement outside the esophagus (as from lymphadenopathy).

Interference with esophageal groove function in vagal indigestion and diaphragmatic hernia may cause chronic ruminal tympany. This also occurs in tetanus.

Tumors and other lesions of the esophageal groove or the reticular wall are less common causes of obstructive bloat. There also may be interference with the nerve pathways involved in the eructation reflex. Lesions of the wall of the reticulum (which contains tension receptors and receptors that discriminate between gas, foam, and liquid) may interrupt the normal reflex that is essential for escape of gas from the rumen. Ruminal tympany also can be secondary to the acute onset of ruminal atony that occurs in anaphylaxis and in grain overload;

this causes a reduction in rumen pH and possibly an esophagitis and rumenitis that can interfere with eructation. Ruminal tympany also develops with hypocalcemia.

Chronic ruminal tympany is relatively frequent in calves up to 6 mo old without apparent cause; this form usually resolves spontaneously. Unusual postures, particularly lateral recumbency, are commonly associated with secondary tympany. Ruminants may die of bloat if they become accidentally cast in dorsal recumbency or other restrictive positions in handling facilities, crowded transportation vehicles, or irrigation ditches.

Clinical Findings: Bloat is a common cause of sudden death. Cattle not observed closely, such as pastured and feedlot cattle and dry dairy cattle, usually are found dead. In lactating dairy cattle, which are observed regularly, bloat commonly begins within 1 hr after being turned onto a bloat-producing pasture.

Bloat may develop on the first day after being placed on the pasture but more commonly develops on the second or third day. In primary pasture bloat, the rumen becomes obviously distended suddenly, and the left flank may be so distended that the contour of the paralumbar fossa protrudes above the vertebral column; the entire abdomen is enlarged.

As the bloat progresses, the skin over the left flank becomes progressively more taut and, in severe cases, cannot be "tented." Dyspnea and grunting are marked and are accompanied by mouth breathing, protrusion of the tongue, extension of the head, and frequent urination.

Occasionally, vomiting occurs. Rumen motility does not decrease until bloat is severe. If the tympany continues to worsen, the animal will collapse and die.

Death may occur within 1 hr after grazing began but is more common ~3-4 hr after onset of clinical signs. In a group of affected cattle, there are usually several with clinical bloat and some with mild to moderate abdominal distention. Death rates as high as 20% are recorded in cattle grazing bloat-prone pasture, and in pastoral areas, the annual mortality rate from bloat in dairy cows may approach 1%. There is also economic loss from depressed milk production in nonfatal cases and from suboptimal use of bloat-prone pastures. Bloat can be a significant cause of mortality in feedlot cattle. In secondary bloat, the excess gas is usually free on top of the solid and fluid ruminal contents, although frothy bloat may be seen in vagal indigestion when there is increased ruminal activity. Secondary bloat is seen sporadically.

There is tympanic resonance over the dorsal abdomen left of the midline. Free gas produces a higher pitched ping on percussion than frothy bloat. The distension of the rumen can be detected on rectal examination. In free-gas bloat, the passage of a stomach tube or trocarization releases large quantities of gas and alleviates distention.

Lesions: Necropsy findings are characteristic. Congestion and hemorrhage of the lymph nodes of the head and neck, epicardium, and upper respiratory tract are marked.

The lungs are compressed, and intrabronchial hemorrhage may be present. The cervical esophagus is congested and hemorrhagic, but the thoracic portion of the esophagus is pale and blanched—the demarcation known as the "bloat line" of the esophagus. The rumen is distended, but the contents usually are much less frothy than before death. The liver is pale due to expulsion of blood from the organ.

Diagnosis: Usually, the clinical diagnosis of frothy bloat is obvious. The causes of secondary bloat must be ascertained by clinical examination to determine the cause of the failure of eructation.

Treatment: Cannulation of Rumen, Cow

A trocar and cannula may be used for emergency relief, although the standard-sized instrument is not large enough to allow the viscous, stable foam in peracute cases to escape quickly enough.

A larger bore instrument (2.5 cm in diametre) is necessary, but an incision through the skin must be made before it can be inserted through the muscle layers and into the rumen.

If the cannula fails to reduce the bloat and the animal's life is threatened, an emergency rumenotomy should be performed. If the cannula provides some relief, an antifoaming agent can be administered through the cannula, which can remain in place until the animal has returned to normal, usually within several hours. When the animal's life is not immediately threatened, passing a stomach tube of the largest bore possible is recommended.

A few attempts should be made to clear the tube by blowing and moving it back and forth in an attempt to find large pockets of rumen gas that can be released. In frothy bloat, it may be impossible to reduce the pressure with the tube, and an antifoaming agent should be administered while the tube is in place.

If the bloat is not relieved quickly by the antifoaming agent, the animal must be observed carefully for the next hour to determine if the treatment has been successful or if an alternative therapy is necessary.

A variety of antifoaming agents are effective, including vegetable oils (eg, peanut, corn, soybean) and mineral oils (paraffins), at doses of 250-500 mL.

Dioctyl sodium sulfosuccinate (docusate), a surfactant, is commonly incorporated into one of the above oils and sold as a proprietary antibloat remedy, which is effective if administered early. Poloxalene (25-50 g, PO) is effective in treating legume bloat but not feedlot bloat. Placement of a rumen fistula provides short-term relief for cases of free-gas bloat associated with external obstruction of the esophagus.

Control and Prevention: Prevention of pasture bloat can be difficult. Management practices that have been used to reduce the risk of bloat include feeding hay before turning cattle on pasture, maintaining grass dominance in the sward, or using strip grazing to restrict intake, with movement of animals to a new strip in the afternoon, not the early morning.

For hay to be effective, it must be at least one-third of the diet. Feeding hay or strip grazing may be reliable when the pasture is only moderately dangerous, but these methods are less reliable when the pasture is in the prebloom stage and the bloat potential is high.

Mature pastures are less likely to cause bloat than immature or rapidly growing pastures. The only satisfactory method available to prevent pasture bloating is continual administration of an antifoaming agent during the risk period.

This is widely practiced in grassland countries such as Australia and New Zealand. The most reliable method is drenching twice daily (eg, at milking times) with an antifoaming agent. Spraying the agent onto the bloatprone pasture is equally effective, provided that the animals have access only to treated pasture. This method is ideal for strip grazing but not when grazing is uncontrolled.

The antifoaming agent can be added to the feed or water or incorporated into feed blocks, but success with this method depends on adequate individual intake. The agent can be "painted" on the flanks of the animals, from which it is licked during the day, but animals that do not lick will be unprotected. Available antifoaming agents include oils and fats and synthetic nonionic surfactants.

Oils and fats are given at 60-120 mL/head/day; doses up to 240 mL are indicated during most dangerous periods. Poloxalene, a synthetic polymer, is a highly effective nonionic surfactant that can be given at 10-20 g/head/day and up to 40 g/head/day in high-risk situations.

It is safe and economical to use and is administered daily through the susceptible period by adding to water, feed grain mixtures, or molasses. Alcohol ethoxylate detergents are equally effective and are more palatable than poloxalene.

Ionophores are effective in preventing bloat, and a sustained-release capsule that is administered into the rumen and releases 300 mg of monensin daily for a 100-day period protects against pasture bloat and improves milk production on bloat-prone pastures.

The ultimate aim in control is development of a pasture that permits high production, while keeping incidence of bloat low. The use of pastures of clover and grasses in equal amounts comes closest to achieving this goal.

Bloat potential varies between cultivars of alfalfa, and low-risk LIRD (low initial rate of digestion) cultivars are available commercially.

The addition of legumes with high condensed tannins to the pasture seeding mix (10% sainfoin) can reduce the risk of bloat where there is strip grazing, as can the feeding of sainfoin pellets. To prevent feedlot bloat, rations should contain ≥10-15% cut or chopped roughage mixed into the complete feed. Preferably, the roughage should be a cereal, grain straw, grass hay, or equivalent.

Grains should be rolled or cracked, not finely ground. Pelleted rations made from finely ground grain should be avoided. The addition of tallow (3-5% of the total ration) may be successful occasionally, but it was not effective in controlled trials. The nonionic surfactants, such as poloxalene, have been ineffective in preventing feedlot bloat, but the ionophore lasalocid is effective in control.

Chapter 4

Traumatic Reticuloperitonitis

Traumatic reticuloperitonitis develops as a consequence of perforation of the reticulum. It is important in differential diagnosis of other diseases marked by stasis of the GI tract because it causes similar signs. It is most common in mature dairy cattle, occasionally seen in beef cattle, and rarely reported in other ruminants.

Cattle commonly ingest foreign objects because they do not discriminate against metal materials in feed and do not completely masticate feed before swallowing. The disease is common when greenchop, silage, and hay are made from fields that contain old rusting fences or baling wire, or when pastures are on areas or sites where buildings have recently been constructed, burned, or torn down. The grain ration may also be a source due to accidental addition of metal.

Etiology

Swallowed metallic objects, such as nails or pieces of wire, fall directly into the reticulum or pass into the rumen and are subsequently carried over the ruminoreticular fold into the cranioventral part of the reticulum by ruminal contractions. The reticulo-omasal orifice is elevated above the floor, which tends to retain heavy objects in the reticulum, and the honeycomb-like reticular mucosa traps sharp objects.

Contractions of the reticulum promote penetration of the wall by the foreign object. Compression of the ruminoreticulum by the uterus in late pregnancy, straining during parturition, and mounting during estrus increase the likelihood of an initial penetration of the reticulum and may also disrupt adhesions caused by an earlier penetration. Perforation of the wall of the reticulum allows leakage of ingesta and bacteria, which contaminates the peritoneal cavity.

The resulting peritonitis is generally localised and frequently results in adhesions. Less commonly, a more severe peritonitis develops. Diffuse peritonitis is rare. The object can penetrate the diaphragm and enter the thoracic cavity (causing pleuritis and sometimes pneumonitis) and the pericardial sac (causing pericarditis, sometimes followed by myocarditis, endocarditis, and septicemia). Occasionally, the liver or spleen may be pierced and become infected.

Clinical Findings: The initial attack is characterized by sudden onset of ruminoreticular atony and a sharp fall in milk production. Fecal output is decreased. The rectal temperature is often mildly increased.

The heart rate is normal or slightly increased, and respiration is usually shallow and rapid. Initially, the cow exhibits an arched back; an anxious expression; a reluctance to move; and an uneasy, careful gait. Forced sudden movements as well as defecating, urinating, lying down, getting up, and stepping over barriers may be accompanied by groaning.

A grunt may be elicited by applying pressure to the xiphoid or by elevating this area firmly and then pinching the withers, which causes extension of the thorax and lower abdomen. The grunt can be detected by placing a stethoscope over the trachea and applying pressure or pinching the withers at the end of an inspiration.

Tremor of the triceps and abduction of the elbow may be seen. In chronic cases, feed intake and fecal output are reduced, and milk production remains low. Signs of cranial abdominal pain become less apparent, and the rectal temperature usually returns to normal as the acute inflammation subsides and peritoneal contamination is walled off.

Some cattle develop chronic vagal indigestion, possibly due to the adhesions that form after foreign body perforation, particularly those on the ventromedial reticulum. Cows with pleuritis or pericarditis due to foreign body perforation usually are depressed, tachycardic (>90 bpm), and pyrexic (104°F [40°C]). Pleuritis is manifest by fast, shallow respiration; muffled lung sounds; and possibly pleuritic friction rubs. Thoracentesis may yield several litres of fluid. Traumatic pericarditis usually is characterized by muffled heart sounds, possibly with pericardial friction rubs, and occasionally by gas and fluid splashing sounds on auscultation.

This has been described as a washing machine murmur. Jugular vein distention with a pronounced jugular pulse is present early in the course, and congestive heart failure with marked submandibular and brisket edema is a frequent sequela. Prognosis is grave with these complications. Penetration through the myocardium usually results in extensive hemorrhage into the pericardial sac and sudden death.

Diagnosis: This can be based on history (when available) and clinical findings if the cow is examined when signs initially appear. Without an accurate history and when the condition has been present for several days or longer, diagnosis is more difficult. Other causes of peritonitis, particularly perforated abomasal ulcers, can be difficult to distinguish from traumatic reticuloperitonitis.

Differential diagnoses should include conditions that can produce variable or nonspecific GI signs, eg, indigestion, lymphosarcoma, or intestinal obstruction. Abomasal displacement or volvulus should be ruled out by simultaneous auscultation and percussion. Pleuritis or pericarditis of nontraumatic origin produces signs similar to those associated with foreign body perforation.

Although not always necessary, laboratory tests may be helpful. In many cases, there is a neutrophilia with a left shift. Fibrinogen and, in chronic cases, total plasma protein concentrations may be high.

The acid-base status and serum electrolyte levels are typically normal because abomasal and small-intestinal absorption can remain normal. However, marked hypokalemic, hypochloremic metabolic alkalosis can be seen, presumably because adynamic ileus from peritonitis can affect abomasal and GI motility and resorption of abomasal secretions. The metabolic alkalosis can be created or exacerbated by treatment with alkalinizing agents such as magnesium hydroxide used as a laxative. Peritoneal fluid analysis can be helpful in determining if peritonitis is present. However, the nucleated cell count and the protein level return to normal as the contamination is walled off. Radiographs may detect metallic material in the reticulum.

To determine whether the reticulum has been perforated, the foreign body must be visible beyond the border of the reticulum or be positioned off the floor of the reticulum. Depression in the cranioventral aspect of the reticulum or identification of an abscess (by gas accumulation outside a viscus), soft-tissue masses, or a fluid line in the cranial abdomen are also reliable radiographic findings.

Portable radiographic units cannot penetrate the reticular area of standing adult cattle, and the cow may need to be transported to where there is equipment with sufficient power. The area can be radiographed using portable equipment if the systemic condition does not preclude placing the cow in dorsal recumbency.

A perforating foreign body will remain in the ventral aspect of the reticulum and be surrounded by gas. Electronic metal detectors can identify metal in the reticulum but do not distinguish between perforating and nonperforating foreign bodies. Ultrasonography of the heart and thorax is useful in the diagnosis of pleuritis and pericarditis.

Treatment: Treatment of the typical case seen early in its course may be surgical or medical. Either approach improves the chances of recovery from ~60% in untreated cases to 80-90%. Surgery involves rumenotomy with manual removal of the object or objects; if an abscess is adhered to the reticulum, it should be aspirated (to confirm that it is an abscess) and then drained into the reticulum.

Antibiotics should be administered perioperatively. Medical treatment involves administration of antibacterials to control the peritonitis and a magnet to prevent recurrence. Because of the mixed bacterial flora in the lesion, a broad-spectrum antimicrobial agent such as oxytetracycline (6.6-11 mg/kg) should be used. Penicillin (22,000 IU/kg, IM, bid) is used widely and is effective in many cases despite its limited spectrum. Affected cows should be confined for 1-2 wk; placing them on an inclined plane (elevated in front) may limit further penetration of the foreign object. Supportive therapy, such as oral or occasionally IV fluids and SC calcium borogluconate, should be administered as needed. Rumen inoculation is beneficial in some cases with prolonged ruminal stasis and loss of normal flora. More advanced cases, those with obvious secondary complications, or those that do not respond to initial medical or surgical therapy should be evaluated from an economic perspective; if the cow is of limited value, slaughter should be considered if the carcass is likely to pass inspection.

Prevention: Preventive measures include avoiding the use of baling wire, passing feed over magnets to remove metallic objects, keeping cattle away from sites of new construction, and completely removing old buildings and fences. Additionally, bar magnets may be administered PO, preferably after fasting for 18-24 hr. Usually, the magnet remains in the reticulum and holds any ferromagnetic objects on its surface. There is good evidence that giving magnets to all herd replacement heifers and bulls at ~1 yr of age minimizes incidence of traumatic reticuloperitonitis.

Vagal Indigestion (Chronic Indigestion)

Vagal indigestion is characterized by gradual development of rumenoreticular and abdominal distention thought to be the result of lesions affecting the vagus nerve. However, vagal nerve involvement is not present in all cases. The most common cause is traumatic reticuloperitonitis. Vagal indigestion is seen in cattle and has been reported in sheep.

Etiology and Pathogenesis: Various diseases can cause vagal indigestion due to injury, inflammation, or pressure on the vagal nerve. However, conditions resulting in mechanical obstruction of the cardia or reticulo-omasal orifice (eg, papillomas or ingested placenta) also have been included in the syndrome if ruminoreticular distention is present and the condition is subacute to chronic. There are 4 types of vagal indigestion based on the site of the functional obstruction. Type I is failure of eructation or free-gas bloat, Type II is a failure of omasal transport, type III is abomasal impaction, and type IV is partial obstruction of the forestomach. Type I vagal indigestion, or failure of eructation, results in free-gas bloat. It is most commonly due to inflammatory lesions in the vicinity of the vagus nerve, such as localised peritonitis, adhesions (usually after an episode of traumatic reticuloperitonitis), or chronic pneumonia. Less common causes include pharyngeal trauma, which affects a more proximal part of the vagus nerve, and esophageal compression by abscesses or neoplasia, such as lymphosarcoma. Free-gas bloat can also be seen with esophageal obstruction by intraluminal foreign bodies or masses. However, this typically is an acute condition, which does not fit the definition of vagal indigestion.

Type II vagal indigestion, or failure of omasal transport, develops as a result of any condition that prevents ingesta from passing through the omasal canal into the abomasum. Adhesions and abscesses (reticular or single liver abscesses) are the most common causes.

They are usually on the right or medial wall of the reticulum near the route of the vagus nerve. Reticular abscesses and adhesions are almost invariably the result of traumatic reticuloperitonitis.

Mechanical obstruction of the omasal canal by ingested material (eg, placenta) or masses (eg, lymphosarcoma, squamous cell carcinoma, granulomas, or papillomas) can also cause chronic ruminoreticular distention due to failure of omasal transport. Type III vagal indigestion is abomasal impaction, which tends to develop due to feeding of dry, course roughage, such as straw, in a chopped or ground form with restricted access to water and usually during extremely cold temperatures.

Secondary impactions are seen after an episode of traumatic reticuloperitonitis or as a sequela of right abomasal displacement or abomasal volvulus or, less commonly, of obstruction of the pylorus (eg, by placenta or trichobezoars).

Vagal indigestion can develop in cattle after abomasal volvulus without abomasal impaction. These cases would presumably fall into the category of failure of omasal transport (type II) with damage to the vagal nerve found more cranial in its course. Type IV vagal indigestion, or partial forestomach obstruction, is poorly defined. It typically develops in cattle during gestation. It may be related to the enlarging uterus shifting the abomasum to a more cranial position, which inhibits normal motility.

Clinical Findings: The clinical signs vary to some extent with the location of the obstruction. In all cases, there is a gradual development (over days to weeks) of ruminoreticular and abdominal distention. Distention of the dorsal and ventral sacs of the rumen result in an "L-shaped" rumen on rectal examination. Left dorsal and left and right ventral distention of the abdomen causes a "papple" (pear plus apple) shape. Cattle with vagal indigestion have a diminished appetite, which typically improves temporarily if distention is relieved. Milk production gradually decreases, fecal output is reduced and often contains long hay particles, and the rumen develops a "splashy" fluid consistency.

The feces are characteristically very scant and sticky. The strength of rumen contractions is decreased; however, rumen motility is often increased (3-4 contractions/min). It is commonly possible to see movements of the left abdominal wall that mirror the movements of the hyperactive rumen. However, rumen contraction sounds are not audible because the contents have become frothy due to the prolonged contractions and failure of the rumen to empty.

Temperature and respiratory rate are usually normal; however, these can be increased depending on the cause. Bradycardia is present in 25-40% of cases. Because bradycardia is uncommonly associated with other conditions, vagal indigestion should be considered in the differential diagnosis in any case in which bradycardia is present.

Tachycardia develops as the disease progresses. Over time, the animal develops a rough hair coat, loses condition, and becomes weak (in some cases to the point of recumbency) and dehydrated.On rectal palpation, the rumen is distended with gas or froth that occupies the entire left abdomen, pushing the left kidney to the right of the midline. The ventral sac of the rumen is enlarged and palpable to the right of the midline (the characteristic "L-shaped" rumen). Palpation of the lower half of the right side of the abdomen below the costochondral junction may detect an impacted abomasum that feels doughy. Hematologic findings vary. The PCV can be increased because of dehydration or decreased because of bone marrow depression (anemia of chronic disease). The WBC may be normal, increased, or decreased. If an inflammatory condition such as peritonitis is present, the neutrophil to lymphocyte ratio is typically reversed, and a neutrophilia may be present. Lymphocytosis can be seen with vagal indigestion due to lymphosarcoma. Leukopenia may be present with diffuse peritonitis. Increased serum globulin and total protein can be seen with abscesses. Metabolic status is normal, or metabolic alkalosis may be present.

The chloride level varies with the site of the obstruction. Low chloride indicates reflux of chloride from the abomasum into the rumen and obstruction at the level of the abomasum. The chloride levels of the rumen fluid may be increased. Metabolic alkalosis is typically present if serum chloride is decreased. The chloride is usually normal if the lesion is cranial to the abomasum. Potassium is usually low due to decreased potassium intake in the feed. Calcium is often moderately decreased because of ongoing milk production; however, it can be low enough to cause recumbency. BUN and creatinine increase with dehydration due to prerenal azotemia.

Diagnosis: Diagnosis is based on the presence of subacute to chronic ruminoreticular and abdominal distention. Because vagal indigestion is by definition a subacute to chronic disease, this diagnosis should not be made in cattle that have not been sick for at least several days, which rules out acute rumen tympanites and acute frothy bloat.

Other causes of abdominal distention, such as ascites and uterine enlargement, are included in the differential diagnosis and can almost invariably be ruled out by rectal palpation due to the absence of ruminoreticular distention.

Occasional cases of longstanding obstruction of the cecum or small intestine can cause severe ruminoreticular and abdominal distention; however, palpable cecal or small-intestinal distention is also palpable rectally. In addition, the rumen is distended but not L-shaped, and a characteristic ping is present in the case of cecocolic volvulus. Diagnosing the specific cause of vagal indigestion is more difficult but is important because of differences in treatment and prognosis. Physical examination, rectal examination, CBC, blood acid-base determination, and serum chemistry values are often useful. Peritoneal fluid analysis can support the diagnosis of peritonitis if total protein or nucleated cells are increased. Radiographs of the reticulum should be taken to identify a radiopaque linear foreign body (eg, wire) or reticular abscess. Definitive diagnosis often requires exploratory surgery (left paralumbar fossa laparotomy and rumenotomy).

Treatment and Prognosis: If the value of the animal justifies treatment, surgery is almost always needed to identify the underlying cause. Medical management alone is ineffective. A left paralumbar fossa laparotomy and rumenotomy provides the opportunity for definitive treatment in some cases. Emptying the rumen at the time of surgery may help restore normal rumen motility.

Stimulation of low-threshold tension receptors in the reticulum occurs under normal circumstances and causes reflex reticuloruminal contractions. However, severe distention causes stimulation of high-threshold receptors that have the opposite effect and inhibit contractions.

Supportive or symptomatic therapy should be provided in all cases, which typically involves correcting dehydration as well as calcium and electrolyte deficits, commonly with oral fluids and electrolytes. Severely dehydrated animals and those with longstanding disease require IV fluids. Fresh water and normal feed should be available.

Transfaunation at surgery and/or via stomach tube may help reestablish normal rumen flora in cattle with chronic anorexia. Antibiotics should be given if the underlying cause is infectious or if a rumen fistula is created. Choice of antibiotic should be based on culture results if possible.

Treatment of type I vagal indigestion (failure of eructation) also typically involves creating a rumen fistula to allow free gas to escape. If surgery is not economically feasible and the underlying cause of vagal indigestion has been identified and treated, a rumen trocar can be placed temporarily. Such trocars are commercially available and must be secure and self-retaining to prevent potentially fatal leakage of rumen contents into the peritoneal cavity. The trocar should not be removed for at least 2 wk to allow firm adhesions to form between the rumen and body wall. The prognosis for animals with type I vagal indigestion is usually favourable. After creation of a rumen fistula, the signs of vagal indigestion resolve in nearly all cases.

However, animals with chronic respiratory disease or pharyngeal trauma may not recover from the underlying condition. Leakage of ingesta from fistulas can cause off-flavoured milk. Peritonitis can develop from leakage around the fistula or as a sequela of rumenotomy; however, this should not happen with good surgical technique. Type II vagal indigestion (failure of omasal transport) rarely responds to supportive or symptomatic therapy without surgical intervention.

Left paralumbar fossa laparotomy and rumenotomy can be used to identify adhesions in the vicinity of the reticulum, reticular or hepatic abscesses, or obstruction of the omasal canal. Removal of foreign bodies, wires, and some masses at surgery affords an excellent prognosis.

A diagnosis of lymphosarcoma at surgery warrants a grave prognosis. Reticular abscesses identified at surgery should be cautiously drained into the reticulum, and antibiotics given for 10-14 days. Reportedly, 83% of cattle with reticular abscesses respond favourably to treatment. Identification of adhesions in the vicinity of the reticulum warrants a fair to good prognosis with surgery, antibiotic therapy, and appropriate supportive treatment.

Hepatic abscesses must be drained by a second surgery. Large-bore cannulas placed through the body wall, through the adhesions, and into the abscess will drain the pus. However, recurrence is more of a problem with hepatic abscesses than with reticular abscesses.

Animals with type III vagal indigestion (abomasal impaction) diagnosed without surgery usually do not receive further treatment because of the poor prognosis, particularly if there is a history of traumatic reticuloperitonitis or abomasal volvulus. If the diagnosis is made at surgery or if the abomasal impaction is thought to be dietary, dioctyl sodium sulfosuccinate or magnesium sulfate can be infused directly into the abomasum via the reticulo-omasal orifice after emptying the rumen. A nasogastric tube can be passed into the abomasum at surgery and left in place for continued treatment. If possible, impacted material should be removed manually through the reticulo-omasal orifice. Other lesions, such as abscesses, should be identified and drained. Abomasotomy and removal of abomasal contents, using a right paracostal approach with the cow in left lateral recumbency, can be performed as a last resort. However, recurrence of the impaction is common. Pyloric obstruction in cattle is rare and is most often due to a foreign body obstructing the lumen. Pyloromyotomy is almost never effective in resolving abomasal impactions. Type III vagal indigestion has a poor prognosis regardless of the cause or the treatment. However, some cattle with primary abomasal impactions will respond to therapy, although severely affected animals will not. Cattle with secondary impactions due to traumatic reticuloperitonitis or as a sequela of right abomasal displacement or abomasal volvulus seldom recover. Animals with foreign bodies (eg, trichobezoars) obstructing the pylorus have a good prognosis if the obstruction is removed. Therapeutic abortion has been recommended for treatment of cattle with type IV vagal indigestion (partial forestomach obstruction), and some cows have improved with this treatment; however, because type IV vagal indigestion is a poorly defined condition, the prognosis is always guarded. A more specific prognosis is based on response to therapy and identification of a specific lesion at exploratory celiotomy and rumenotomy.

Prevention: The most common cause of vagal indigestion is traumatic reticuloperitonitis, which causes adhesions and abscesses that interfere with vagal nerve function. Therefore, prevention of traumatic reticuloperitonitis is important. Good management practices will prevent some cases of vagal indigestion resulting from chronic pneumonia. Early diagnosis of right-sided abomasal displacements and abomasal volvulus, and surgical correction the day the diagnosis is made, may prevent some cases. Prompt removal of the placenta from the cow's enclosure after parturition will keep it from obstructing the cardia, reticulo-omasal orifice, or pylorus.

Ruminal Drinkers (Ruminal Drinking)

Ruminal drinkers refers to calves that develop chronic indigestion because milk is deposited into the rumen as a result of failure of the reticular groove reflex during drinking. The disease is most common in bucket-fed calves, especially veal calves 2-8 wk old. Calves that "gulp" rather than sip milk are at greatest risk. The milk retained in the rumen ferments and produces acetic acid, butyric acid, and lactate; the pH in the rumen falls; and dyskeratosis of the ruminal mucosa develops. Secondary changes include villous atrophy in the small intestine and reduced disaccharidase activity of the brush border. Affected calves show inappetence, ventral abdominal distention, and poor growth. They pass sticky, clay-like feces that may adhere to the tail, perineum, and hindlegs. Chronically affected calves are small for their age and have a poor prognosis. Fluid-splashing sounds, audible on auscultation over the left flank while the calf is drinking, are diagnostic. Rancid-smelling fermented material can be obtained by stomach tube from the rumen. A ruminal pH of <6 leads to systemic acid-base disturbance. Treatment consists of removing the fermented material and flushing the rumen with saline. With subsequent feedings, an attempt is made to induce reticular groove closure by inducing vigorous sucking activity with the fingers before feeding milk. Calves that relapse should be fed by nipple-bottle or weaned. A rubber nipple floating on the surface of bucket-fed milk may prevent the syndrome. Failure of the reticular groove reflex and putrefactive rumenitis also is seen in calves <2 wk old and can be an important cause of sporadic cases of diarrhea in this age group.

Ruminal Parakeratosis

Ruminal parakeratosis is a disease of cattle and sheep characterized by hardening and enlargement of the papillae of the rumen. It is most common in animals fed a high-concentrate ration during the finishing period. It also is seen in cattle fed rations of heat-treated alfalfa pellets. It does not appear to be related to the feeding of antibiotics or protein concentrates. Incidence in a group may be as high as 40%. The lesions are thought to be caused by the lowered pH and the increased concentration of volatile fatty acids (VFA) in the rumen juice. The lesions usually do not develop in cattle fed unprocessed whole grain (on which animals gain weight as readily), which may be related to the higher pH and higher concentration of acetic acid compared with the longer chain VFA in the rumen juice. Many of the papillae are enlarged and hardened, and several may adhere together to form bundles. The papillae of the anterior ventral sac are commonly affected. In cattle, the roof of the dorsal sac may show multiple foci (each 2-3 cm^2) of parakeratosis. In sheep, abnormal papillae may be visible and palpable through the wall of the intact rumen. Affected papillae contain excessive layers of keratinized epithelial cells, particles of food, and bacteria. The rumens of affected cattle are difficult to clean in the preparation of tripe. The abnormal epithelium, by interfering with absorption, may reduce efficiency of feed utilisation and rate of gain, although there is little evidence to support this theory. Ruminal parakeratosis may be prevented by finishing animals on rations that contain unground ingredients in the proportion of 1 part roughage to 3 parts concentrate. The necessity and economics of prevention are not well defined.

Diseases of the Abomasum: Introduction

Abomasal disorders include left displaced abomasum (LDA), right displaced abomasum (RDA), abomasal volvulus, ulcers, and impaction. Displacement or volvulus is seen most commonly in dairy cows, but can also be seen in dairy bulls and calves. Except for abomasal volvulus, abomasal displacement is rare in beef cattle and essentially undiagnosed in small ruminants. Ulcers are seen in dairy and beef cattle and in calves and lambs; they are rarely diagnosed in small ruminants. Impactions can be primary, which is most frequent in beef cattle, or secondary, which develop most often in dairy cows as a form of vagal indigestion. Impactions may have a hereditary basis in some black-faced sheep.

Left or Right Displaced Abomasum and Abomasal Volvulus

Because the abomasum is suspended loosely by the greater and lesser omenta, it can be moved from its normal position on the right ventral part of the abdomen to the left or right side (LDA, RDA), or it can rotate on its mesenteric axis while displaced to the right (abomasal volvulus). It can shift from its normal position to left displacement or to right displacement over a relatively short period. Abomasal volvulus can develop rapidly or slowly from an uncorrected RDA.

Etiology: Although LDA, RDA, and abomosal volvulus (previously referred to as RTA for right torsion of the abomasum) are often considered separately, there is evidence of a common underlying etiology; they may be different manifestations of the same or a similar disease process. The etiology is multifactorial, although abomasal hypomotility and gas production contribute to development of displacement or volvulus. Important contributing factors include abomasal hypomotility associated with hypocalcemia and concurrent diseases (mastitis, metritis) associated with endotoxemia and decreased rumen fill, periparturient changes in the position of intra-abdominal organs, and genetic predisposition, particularly in deep-bodied cows. Hypomotility is also related to ingestion of high-concentrate, low-roughage diets, which reduce abomasal motility through a poorly defined mechanism that may involve increased concentrations of volatile fatty acids.

In addition, high-concentrate diets result in a linear increase in gas production (mostly carbon dioxide, methane, and nitrogen). Finally, subclinical and clinical ketosis increase the risk of abomasal displacement through an unknown mechanism that may be associated with decreased rumen fill. About 80% of displacements are seen within 1 mo of parturition; however, they can be seen at any time. LDA is much more common than RDA (30:1); cases of volvulus are also more common than RDA (10 LDA to 1 volvulus). Abomasal volvulus is preceded by RDA.

Pathogenesis: In LDA, as a result of abomasal hypomotility and gas production, the partially gas-distended abomasum becomes displaced upward along the left abdominal wall lateral to the rumen.

It is primarily the fundus and greater curvature of the abomasum that become displaced, which in turn causes displacement of the pylorus and duodenum. The omasum, reticulum, and liver are also rotated to varying degrees. The abomasal obstruction is partial, and although the segment contains some gas and fluid, a certain amount can still escape, and the distention rarely becomes severe. Because there is no interference with blood supply, the effects of displacement are entirely due to interference with digestion and passage of ingesta, which lead to decreased appetite and dehydration. A mild metabolic alkalosis with hypochloremia and hypokalemia are common. The hypochloremic metabolic alkalosis is due to abomasal hypomotility, continued secretion of hydrochloric acid into the abomasum, and the partial abomasal outflow obstruction, with sequestration of chloride in the abomasum and reflux into the rumen. Hypokalemia is due to decreased intake of feeds high in potassium, sequestration of potassium in the abomasum, and dehydration. Secondary ketosis is common and may be complicated by development of fatty liver disease (*Fatty Liver Disease of Cattle). In* RDA, hypomotility, gas production, and displacement of the partially gas-filled abomasum occur as in LDA.

Mild hypokalemic, hypochloremic, metabolic alkalosis develops as well. After this dilatation phase, rotation of the abomasum on its mesenteric axis leads to volvulus and local circulatory impairment and ischemia (hemorrhagic strangulating obstruction).

The volvulus is usually in a counterclockwise direction when viewed from the rear and the right side of the animal. The omasum is displaced medially and can be involved in the volvulus with occlusion of its blood supply (called an omasal-abomasal volvulus). The liver and reticulum usually are displaced also. In rare cases, the reticulum can be involved (called a reticular-omasal-abomasal volvulus). A large quantity of fluid accumulates in the abomasum; chloride is sequestered there as well. Hypochloremic, hypokalemic metabolic alkalosis develops. The blood supply to the abomasum, and often the omasum and proximal duodenum, is compromised, eventually resulting in ischemic necrosis of the abomasum as well as dehydration and circulatory failure. As this progresses, a metabolic acidosis is superimposed on the metabolic alkalosis.

Clinical Findings: The typical history of displacement includes anorexia (most commonly a lack of appetite for grain with a decreased or normal appetite for roughage) and decreased milk production (usually significant but not as dramatic as with traumatic reticuloperitonitis or other causes of peritonitis). In abomasal volvulus, anorexia is complete, milk production is more markedly and progressively reduced, and clinical deterioration is rapid. In abomasal displacement, temperature, heart rate, and respiratory rate are usually normal. The caudal part of the rib cage on the side of the displacement may appear "sprung." Hydration appears subjectively normal with displacements except in some chronic cases. Rumen motility may be normal but often is reduced in frequency and strength of contraction. Feces are usually reduced in quantity and more fluid than normal. The most important diagnostic physical finding is a ping on simultaneous auscultation and percussion of the abdomen, which should be performed in the area marked by a line from the tuber coxae to the point of the elbow, and from the elbow toward the stifle.

The ping characteristic of an LDA is most commonly located in an area between ribs 9 and 13 in the middle to upper third of the abdomen; however, the ping can be more ventral or more caudal, or both. Pings associated with a rumen gas cap are usually more dorsal, less resonant, and extend more caudally through the paralumbar fossa.

Rectal examination can confirm a gas-filled rumen or an extremely empty rumen that correlates with the rumen ping in these cases. Pings associated with pneumoperitoneum typically are less resonant, present on both sides of the abdomen, and inconsistent in location on repeated evaluation. Frequently, secondary ketosis develops and ketones are present in the urine or milk. Ketosis that develops in association with abomasal displacement responds only transiently to treatment and recurs (as compared with primary ketosis, which develops early in lactation in high-producing cows and responds to therapy permanently if instituted early).

See also ketosis, *Ketosis in Cattle: Introduction*.The ping associated with RDA also is most commonly located in the area between ribs 10 and 13. Differentiation between various causes of a right-sided ping is difficult in some cases.

A small ping underlying ribs 12 or 13 and extending as far forward as rib 10 is common in cows with functional ileus from a number of causes. It is most often associated with gas in the ascending colon and resolves with correction of the underlying condition. Cecal dilatation and rotation are characterized by a right-sided ping. The ping extends through the dorsal paralumbar fossa in cecal dilatation and usually is located more caudally (well into the paralumbar fossa) in cecal rotation compared with the ping of RDA. Palpation per rectum is helpful in differentiating an RDA from cecal dilatation or rotation. Other right-sided pings are produced by pneumoperitoneum or gas in the rectum, descending colon, duodenum, or uterus. Spontaneous fluid splashing or gas tinkling sounds may be heard on auscultation of the area of the ping or on simultaneous ballottement and auscultation of the abdomen (succussion). The characteristic rectal examination findings with LDA include a medially displaced rumen and left kidney. The abomasum is rarely palpable in LDA and only occasionally in RDA. The clinical signs associated with abomasal volvulus are more severe than with simple displacements because of the vascular compromise. However, an early abomasal volvulus can be difficult to distinguish from an RDA except by the presence of a right-sided ping cranial to rib 10 (indicating medial displacement of the liver by the abomasal volvulus) and the anatomic position identified at surgery. In contrast to cases of displacement, an animal with abomasal volvulus has tachycardia proportional to the severity of the condition. The area of the ping is usually larger (extending as far forward as rib 8), and the amount of succussible fluid is greater. The animal is more depressed, and signs of weakness, toxemia, and dehydration develop as the disease progresses. The caudal extent of the abomasum is usually palpable per rectum. Without therapy, the animal often becomes recumbent within 48-72 hr after developing volvulus. Death occurs from shock and dehydration and is sudden if the ischemic abomasum ruptures.

Diagnosis: For displacement or volvulus, diagnosis is based on the presence of the characteristic ping on simultaneous auscultation and percussion and excluding other causes of left- or right-sided pings. Recent parturition, partial anorexia, and decreased milk production suggest displacement. A ketosis that is only temporarily responsive to treatment is consistent with abomasal displacement, which may be intermittent. The typical signs on physical examination (in addition to the ping), rectal examination, and laboratory evaluation also support the diagnosis. Melena or signs of peritonitis (eg, fever, tachycardia, localised abdominal pain, pneumoperitoneum) with an LDA may indicate a bleeding or perforated abomasal ulcer, respectively.

Treatment: Open (surgical) and closed (percutaneous) techniques can be used to correct displacements. Rolling a cow through a 70° arc after casting her on her right side corrects most LDA; however, recurrence is very likely. LDA can be corrected surgically using right flank pyloric omentopexy, right paramedian abomasopexy, left paralumbar abomasopexy, or combined left flank and right paramedian laparoscopy. Blind suture techniques (toggle-pin fixation or the "big needle" [blind-stitch] method), performed in the right paramedian area, are percutaneous methods for correction of LDA; however, the exact location of the suture is not known. Potentially fatal complications following blind suture techniques can develop, although the reported success is similar to that of surgical correction.

With toggle-pin fixation, the pH can be checked to confirm that the pin is in the abomasum, which reduces the likelihood of attaching rumen, small intestine, or omentum to the body wall rather than the abomasum. RDA and abomasal volvulus are corrected surgically (using right paralumbar fossa omentopexy or right paramedian abomasopexy) when economically feasible.

The right paramedian abomasopexy should be used only for correcting RDA and abomasal volvulus in cattle that are unable to stand. Ancillary treatment of animals with displacements include treating any concurrent disease (eg, metritis, mastitis, ketosis). Calcium borogluconate SC or calcium gels PO help restore normal abomasal motility in many cases. In simple displacement, fluid and electrolyte abnormalities correct spontaneously with access to water and a salt block. Providing electrolyte water (60 g sodium chloride and 30 g potassium chloride in 19 L of water) via stomach tube is helpful in cases of longer duration.

Animals with significant dehydration and metabolic derangement require IV therapy, which is typically administered as hypertonic saline (7.2% NaCl, 5 mL/kg, IV over 5 min). Occasionally, animals with abomasal displacement or volvulus have atrial fibrillation, thought to be of metabolic origin. Correction of the displacement or volvulus almost always results in correction of the atrial fibrillation within 1 wk. Aggressive treatment of ketosis plays an important role in the successful treatment of abomasal displacement, as most of the cattle that die following surgical correction of LDA and RDA do so from the metabolic consequences of prolonged anorexia. The prognosis after correction of simple LDA or RDA is good, with survival rates of 95%. Abomasal volvulus has a variable and less favourable prognosis (average survival rate of 70%); a high heart rate, moderate to severe dehydration, a longer period of illness, a large quantity of fluid in the abomasum, and the presence of omasal-abomasal or reticulo-omasal-abomasal volvulus are associated with a poor prognosis.

Prevention: The incidence of displacements can be decreased by ensuring a rapid increase in rumen volume following calving, feeding a total mixed ration rather than feeding grain twice daily ("slug feeding"), avoiding rapid dietary changes, maintaining adequate roughage in the diet, avoiding postparturient hypocalcemia, and minimizing and promptly treating concurrent disease and ketosis.

Abomasal Ulcers

Abomasal ulcers affect mature cattle and calves and have several different manifestations.

Etiology and Pathogenesis: Except for lymphosarcoma of the abomasum and the erosions of the abomasal mucosa that develop in viral diseases such as bovine viral diarrhea, rinderpest, and bovine malignant catarrhal fever, the causes of abomasal ulceration are not well understood. Many different causes have been suggested. Although abomasal ulcers can be seen any time during lactation, they are common in high-producing, mature dairy cows within the first 6 wk after parturition. The most likely cause is prolonged inappetence, which results in sustained periods of low abomasal pH. Abomasal ulcers may also arise in association with lymphosarcoma, abomasal disorders (displacement or volvulus), or increased intraluminal pressure causing ischemia of abomasal mucosa; they may also appear to be unrelated to other disease. Abomasal ulcers are very common in milk-fed calves after they have consumed milk or milk replacer for 4-12 wk. Most of these are subclinical and nonhemorrhagic. Occasionally, milk-fed calves <2 wk old are affected by acute, hemorrhagic abomasal ulcers that may perforate and cause rapid death. Well-nourished suckling beef calves, 2-4 mo old, may be affected by acute abomasal ulcers. Abomasal trichobezoars are common in these calves, but do not appear to increase the risk of ulcer formation.

Clinical Findings: The syndrome varies, depending on whether ulceration is complicated by hemorrhage or perforation and by the severity of such hemorrhage or peritonitis. A system of classification is based on the depth of penetration or the degree of hemorrhage or peritonitis caused by the ulcer: Type I is an erosion or ulcer without hemorrhage, Type II is hemorrhagic, Type III is perforated with acute localised peritonitis, and Type IV is perforated with acute diffuse peritonitis. There may be only a single ulcer or many acute and chronic ulcers.

Cattle with bleeding abomasal ulcers may be asymptomatic except for intermittent occult blood in the feces, or they can die acutely from massive hemorrhage. Common clinical signs include mild abdominal pain, bruxism, sudden onset of anorexia, tachycardia (90-100 bpm), and fecal occult blood or melena that may be intermittent.

Signs of blood loss are seen with major hemorrhage and may include tachycardia (100-140 bpm), pale mucous membranes, weak pulse, cool extremities, shallow breaths, tachypnea, and melena. More severe signs include acute rumen stasis, generalized abdominal pain with a reluctance to move and an audible grunt or groan with each breath, weakness, and dehydration. Melena may not be present in peracute cases because it takes at least 8 hr for abomasal blood to be detected in the feces.

As the condition progresses, body temperature drops, and the animal becomes recumbent and dies within 6-8 hr. In general, bleeding ulcers do not perforate, and perforating ulcers do not bleed into the GI tract sufficiently to produce melena. However, hemorrhage and perforation are seen together occasionally, usually in cases that are chronic or associated with abomasal displacement. Calves with abomasal ulceration and hairballs may have a distended gas- and fluid-filled abomasum that is palpable behind the right costal arch. Deep palpation may reveal abdominal pain associated with local peritonitis due to a perforated ulcer. In calves, perforating ulcers are more common than bleeding ulcers.

Lesions: Ulceration is most common in the fundic region in adult cattle and in the pyloric antrum in milk-fed calves. The single or multiple ulcers measure from a few millimetres to 5 cm in diametre. The affected artery is usually visible after ingesta and necrotic tissue are removed from a bleeding ulcerated area. Most cases of perforation are walled off by the omentum, which forms a cavity 12-15 cm in diametre that contains degenerated blood and necrotic debris. Material from this cavity may infiltrate widely through the omental fat. Adhesions may form between the ulcer and surrounding organs or the abdominal wall.

Diagnosis: In cases with only slight bleeding and mild clinical signs, diagnosis is difficult and may require repeated fecal evaluations for occult blood. Other conditions that can cause partial anorexia and decreased milk production should be excluded by physical examination and laboratory tests, including abdominocentesis. In cases with melena, the diagnosis can be based on physical examination alone.

The PCV can help to determine the degree of hemorrhage. An occult blood test of the feces can confirm melena. Other conditions that result in blood in the feces should be eliminated. Blood from portions of the GI tract distal to the abomasum reacts on fecal occult blood tests; it is usually bright red if from the large intestine or raspberry-coloured if from the small intestine.

Animals with abomasal lymphosarcoma can have a bleeding syndrome similar to that associated with abomasal ulcers but do not respond to therapy. Occasionally, oral, pharyngeal, and laryngeal lesions bleed, and the swallowed blood appears in the feces. Similarly, pulmonary abscesses that form as a sequela of rumenitis by embolization to the lungs and liver can erode blood vessels and result in hemoptysis; if the blood is swallowed, this can also result in melena.

Fecal occult blood may also be due to abomasal volvulus or to bloodsucking helminths. Diagnosis of perforating abomasal ulcers is based on physical examination and excluding other causes of peritonitis. Abomasal ulceration with perforation and local peritonitis may be indistinguishable from chronic traumatic reticuloperitonitis. A magnet in the reticulum (confirmed by use of a compass) or an accurate history of having given the cow a magnet before the onset of signs decreases the likelihood of traumatic reticuloperitonitis. Reticular radiographs may confirm or exclude the presence of radiopaque foreign bodies in the reticulum. In some cases, there is a neutrophilia, possibly with a left shift. Evaluation of peritoneal fluid will confirm peritonitis if total protein and nucleated cell count are increased. Intracellular bacteria or degenerate neutrophils are rarely seen because, in most cases, the infection is rapidly walled off.

The diagnosis of diffuse peritonitis due to perforation is based on physical examination and excluding other causes. Rupture of a distended viscus, such as can occur with abomosal volvulus or cecal rotation, produces similar signs. Regardless of the cause of diffuse peritonitis, the prognosis is grave because of overwhelming infection and cardiovascular deterioration. There is neutrophilia with a marked left shift and hemoconcentration. Abdominal fluid is usually readily obtainable in large quantities, and the protein level is increased; the nucleated cell count may be increased, or it may be normal due to dilution or utilisation.

Treatment: Most cases of abomasal ulcers are undiagnosed and therefore untreated. Occasionally, a presumptive diagnosis is made and medical treatment instituted.

The most important treatment is to get the animal to eat, as food is an excellent buffer and continual flow of forestomach contents (pH 6.0-7.0) into the abomasum helps increase abomasal pH. Broad-spectrum antibiotic therapy (given for ^{3}5 days or until the rectal temperature is normal for 48 hr) is indicated for perforating ulcers.

Antacids are effective in increasing abomasal pH in milk-fed calves when administered at 4- to 6-hr intervals in a manner that induces esophageal groove closure; however, their efficacy is extremely questionable in adult ruminants because of ruminal dilution. H_2 -receptor antagonists are effective in increasing abomasal pH in milk-fed calves; however, the oral doses required for cimetidine (100 mg/kg, tid) and ranitidine (50 mg/kg, tid) are high. Because NSAID can contribute to ulceration, their use is contraindicated. The prognosis for localised peritonitis associated with perforating abomasal ulcers is good with medical therapy and dietary alteration. Recovery generally takes 1-2 wk, and animals that are fully recovered for 1-2 wk generally do not experience recurrence. Surgery is indicated for perforating abomasal ulcers only when the abomasum is displaced; however, significant abdominal contamination can occur in the process of breaking down adhesions and resecting or oversewing the ulcer. Animals in which the ulcerated area is resected or oversewn usually recover. Animals with diffuse peritonitis after perforation of an abomasal ulcer rarely respond to therapy, and the prognosis is grave. Treatment consists of rapid and continued IV fluid therapy (based on the current metabolic status) and IV broad-spectrum antibiotics. The few animals that recover from diffuse peritonitis usually have massive abdominal adhesions. For bleeding ulcers, blood transfusions and fluid therapy may be necessary in addition to dietary management, stall confinement, and oral antacids. If hemorrhage is acute, the PCV may not reflect the severity because equilibration between intravascular and extravascular fluid after blood loss takes at least 4 hr. Generally, a blood transfusion is required whenever weakness and lethargy are present; a decision regarding transfusion should be based on clinical signs rather than PCV. Cross-matching is not usually necessary; a single transfusion of 4-6 L of blood is required. Some cattle require more than one transfusion over the course of several days. Complete recovery usually takes 1-2 wk. The prognosis is good if weakness and lethargy have not developed before treatment is started.

Prevention: Animals should be encouraged to keep eating to avoid prolonged periods of inappetence and low abomasal pH.

Dietary Abomasal Impaction

Impaction of the abomasum develops in pregnant beef cows during cold winter months when cattle have decreased water intake and are fed poor-quality roughage. It also has been seen in feedlot cattle fed a variety of mixed rations containing chopped or ground roughage (straw, hay) and cereal grains and in late-pregnancy dairy cows on similar feeds.

Etiology: The cause is unknown but considered to be consumption of excess roughage that is low in both digestible protein and energy. Impaction with sand can occur if cattle are fed hay or silage on sandy soils, or root crops that are sandy or dirty. Outbreaks may affect up to 15% of all pregnant cattle on individual farms when the ambient temperature drops to -14°F (-26°C) or lower for several days.

Pathogenesis: The pathogenesis is unknown but is related to diet. Once the abomasum becomes impacted, subacute obstruction of the upper GI tract develops. Ions of hydrogen and chloride are continually secreted into the abomasum in spite of the impaction, and atony and alkalosis with hypochloremia result. Varying degrees of dehydration develop because fluids are not moving beyond the abomasum into the duodenum for absorption. Sequestration of potassium ions in the abomasum results in hypokalemia. Dehydration, alkalosis, electrolyte imbalance, and progressive starvation are seen. Impaction of the abomasum may be severe enough to cause irreversible abomasal atony.

Clinical Findings and Lesions: Complete anorexia, scant feces, moderate distention of the abdomen, weight loss, and weakness are usually the initial signs. Body temperature is usually normal but may be subnormal during cold weather. A mucoid nasal discharge tends to collect at the external nares and on the muzzle; the muzzle is usually dry and cracked due to the failure of the animal to lick its nostrils and to the effects of dehydration.

The heart rate may be increased, and mild dehydration is common. Most often, the rumen is static and distended with dry contents, but it may contain excess fluid if the cow has been fed finely ground feed. The pH of the ruminal fluid is usually normal (6.5-7). Protozoal activity in the rumen ranges from normal to a marked reduction in numbers and activity (assessed microscopically under low power).

The impacted abomasum is usually in the right lower quadrant on the floor of the abdomen. Deep palpation and strong percussion of the right flank may indicate the presence of a large, firm mass (impacted abomasum) and elicit a grunt (as is common in acute traumatic reticuloperitonitis), probably because of distention of the abomasum and stretching of its serosa. Severely affected cattle die 3-6 days after the onset of signs. The abomasum ruptures in some cases, and death from acute, diffuse peritonitis and shock occurs precipitously in a few hours. In sand impaction, there is considerable weight loss, chronic diarrhea with sand in the feces, weakness, recumbency, and death in a few weeks. Metabolic alkalosis, hypochloremia, hypokalemia, and hemoconcentration are common, as are total and differential WBC counts within the normal range. At necropsy, the abomasum is commonly enlarged (up to 8 times normal size) and impacted with dry rumen-like contents. The omasum may be similarly enlarged and impacted. The rumen is grossly enlarged and filled with dry contents or fluid. The GI tract beyond the pylorus is characteristically empty and has a dry appearance. Varying degrees of dehydration and emaciation are also present. If the abomasum has ruptured, lesions of acute diffuse peritonitis are present.

Diagnosis: Clinical diagnosis is based on the nutritional history, clinical evidence of impaction, and laboratory results. The disease must be differentiated from secondary abomasal impaction as a form of vagal indigestion. Impaction of the abomasum as a complication of traumatic reticuloperitonitis usually is seen in late pregnancy, and commonly only in one animal. A mild fever may or may not be present, and there may be a grunt on deep palpation of the xiphoid. The rumen is enlarged and may be hypermotile (early) or atonic (late). In many cases, it is impossible to distinguish between the 2 causes of impacted abomasum, and a right flank laparotomy may be necessary to explore the abdomen for peritoneal lesions.

Treatment: The challenge is to recognise the cases that will respond to treatment and those that will not, ie, to determine those that should be slaughtered immediately for salvage. Cows that are weak, have a severely impacted abomasum, and have a marked tachycardia (100-120 bpm) are poor treatment risks. In cows that are treated, the metabolic alkalosis, hypochloremia, hypokalemia, and dehydration should be corrected. Lubricants and cathartics can be used in an attempt to move the impacted material, or the abomasum should be emptied surgically. Balanced electrolyte solutions are infused IV continuously for up to 72 hr at a daily rate of 80-120 mL/kg. Some cows respond well to this therapy and begin ruminating and passing feces in 48 hr. Mineral oil can be administered at 4L/day for 3 days. Alternatively, dioctyl sodium sulfosuccinate (DSS) can be given by stomach tube at 120-180 mL of a 25% solution for a 1,000-lb (450-kg) animal mixed with ~20 L of warm water and repeated daily for 3-5 days. This dose rate will kill rumen protozoa. Mineral oil and DSS should not be administered simultaneously because DSS may potentiate the absorption of mineral oil. A beneficial response cannot be expected in <24 hr; in cattle that respond, improvement is usually seen by the end of day 3 after treatment begins. Surgery may be considered, but results are often unsuccessful, probably because of abomasal atony, which appears to worsen after surgery. An alternative may be a rumenotomy to empty the rumen and infuse mineral oil directly into the abomasum through the reticulo-omasal orifice in an attempt to soften and promote the evacuation of the abomasal contents. Cattle with secondary impactions that develop as a sequela of traumatic reticuloperitonitis or abomasal volvulus usually show signs of vagal indigestion, and abomasal impaction may be diagnosed at the time of exploratory surgery. The induction of parturition using dexamethasone (20 mg, IM) may be indicated in affected cattle within 2 wk of term and in which the response to treatment for a few days has been unsuccessful. Parturition may assist recovery because of a reduction in intra-abdominal volume. For sand impaction, affected cattle should be moved off the sandy soil and fed good hay and a grass mixture containing molasses and minerals. Severely affected cattle should be treated with mineral oil (4 L/day for 3 days).

Prevention and Control: Prevention is possible by providing the necessary nutrient requirements for wintering pregnant beef cattle. When low-quality roughage is used, it should be analyzed for crude protein and digestible energy. Based on the analysis, grain is usually added to the ration to meet energy and protein requirements. The nutrient requirements of beef cattle (*Nutritional Requirements*) are guidelines for use under average conditions; higher nutrient levels than those indicated may be necessary, particularly during periods of severe cold stress. Adequate fresh drinking water should be supplied at all times; the practice of forcing wintering cows to obtain their water requirements by eating snow while on low-quality roughage is hazardous.

Acute Intestinal Obstructions in Large Animals: Introduction

Intestinal obstructions are seen in all large animal species but are most common in horses. Cattle are the most commonly affected ruminants; diagnosis in sheep and goats is rare. Other than inguinal hernias, obstructions are infrequently recognised in pigs. In general, obstructions are mechanical or functional, and can be seen in any part of the intestinal tract. They can interrupt the flow of ingesta, and vascular integrity may or may not be compromised (strangulating or simple obstruction, respectively).

Etiology and Pathogenesis: The inciting cause of an intestinal obstruction often is not determined. Functional obstructions are associated with altered intestinal motility, often due to dietary or management factors, parasite infection, enteritis, or peritonitis. Mechanical obstructions (physical blockage of ingesta) occur due to abnormalities in the bowel lumen, in the wall, or outside the tract. Congenital obstructions (atresia jejuni, coli, recti, and ani in calves, atresia ani in lambs and pigs) result in the lack of passage of feces since birth.

In horses, transient functional obstructions are common, as are feed impactions, which usually involve the pelvic flexure. Parasite infection or migration, dental abnormalities, and dietary or management factors are often implicated. Impactions and other luminal obstructions can result from coarse feeds, reduced water intake, enteroliths, or ingested foreign material. Sites of impaction other than the pelvic flexure are the small colon, transverse colon, right dorsal colon, cecum, and ileum. Other causes of intestinal obstruction in horses are volvulus (twist on the mesenteric axis), torsion (twist along the long axis of the bowel), displacement of the ascending (large) colon, and volvulus of part or all of the small intestine.

Altered motility and possibly strenuous exercise and rolling may be initiating causes. Broodmares may be predisposed to volvulus, torsion, or displacement of the ascending colon during gestation and shortly after parturition. Obstruction occurs either due to incarceration of the intestine (usually small) by herniation through the inguinal canal, diaphragm, mesenteric defects, umbilicus, or epiploic foramen; or because of fibrous bands (adhesions, mesodiverticular bands, or stalks of pedunculated lipomas). Standardbred stallions and colts develop inguinal and scrotal hernias more commonly than other breeds. Diaphragmatic hernias and mesenteric defects may be congenital or traumatically induced. Adhesions in horses are most often the sequela of parasite migration or abdominal surgery; however, most adhesions are clinically silent. Pedunculated lipomas are common in older horses. Ileocecal, cecocecal, cecocolic, and small-intestinal intussusceptions also are seen. Lymphosarcoma and other abdominal neoplasms as well as abdominal abscesses can cause intestinal obstruction. In cattle, specific causes include intussusception; volvulus of the jejunoileal flange of the small intestine; volvulus at the root of the mesentery; cecocolic volvulus; and atresia coli, recti, and ani. Intussusceptions are thought to be the result of irregular peristaltic movements related to enteritis, intestinal parasitism, dietary disorders, and mural masses.

Altered intestinal motility may also cause intestinal volvulus. Obstructions of the small intestine can develop due to a variety of fibrous bands (eg, adhesions, parovarian bands, falciform ligament, spermatic cord retraction into the abdomen after surgical castration), mural thickening (eg, intestinal adenocarcinoma), extramural masses (eg, lymphosarcoma, fat necrosis, abdominal abscesses), herniation (inguinal or umbilical), or hemorrhagic jejunitis (which results in luminal blood clots and obstruction).

Adhesions and abdominal abscesses can form subsequent to peritonitis, intraperitoneal injections, or previous abdominal surgery. Decreased motility caused by accumulation of volatile fatty acids, possibly related to high-concentrate rations or an abrupt increase in the concentrate: forage ratio, have been suggested as causes of cecocolic volvulus in cattle. They also are associated with advanced pregnancy and ileus from concurrent disease. Atresia coli develops most commonly in Holstein calves secondary to in utero ischemia of the developing spiral colon.

Clinical Findings and Diagnosis: Intestinal obstruction in horses generally manifests as abdominal pain. In cattle, signs of abdominal pain include treading, stretching, and kicking at the abdomen, and less commonly rolling and bellowing. These signs are generally more subtle than in horses and are usually referable to small-intestinal distention, tension on the intestinal mesentery (by the weight of distended bowel), or vascular impairment. Signs of pain are relatively consistent but often transient with intussusceptions and are seen in some cases of cecocolic volvulus. Cattle with volvulus of the small intestine at the root of the mesentery are severely affected. Usually, cattle with intestinal obstruction are anorectic and pass few or no feces, and milk production in lactating cows drops suddenly. The feces that are passed may be covered with mucus, or mixed or coated with blood. Thick, raspberry-coloured blood mixed with scant feces is characteristic of small-intestinal bleeding, particularly that associated with intussusception. Blood from the colon or rectum is generally brighter red. Melena is typical of abomasal bleeding.

Calves with atresia coli are normal at birth but have progressive abdominal distention and decreased appetite over the first few days of life. *Abdominal* distention, usually with a ping on simultaneous auscultation and percussion, in the upper right caudal abdominal quadrant occurs with cecocolic volvulus. Cecal dilatation does not produce abdominal distention, but a ping is generally present in the caudal dorsal paralumbar fossa. In cecocolic volvulus, one or more large distended loops of large intestine are present.

Rumen motility is usually present, and metabolic and cardiovascular derangement tend to be mild except in cecocolic volvulus of long duration. Abdominal distention in the lower right abdominal quadrant is sometimes seen with small-intestinal distention.

Distended loops of bowel may be palpable on rectal examination, and fluid may be heard on simultaneous ballottement and auscultation of the right side of the abdomen. Small areas of tympanic resonance may be heard on simultaneous auscultation and percussion. Intussusceptions and fibrous bands that cause small-intestinal obstruction can be palpated rectally in some cases.

Profound changes in cardiovascular parameters, such as tachycardia, abnormal colour of the mucous membranes, prolonged capillary refill time, and dehydration, are most commonly associated with hemorrhagic strangulating obstructions such as volvulus of the jejunal-ileal flange of the small intestine. Volvulus of the jejunal-ileal flange and volvulus at the root of the mesentery are characterized by acute onset and rapid cardiovascular deterioration. This is in contrast with cecocolic volvulus or intussusception, which can continue for several days. Metabolic derangements range from hypokalemic, hypochloremic metabolic alkalosis in longstanding small-intestinal and duodenal obstructions to severe metabolic acidosis with hemorrhagic strangulating obstructions. Usually, there are no metabolic derangements in mild functional obstructions and early (simple) mechanical obstructions, particularly if a relatively distal part of the intestinal tract is involved. Hypocalcemia can develop, presumably due to decreased calcium absorption from the duodenum. Peritoneal fluid changes reflect the degree of peritonitis and may aid in the diagnosis in both cattle and horses, although results are more variable in cattle. Hemorrhagic strangulating obstructions are characterized by an increase in RBC, with subsequent increases in total protein and nucleated cell counts due to extravasation through the bowel wall. Neutrophils become degenerative, and intracellular gram-positive and gram-negative bacteria are seen as the integrity of the bowel wall is lost. Plant material in the peritoneal cavity is indicative of bowel rupture or inadvertent enterocentesis. Simple obstructions with severe dilatation of the bowel can be associated with increases in total protein and, less commonly, nucleated cell counts. Peritoneal fluid analysis is normal with most simple mechanical and functional obstructions. When neoplasms are present, neoplastic cells are sometimes identified in peritoneal fluid.

Treatment: For treatment of obstruction in horses, *see* colic, *Colic in Horses: Introduction*. Treatment of functional obstructions in cattle is generally symptomatic and supportive after identifying and eliminating the inciting cause (eg, excessive grain intake) and allowing time for normal intestinal motility to return. If present, dehydration and electrolyte imbalances should be corrected by appropriate fluid therapy (PO or IV). Lactating cows often benefit from calcium gels administered orally or calcium borogluconate administered SC, and secondary ketosis should be treated if present. Occasionally, surgical decompression is required in cases of functional obstruction. Mechanical obstructions almost always require surgery. Antibiotic therapy should be started preoperatively; supportive therapy, such as fluids, electrolytes, and calcium, should be administered if needed. The prognosis with most functional obstructions is good with appropriate supportive therapy, particularly if the inciting cause is identified and eliminated. Horses that require exploratory celiotomy to correct an intestinal obstruction have an overall longterm survival rate of 50%. The survival rate is lower for horses with hemorrhagic strangulating obstructions than for horses with simple obstructions, but early surgical intervention can improve the prognosis. In cattle, 70-80% of those with cecocolic volvulus survive, although 10% of cases recur. For cows with small-intestinal obstruction amenable to resection and anastomosis, 30-40% survive and lead a productive life. For cows with volvulus of the jejunal-ileal flange of the small intestine or at the root of the mesentery, ~50% survive if surgical correction is performed within a few hours of onset. Only 30% of calves with atresia coli survive to adulthood. Surgical correction is not recommended in Holstein calves because the condition is probably inherited in this breed, although vascular damage secondary to amniotic vesicle palpation in the first 6 wk of embryonic development can also lead to intestinal ischemia and atresia in calves.

Prevention: Prevention of all, or even most, cases of intestinal distention is not possible. However, abrupt changes in feeding and management, inadequate water intake, parasite infection, dental abnormalities, and access to coarse feeds and foreign material should be avoided or corrected.

Campylobacteriosis: Introduction

Gastrointestinal campylobacteriosis, caused by Campylobacter jejuni or C coli, is associated with diarrhea in various animal hosts, including dogs, cats, calves, sheep, ferrets, mink, several species of laboratory animals, zoo animals, and humans. In humans, it is a leading cause of diarrhea. C jejuni and C coli are also recovered from feces of asymptomatic carriers. Animals, including dogs and cats (especially those recently purchased from shelters), and wild animals maintained in captivity can serve as sources of human infection. The agents also are isolated frequently from the feces of chickens, turkeys, pigs, and other species.

The organism commonly contaminates poultry meat, which serves as one of the major vehicles of spread of C jejuni to humans.The disease is found worldwide; its prevalence appears to be increasing as proper culture techniques for C jejuni and C coli are refined and updated. Clinical manifestations may be more severe in younger animals. In studies using monoclonal and polyclonal antibodies, Campylobacter spp (including C jejuni) have been associated with proliferative ileitis in hamsters and proliferative colitis in ferrets. A cause and effect relationship has not been proved experimentally, however. Proliferative bowel disease in these animals is now known to be caused by Lawsonia intracellularis .

Etiology: Campylobacter is a gram-negative, microaerophilic, slender, curved, motile bacterium with a polar flagellum. C jejuni is routinely associated with diarrheal disease; however, C coli, distinguished from C jejuni on the basis of hippurate hydrolysis, is occasionally isolated from diarrheic animals and is routinely recovered from asymptomatic pigs. Other intestinal, catalase-negative campylobacters, C upsaliensis and C helveticus, have been isolated from diarrheic dogs and cats as well as asymptomatic dogs and cats. Campylobacter was once associated with swine dysentery (*Swine Dysentery*), but this is now recognised as being caused by Treponema hyodysenteriae . Most believe that Campylobacter spp do not produce porcine proliferative enteritis (*Porcine Proliferative Enteritis*), even though a new organism, C hyoilei, isolated from swine in Australia, has been associated with porcine proliferative enteritis. Its role in this disease, however, is not clearly established. C mucosalis and C hyointestinalis have also been isolated from swine but are not considered enteric pathogens. Because of slow growth and microaerobic requirements, standard culture methods require selective media that incorporate various antibiotics to suppress competing fecal microflora. C jejuni and C coli grow well at 42°C in an atmosphere of 5-10% carbon dioxide and an equal amount of oxygen. Cultures are incubated 48-72 hr; colonies are round, raised, translucent, and sometimes mucoid. The organism can be identified by a series of biochemical tests readily available in any diagnostic laboratory. Recently, PCR assays have been used to identify Campylobacter spp . Identification is important to distinguish campylobacters from the growing number of novel enterohepatic helicobacters being isolated from a variety of animals.

Transmission and Epidemiology: As with most intestinal pathogens, fecal-oral spread and food- or waterborne transmission appear to be the principal avenues of infection.

One suspected source of infection for pets, as well as mink and ferrets raised for commercial purposes, is ingestion of undercooked poultry and other raw meat products. Asymptomatic carriers can shed the organism in their feces for prolonged periods and contaminate food, water, milk, and fresh processed meats (including pork, beef, and poultry products). The organism can survive in vitro at 41°F (5°C) for 2 mo and can survive in feces, milk, water, and urine. Wild birds also may be important sources of water contamination. Unpasteurized milk has been cited as a principal source of infection in several human outbreaks. Strain identification to study the epizootiology of C jejuni and C coli, in addition to Penner serotyping, is now done using molecular techniques such as restriction fragment length polymorphism and ribotyping.

Clinical Findings: The diarrhea appears to be most severe in young animals. Typical signs in dogs include mucus-laden, watery, and/or bile-streaked diarrhea (with or without blood) that lasts 3-7 days; reduced appetite; and occasional vomiting. Fever and leukocytosis may also be present. In certain cases, intermittent diarrhea may persist >2 wk; in some, it may be present for months. Gnotobiotic puppies inoculated with C jejuni developed malaise, loose feces, and tenesmus within 3 days of inoculation. In calves, signs vary from mild to moderate. The diarrhea is thick and mucoid with occasionally visible blood flecks; body temperature may be normal. Diarrhea with mucus and blood also has been observed in primates, ferrets, mink, and cats. Organisms with ultrastructure similar to that of Campylobacter spp have been seen in hyperplastic ileal epithelial mucosa of hamsters with proliferative ileitis; C jejuni has been isolated from these lesions but has failed to reproduce the syndrome. Organisms with Campylobacter -like morphology also have been associated with proliferative colitis in ferrets and with hyperplastic intestinal lesions in guinea pigs and rats. Campylobacter -like organisms have been described in young rabbits with acute typhlitis. It is now known that these organisms are Lawsonia intracellularis, an organism closely related to Desulfovibrio spp .

Lesions: In 3-day-old chickens infected with C jejuni, the organisms were detected within epithelial cells and mononuclear cells of the lamina propria; the jejunum and ileum were the most severely affected. Congested and edematous colons were found in dogs 43 hr after inoculation; microscopically, epithelial height, brush border, and numbers of goblet cells in the colon and cecum were all reduced. Hyperplastic epithelial glands resulted in a thickened mucosa. Histologic changes in calves primarily involve the jejunum but also can involve the ileum and colon. The lesions vary from mild changes to severe hemorrhagic enteritis. The mesenteric lymph nodes are edematous. Experimentally, some strains of C jejuni produce a hepatitis in mice, and the organism has been isolated from inflamed livers of dogs. A cytotoxin, referred to as cytolethal distending toxin, has been identified in C jejuni ; however, its role in production of intestinal disease is not known. In vitro, the cytotoxin causes distention of cell lines and cell cycle arrest in the G_2M1 phase of the cell cycle.

Diagnosis: The standard method for diagnosis is microaerobic culture of feces at 42°C; a special medium is commercially available. Diagnosis is also possible by using darkfield or phase-contrast microscopy, by which fresh fecal samples are examined for the characteristic darting motility of C jejuni . This method is especially useful during the acute stage of diarrhea when large numbers of organisms are more likely to be shed in the feces. Various techniques can detect serum antibodies to various antigens of Campylobacter spp . Heat-stable or heat-labile antigen schemes are used routinely to serotype various strains. Serial serum samples to demonstrate rising antibody titers are helpful in diagnosis. Intestinal viruses and other intestinal bacterial pathogens must be ruled out as primary or copathogens in animals with Campylobacter - associated diarrhea.

Treatment and Control: Isolation of C jejuni or C coli from diarrheic feces is not, in itself, an indication for antibiotic therapy. Because C jejuni and C coli are not routinely cited as potential intestinal pathogens in animals (except for diarrhea in young cats and dogs and in several species of primates), efficacy of antibiotic therapy has been reported infrequently. In certain cases in which animals are severely affected or are a zoonotic threat, antibiotic treatment may be indicated. In general, C jejuni and C coli isolates from animals are similar to isolates obtained from human populations. Erythromycin, the drug of choice for Campylobacter diarrhea in humans, is also effective in other animals, although erythromycin-resistant strains of Campylobacter spp have been recovered from swine. Gentamicin, furazolidone, and doxycycline also can be used. Ampicillin is relatively inactive against most strains of Campylobacter, and most strains are also resistant to penicillin. Tetracycline and kanamycin resistance in certain C jejuni strains is reported to be plasmid-mediated and transmissible within C jejuni serotypes. Efficacy of sulfadimethoxine and sulfa combinations is variable. Before therapy is instituted, isolation and sensitivity tests should be done. Some animals continue to shed the organism despite antibiotic therapy. Quinolone antibiotics may be useful in eliminating C jejuni and C coli in asymptomatic carriers, but drug resistance may develop.

Salmonellosis: Introduction Salmonellosis is caused by many species of salmonellae and characterized clinically by one or more of 3 major syndromes—septicemia, acute enteritis, and chronic enteritis. The disease is seen worldwide and in all animals. The incidence has increased with the intensification of livestock production. Young calves, piglets, lambs, and foals usually develop the septicemic form. Adult cattle, sheep, and horses commonly develop acute enteritis, and chronic enteritis may develop in growing pigs and occasionally in cattle. Pregnant animals may abort. The clinically normal carrier animal is a serious problem in all host species. Salmonellosis is seen infrequently in dogs and cats and is characterized by acute diarrhea with or without septicemia. The incidence of human salmonellosis has increased in recent years, and animals have been incriminated as the principal reservoir. Transmission to humans occurs via contaminated drinking water, milk, meat, and foods such as cake mixes that use contaminated ingredients; poultry and eggs (*Salmonelloses: Introduction*) are particularly important sources of infection.

Etiology, Epidemiology, and Pathogenesis: While many other Salmonella spp may cause disease, the more common ones in each species are as follows: Cattle— Salmonella serovar typhimurium, Salmonella serovar dublin, and Salmonella serovar newport ; Sheep and goats— S typhimurium, S dublin, Salmonella serovar anatum, and Salmonella serovar montevideo; Pigs— S typhimurium and Salmonella serovar choleraesuis;

Horses— S typhimurium, S anatum, S newport, Salmonella serovar enteritidis, and Salmonella serovar IIIa 18:z_4z_{23}. Although their resulting clinical patterns are not distinct, different species of salmonellae tend to differ in their epidemiology.

Plasmid profile and drug-resistance patterns are sometimes useful markers for epidemiologic studies. Feces of infected animals can contaminate feed and water, milk, fresh and processed meats from abattoirs, plant and animal products used as fertilizers or feedstuffs, pasture and rangeland, and many inert materials.

The organisms may survive for months in wet, warm areas such as in feeder pig barns or in water dugouts but survive <1 wk in composted cattle manure. Rodents and wild birds also are sources of infection. Pelleting of feeds reduces the level of contamination by salmonellae. The prevalence of infection varies among species and countries and is much higher than the incidence of clinical disease, which is commonly precipitated by stressful situations such as sudden deprivation of feed, transportation, drought, crowding, parturition, and the administration of some drugs.

Salmonellosis is common in hospitalized horses that have been subjected to prolonged surgical procedures. Use of oral antimicrobial agents is sometimes a risk factor for the disease. The usual route of infection is oral and, after infection, the organism multiplies in the intestine and causes enteritis.

Greater susceptibility of the young may be due to high gastric pH, absence of a stable intestinal flora, and limited immunity. Penetration of bacteria into the lamina propria likely contributes to gut damage and diarrhea.

The inflammatory response is marked, and salmonellae are engulfed by phagocytic cells; however, the bacteria can survive and multiply in these cells. Septicemia may follow with subsequent localisation in brain and meninges, pregnant uterus, distal aspects of the limbs, and tips of the ears and tails, which can result, respectively, in meningoencephalitis, abortion, osteitis, and dry gangrene of the feet, tail, or ears. The organism also frequently localises in the gallbladder and mesenteric lymph nodes, and survivors intermittently shed the organism in the feces. Calves rarely become carriers but virtually all adults do for variable periods—up to 10 wk in sheep and cattle and up to 14 mo in horses.

Adult cattle infected with S dublin excrete the organism for years. Infection may persist in lymph nodes or tonsils, with no salmonellae in the feces. Latent carriers may begin shedding the organism or even develop clinical disease under stress. A passive carrier acquires infection from the environment but is not invaded, so that if removed from the environment, it ceases to be a carrier.

Cattle and Sheep: In calves and lambs, the disease is usually endemic on a particular farm, with sporadic explosive outbreaks. Subclinical infection with occasional herd outbreaks may be seen in adult cattle. Stressors that precipitate clinical disease include deprivation of feed and water, minimal levels of nutrition, long transport times, calving, and mixing and crowding in feedlots.

Pigs: Outbreaks of septicemic salmonellosis in pigs are rare and usually can be traced to a purchased, infected pig. Purchase of feeder pigs from salmonellae-free herds and use of the "all-in/all-out" policy in finishing units minimize exposure.

Horses: Many horses may be carriers. In adults, most cases develop after the stress of surgery or transport, especially when horses are moved through sales yards, deprived of feed and water, and then overfed at their destination.

Mares may be inapparent shedders and, despite several negative cultures before foaling, may shed the bacteria at parturition and infect the newborn foal. Salmonellosis in horses hospitalized for other causes is a major problem for equine clinics and stud farms. In these circumstances, carriers are constantly reintroduced, the environment is persistently contaminated, and a large population of vulnerable horses is at risk. Septicemic salmonellosis is also common in foals; it may be endemic on a given premises or there may be outbreaks. *Dogs* and Cats: Many dogs and cats are asymptomatic carriers of salmonellae. Clinical disease is uncommon, but when it is seen, it is often associated with hospitalization, another infection or debilitating condition in adults, or exposure to large numbers of the bacteria in puppies and kittens.

Clinical Findings: Septicemia is the usual syndrome in newborn calves, lambs, foals, and piglets, and outbreaks may occur in pigs up to 6 mo old. Illness is acute, depression is marked, fever (105-107°F [40.5-41.5°C]) is usual, and death occurs in 24-48 hr. In pigs, a dark red to purple discolouration of the skin is common, especially of the ears and ventral abdomen.

Nervous signs may be seen in calves and pigs; these animals may also suffer from pneumonia. Mortality may reach 100%. Acute enteritis is the common form in adults as well as in calves that are usually ≥1 wk old.

Initially, there is fever (105-107°F [40.5-41.5°C]), followed by severe watery diarrhea, sometimes dysentery, and often tenesmus. In a herd outbreak, several hours may lapse before the onset of diarrhea, at which time the fever may disappear. The feces, which vary considerably, may have a putrid odor and contain mucus, fibrinous casts, shreds of mucous membrane, and in some cases, large blood clots.

Rectal examination causes severe discomfort, tenesmus, and commonly dysentery. Milk production often declines precipitously in dairy cows. Abdominal pain is common and severe in horses. Affected horses are severely dehydrated and may die within 24 hr of the onset of diarrhea; mortality may reach 100%.

A marked leukopenia and neutropenia are characteristic of the acute disease in horses. In dogs and cats, clinical disease takes the form of acute diarrhea with septicemia and is seen occasionally in puppies and kittens or in adults stressed by concurrent disease.

Pneumonia may be evident. Abortion is likely to occur in pregnant bitches or queens. Conjunctivitis is sometimes seen in affected cats. Subacute enteritis may develop in adult horses and sheep on farms where the disease is endemic. The signs include mild fever (103-104°F [39-40°C]), soft feces, inappetence, and some dehydration. There may be a high incidence of abortion in cows and ewes, some deaths in ewes after abortion, and a high mortality rate due to enteritis in lambs younger than a few weeks of age. In cattle, the first signs may be fever and abortion, followed several days later by diarrhea. Chronic enteritis is a common form in pigs and adult cattle. There is persistent diarrhea, severe emaciation, intermittent fever, and poor response to treatment. The feces are scant and may be normal or contain mucus, casts, or blood. In growing pigs, rectal stricture may be a sequela if the terminal part of the rectum is involved. Affected pigs are anorectic and lose weight; the abdomen becomes grossly distended. The stricture is obvious on digital palpation and necropsy. A number of Salmonella spp are found in foxes, especially kits, and produce a peracute enteritis. Fur-bearing and zoo carnivores may be affected. Contaminated feed is often the source of infection. Several rodents (eg, guinea pigs, hamsters, rats, and mice) and rabbits are susceptible. Rodents commonly act as a source of infection on farms where the disease is endemic. Pet turtles were once a common source of infection in humans that has been virtually eliminated by the curtailment of commercial trafficking in turtles.

Diagnosis: This depends on the clinical signs and on the laboratory examination of feces, tissues from affected animals, feed (including all mineral supplements used), water supplies, and feces from wild rodents and birds that may inhabit the premises. The clinical syndromes usually are characteristic but must be differentiated from several similar diseases in each species as follows: Cattle—diarrhea due to enterotoxigenic Escherichia coli, dysentery due to verotoxigenic E coli, coccidiosis, cryptosporidiosis, the alimentary tract form of infectious bovine rhinotracheitis, bovine viral diarrhea, hemorrhagic enteritis due to Clostridium perfringens types B and C, arsenic poisoning, secondary copper deficiency (molybdenosis), winter dysentery, paratuberculosis, ostertagiasis, and dietetic diarrhea; Sheep—enteric colibacillosis, septicemia due to Haemophilus sp or pasteurellae, and coccidiosis; Pigs—enteric colibacillosis of newborn pigs and weanlings, swine dysentery, campylobacteriosis, and the septicemias of growing pigs (which include erysipelas, classical swine fever, and pasteurellosis); Horses—septicemia (due to E coli, Actinobacillus equuli, or streptococci) and colitis-X.

Treatment: Early treatment is essential for septicemic salmonellosis, but there is controversy regarding the use of antimicrobial agents for intestinal salmonellosis. Oral antibiotics may deleteriously alter the intestinal microflora, interfere with competitive antagonism, and prolong shedding of the organism. There is also concern that antibiotic-resistant strains of salmonellae selected by oral antibiotics may subsequently infect humans. Broad-spectrum antibiotics are used parenterally to treat the septicemia.

Initial antimicrobial therapy should be based on knowledge of the drug resistance pattern found in the area. Nosocomial infections often involve highly drug-resistant organisms. Trimethoprim-sulfonamide combinations are often effective. Alternatives are ampicillin, fluoroquinolones, or third-generation cephalosporins.

Treatment should be continued daily for up to 6 days. Oral medication should be given in drinking water because affected animals are thirsty due to dehydration, and their appetite is generally poor. Fluid therapy to correct acid-base imbalance and dehydration is necessary. Calves, adult cattle, and horses need large quantities of fluids. Antibiotics such as ampicillin or cephalosporins lead to lysis of the bacteria with release of endotoxin. NSAID may be used to reduce the effects of endotoxemia. Horses with acute intestinal salmonellosis are severely acidotic and hyponatremic and may need to be treated initially with 5% sodium bicarbonate, IV, at 5-8 L/450 kg body wt. This is followed by balanced electrolytes containing potassium to correct the hypokalemia that may follow correction of the acidosis. In horses, flunixin meglumine is recommended for its antiendotoxic properties. Corticosteroids are not recommended because of their immunosuppressive effects and their potential to exacerbate laminitis. IV administration of plasma with a high titer of Salmonella lipopolysaccharide core antibodies may be beneficial in horses. Plasma with serotype-specific antibodies is even more beneficial. Septicemic salmonellosis in pigs usually responds favourably if treated early. However, the intestinal form is difficult to treat effectively in all species. Although clinical cure may be achieved, bacteriologic cure is difficult, particularly in adult animals, because the organisms become established in the biliary system and are intermittently shed into the intestinal lumen, which causes chronic relapsing enteritis and contamination of the environment.

Control and Prevention: These are major problems because of carrier animals and contaminated feedstuffs. Drain swabs or milk filters may be cultured to monitor the salmonellae status of a herd. The principles of control include prevention of introduction and limitation of spread within a herd.

Prevention of Introduction: Every effort must be made to prevent introduction of a carrier; animals should be purchased directly only from farms known to be free of the disease and should be isolated for ≥1 wk while their health status is monitored. Ensuring that feed supplies are free of salmonellae depends on the integrity of the source.

Limitation of Spread Within a Herd: In an outbreak, the following procedures should be implemented: 1) Carrier animals should be identified and either culled or isolated and treated vigorously. Treated animals must be rechecked several times before there can be confidence that they are not carriers. 2) The prophylactic use of antibiotics in feed or water supplies may be considered (but the hazards have been mentioned above). 3) Movement of animals around the farm should be restricted to limit infection to the smallest group. Random mixing of animals should be avoided. 4) Feed and water supplies must be protected from fecal contamination. 5) Contaminated buildings must be vigorously cleaned and disinfected. 6) Contaminated material must be disposed of carefully. 7) All persons should be aware of the hazards of working with infected animals and the importance of personal hygiene. 8) Use of a vaccine should be considered, particularly in an outbreak involving pregnant cattle in which a vaccine has been shown to confer some protection in adults and calves. Commercial killed bacterins or autogenous bacterins may be used. Live attenuated vaccines show considerable promise, but they are not available commercially. 9) Stresses should be minimized. 10) Fetal membranes of mares should be placed in a plastic bag until the mare eliminates them, and the foal should be fed colostrum before contact with the mare.

Salmonella Vaccines: Salmonellae are intracellular parasites, and a live vaccine is therefore expected to be necessary for optimal immune protection against disease. Several studies with live attenuated Salmonella vaccines in pigs, cattle, and chickens have shown them to be effective in stimulating a strong cell-mediated immune response and protecting animals against disease. A live attenuated S choleraesuis vaccine that has been licensed for use in swine appears to be effective in reducing colonization of tissues and protecting pigs from disease following challenge with virulent organisms. This vaccine has also been reported to reduce the prevalence of Salmonella infections in pigs under field conditions. This vaccine also protected calves against experimental challenge with S Dublin following intranasal or subcutaneous administration of the vaccine. The administration of the S choleraesuis vaccine to pregnant dairy cows reduced the frequency of shedding of serogroup C1 salmonellae during the peripartum period. Live S enteritidis has been effective in significantly reducing the infection of laying hens challenged with S enteritidis . The commercial vaccines available for use in cattle are bacterins and appear to induce a modest level of protection. When given to pregnant cows, they induce antibodies in colostrum, which provide an important measure of protection to calves, which are most susceptible in the first week of life.

Salmonellosis in Veterinary Teaching Hospitals: The risk of equine salmonellosis epidemics is particularly high in veterinary teaching hospitals. A high case load, the presence of animals with severe illnesses, and the stresses of transportation contribute to this risk. The serotype most commonly implicated is S typhimurium but other serotypes that have been identified include Salmonella serovar heidelberg, Salmonella serovar krefeld, Salmonella serovar infantis, and S anatum . They are frequently resistant to multiple drugs. Contamination of the hospital environment often begins with the introduction of the organisms by a carrier animal. Animals in the hospital (which are often highly susceptible) readily develop diarrhea and contribute to further contamination of the hospital. Infection rates as high as 18% have been reported. Nosocomial infection can be identified by development of salmonellosis ≥3 days after hospitalization and by isolation of hospital-associated Salmonella from cases. The identification of hospital-associated Salmonella involves determination of serotype, drug resistance patterns, and possibly other strain markers such as pulsed field gel electrophoresis patterns, ribotype, and plasmid profiles. Many hospitals have developed protocols designed to minimize the occurrence of these epidemics, including isolating horses with diarrhea, controlling animal traffic patterns, routinely disinfecting the hospital with an agent of known effectiveness, controlling rodents, using footbaths, limiting access to the hospital area, regularly monitoring drains and other areas of the hospital for salmonellae, routinely repeatedly monitoring horses admitted to the hospital to determine whether they are shedding Salmonella, wearing barrier clothing when attending animals at high risk, and educating personnel. Renovations to the hospital may be required to facilitate thorough cleaning. Closing the hospital for a period of time is often necessary to thoroughly clean and disinfect the premises and to break the cycle of transmission. Outbreaks of salmonellosis have been reported among dogs in veterinary teaching hospitals, but these occurrences are uncommon; antibacterial therapy is a predisposing factor.

Tyzzer's Disease: Introduction

Tyzzer's disease is an acute bacterial infection of a wide range of animals that is seen worldwide. Sporadic fatal infection of foals is common, and acute fatal epidemics occur in laboratory animals. The disease is rare in dogs, cats, and calves. It primarily affects young, stressed animals; however, some species appear resistant unless stressed or immunosuppressed, while others are susceptible without immunosuppression. Immunosuppressive drugs and some antibacterials, especially sulfonamides, predispose animals to the disease.

Etiology and Pathogenesis: The cause is Clostridium piliforme (previously Bacillus piliformis), a motile, filamentous, gram-negative, sporeforming, obligate, intracellular bacterium. It does not grow in cell-free media but can be cultured in the yolk sac of chick embryos or tissue culture cells. The vegetative phase is very labile; spores may survive in soiled bedding at room temperature for 1 yr and can also survive at ~133°F (60°C) for 1 hr.The pathogenesis is poorly understood. Infection most likely results from oral exposure. Possible sources include infective spores from the environment, contact with carrier animals, and in foals, ingestion of horse feces. The primary site of infection is the lower intestinal tract with subsequent dissemination via the blood or lymphatics. The bacterium has an affinity for the intestine (epithelial and smooth muscle cells), hepatocytes, and cardiac myocytes. Stress factors such as capture, overcrowding, shipping, and poor sanitation appear to be predisposing. Sulfonamide administration predisposes rabbits to the disease. Mortality is highest at weaning age except in foals, in which the disease is seen between 1 and 6 wk of age, with most cases between 1 and 2 wk. In some species, the disease has been identified concurrently with other diseases, eg, feline infectious peritonitis in cats, distemper and mycotic pneumonia in dogs, and cryptosporidial and coronaviral enteritis in calves. The disease most often affects well-nourished animals during periods of stress. Under laboratory conditions, stress is created by immunosuppressive drugs or other factors that can be easily identified. With many experiments, stress may be involved as part of the protocol, and when the disease develops, it is devastating.

Clinical Findings: After experimental infection, the incubation period in foals is 3-7 days; under natural conditions, the period is unknown. Most foals are found in a coma or dead. Clinical signs, if seen, are of short duration (a few hours to 2 days). Signs are variable, but may include depression, anorexia, pyrexia, jaundice, diarrhea, and recumbency. Terminally, there are convulsions and coma. Signs vary slightly between species. Laboratory animals may show depression, ruffled coat, and varying degrees of watery diarrhea; at the start of an outbreak, they often are found dead. Clinicopathologic tests are of little value in laboratory animals because they die so rapidly. In foals, the serum enzymes sorbitol dehydrogenase, AST, alkaline phosphatase, lactate dehydrogenase, and ã-glutamyltransferase are increased. There is also hyperbilirubinemia, leukopenia, hemoconcentration, and terminally profound hypoglycemia.

Lesions: Characteristic lesions are seen in the liver, myocardium, and intestinal tract. In the liver, white, gray, or yellowish foci of necrosis, 2 mm in diametre, are few to disseminated. The hepatic necrosis is most marked and disseminated in foals in which the multiple necrotic foci with slightly depressed hemorrhagic centres appear to infect almost every hepatic lobule. In addition, there is marked hepatomegaly, and the hepatic lymph nodes are hyperplastic. In rabbits, severe lesions develop in the intestines and heart. The terminal ileum, cecum, and proximal colon are diffusely reddened. Diffuse ("paint-brush") hemorrhage is frequently seen on the serosa of the cecum. Patchy areas of mucosal necrosis are present in the cecum and colon, together with marked edema of the wall of the cecum. Mesenteric lymph nodes may be enlarged and edematous. White streaks in the myocardium may be present, especially near the apex. Intestinal and heart lesions are generally milder or absent in other animals. Microscopically, randomly distributed and coalescing foci of necrosis in the liver are associated with scant to moderate infiltration of neutrophils and macrophages. The causative bacteria are found in a crisscross pattern in viable hepatocytes at the periphery of the necrotic foci. In the cecum and colon of rabbits, patchy areas of necrosis extend as deep as the muscularis externa with associated mucosal and submucosal infiltrates of neutrophils. Organisms may be found in the epithelium, muscularis mucosa, and muscularis externa of the affected intestine. When cardiac lesions are present, they consist of foci of fibre fragmentation, vacuolation, loss of cross-striations, and minimal inflammatory cell infiltration.

Diagnosis: Definitive diagnosis is based on demonstration of organisms in tissue sections with special stains. The organism stains poorly with H&E and Gram's stains. With Giemsa stain, the bacillus stains well in the liver and intestinal epithelium and in smears of infected organs but poorly in smooth muscles and cardiac muscle cells. The Warthin-Starry or Levaditi silver stains are preferable to other stains because the bacillus stains well in the cytoplasm of all infected cells.

Treatment and Control: Little is known about the effectiveness of antibiotics for treatment; some antibiotics are known to aggravate the disease. C piliforme is sensitive to tetracycline and partially sensitive to streptomycin, erythromycin, penicillin, and chlortetracycline; it is resistant to sulfonamides and chloramphenicol. In foals, the disease seems to be nearly 100% fatal, although it is likely that some foals survive. A definitive clinical diagnosis is not possible due to the lack of a definitive diagnostic test. Once the disease is present on a farm, it may be seen sporadically year after year. Animals suspected of being infected may be treated IV initially with 50% dextrose, followed by 10% dextrose (slowly), other fluid therapy, and antibiotics. Most foals respond dramatically to the dextrose therapy but relapse into a coma and die in a few hours. Rarely, an occasional foal appears to survive the disease after prolonged treatment with dextrose given slowly IV with antibiotics. Because the disease in foals is sporadic and not highly contagious, specific preventive measures are usually not indicated. Reducing factors that cause stress and immunosuppression lessens the incidence. When the disease is seen in a colony, treatment is not recommended because it prolongs the disease and possibly produces carrier animals. It is best to destroy all animals in the colony and attempt to restock with disease-free animals.

Amebiasis: Introduction (Amebiosis)

Amebiasis is an acute or chronic colitis, characterized by persistent diarrhea or dysentery, that is prevalent in tropical and subtropical areas worldwide. Its prevalence has declined in the USA over the past several decades, but the disease is still important in many tropical areas, particularly in times of disasters.

It is common in people and nonhuman primates, sometimes seen in dogs and cats, and rare in other mammals. Several species of amebae are found in mammals, but the only known pathogen is Entamoeba histolytica . Humans are the natural host for this species and the usual source of infection for domestic animals. Mammals become infected by ingesting food or water contaminated with feces containing infective cysts. E dispar is a noninvasive, nonpathogenic amoeba that is molecularly distinct but morphologically indistinguishable from the pathogenic species E histolytica . Einvadens of reptiles is also morphologically identical to E histolytica, but it is not transmissible to mammals.

Clinical Findings: E histolytica is a pathogen with variable virulence. It lives in the lumen of the large intestine and cecum and may produce no obvious clinical signs or invade the intestinal mucosa and produce mild to severe, ulcerative, hemorrhagic colitis. In acute disease, fulminating dysentery may develop, which may be fatal, progress to chronicity, or resolve spontaneously. Chronic cases may show weight loss, anorexia, tenesmus, and chronic diarrhea or dysentery, which may be continuous or intermittent. In addition to the colon and cecum, amebae may invade perianal skin, genitalia, liver, brain, lungs, kidneys, and other organs. Signs may resemble those of other colonic diseases (eg, trichuriasis, balantidiasis). Invasive amebiasis is exacerbated by immunosuppression.

Diagnosis: Definitive diagnosis depends on finding E histolytica trophozoites or cysts in feces. Trophozoites are best seen in direct saline smears or in stained sections of affected colonic tissue. These parasites are difficult to find because many animals with extraintestinal amebiasis have no concurrent intestinal infection. Colonoscopy with scraping or biopsy of ulcerations is more effective than fecal examination in diagnosing amebic colitis. In intestinal infections, repeated examinations may be necessary because parasites may be passed periodically in the feces. Trophozoites range in size from 10-60 μm but usually are >20 μm in diametre, have a single vesicular nucleus, (usually with a central karyosome), are motile, and may contain ingested RBC. Feces should be examined promptly because the trophozoites die quickly once outside the body. Fecal leukocytes may be mistaken for amebae, so fixed and stained fecal smears (iodine, trichrome, iron, hematoxylin, or periodic acid-Schiff reaction) may be necessary for identification. Cysts range from 10-20 μm in diametre; the usual size is 12-15 μm. Mature cysts have 4 nuclei, while immature cysts may have 1 or 2. In primates, the cysts may be recovered and identified on zinc sulfate flotations or in fixed and stained preparations (iodine, trichrome, or iron hematoxylin); however, E histolytica cysts are seldom if ever excreted by dogs or cats. An ELISA-based antigen test, available for diagnosis in humans, may also aid diagnosis in other mammals. Immunostaining may also be useful.

Treatment: Scant information on treatment in animals is available. Metronidazole (10-25 mg/kg, PO, bid for 1 wk) or furazolidone (2-4 mg/kg, PO, tid for 1 wk) has been suggested. Dogs may continue to shed trophozoites after therapy.

Giardiasis: Introduction (Giardosis, Lambliasis, Lambliosis)

Giardiasis is a chronic, intestinal protozoal infection that is seen worldwide in most domestic and wild mammals, many birds, and people. Infection is common in dogs and cats, occasional in ruminants, and rare in horses and pigs. The number of different species and the zoonotic potential of Giardia spp are controversial. There is circumstantial evidence that Giardia spp that infect domestic animals can infect people. It appears that some Giardia spp isolates are infective to a variety of mammals, while others are more species specific. Wild animals may also be reservoirs. Giardia spp have been reported to be found in 1-39% of fecal samples from pet and shelter dogs and cats, with a higher rate of infection in younger animals.

Etiology and Transmission: Flagellate protozoa (trophozoites) of the genus Giardia inhabit the mucosal surfaces of the small intestine, where they attach to the brush border, absorb nutrients, and multiply by binary fission. Trophozoites encyst in the small or large intestine and pass in the feces. The cyst is the infective stage, and transmission occurs by the fecal-oral route. Cyst shedding may be continuous over several days and weeks but is often intermittent. Although occasionally passed in the feces, trophozoites are not infective. Incubation and prepatent periods are generally 5-14 days. Cysts can survive in the environment, but trophozoites cannot. Overcrowding and high humidity favour survival of cysts and transmission. Earlier classifications have assigned different species names to the Giardia of various hosts; it is generally agreed that all species infecting mammals (except some rodents) are structurally similar.

Clinical Findings and Lesions: Giardia infections in dogs and cats may be inapparent or may produce weight loss and chronic diarrhea or steatorrhea, which can be continual or intermittent, particularly in puppies and kittens. Clinical disease is also reported in calves. Feces usually are soft, poorly formed, pale, malodorous, contain mucus, and appear fatty. Watery diarrhea is unusual in uncomplicated cases, and blood is not present in feces; typical small-bowel diarrhea is more common. Occasionally vomiting occurs. Giardiasis must be differentiated from other causes of nutrient malassimilation (eg, exocrine pancreatic insufficiency [*Exocrine Pancreatic Insufficiency*], intestinal malabsorption [*Malabsorption Syndromes*]). Clinical laboratory findings usually are normal. Pathogenesis of Giardia spp infections is poorly understood. Gross intestinal lesions are seldom evident, although microscopic lesions, consisting of villous atrophy and cuboidal enterocytes, may be present. Laboratory studies have demonstrated malabsorption of nutrients, decreased quantities of intestinal disaccharides, increased enterocyte turnover, lymphocytic infiltration, and villous atrophy.

Diagnosis: The motile, piriform trophozoites (10-20 × 7-10 μm) are occasionally seen in saline smears of loose or watery feces. They should not be confused with trichomonads, which have a single rather than double nucleus, an undulating membrane, and no concave ventral surface. The oval cysts (9-15 × 7-10 μm) are best detected in feces concentrated by the zinc sulfate (specific gravity 1.18) flotation technique. Sodium chloride, sucrose, or sodium nitrate flotation media are too hypertonic and severely distort the cysts. Staining cysts with iodine aids identification. Because Giardia cysts are excreted intermittently, several fecal examinations should be performed if giardiasis is suspected; eg, 3 samples collected and examined over 3-5 days. About 70% of infected dogs can be identified with a single zinc sulfate flotation; 93% can be identified with 2. In dogs, duodenal aspiration for trophozoite detection is useful; however, in cats, Giardia spp are more prevalent in the mid to lower small intestine. An ELISA that detects Giardia antigen in the feces of dogs and cats is available, but field data on sensitivity and specificity are lacking.

Treatment: No drugs are approved for treating giardiasis in animals. Fenbendazole (50 mg/kg/day) effectively removes Giardia cysts from the feces of dogs; no side effects are reported, and it is safe for pregnant and lactating animals. This dosage is approved for controlling and removing Toxocara canis, Trichuris vulpis, and Ancylostoma caninum in dogs. Recently, a combination product of praziquantel, pyrantel pamoate, and febantel decreased cyst excretion in infected dogs. Fenbendazole is not approved in cats, but may reduce clinical signs and cyst shedding at 50 mg/kg/day, PO, for 3-5 days. Albendazole is effective at 25 mg/kg, PO, bid for 2 days in dogs and for 5 days in cats, but should not be used in these animals because it has led to bone marrow suppression and is not approved for use in these species. Giardia- infected calves may be treated with albendazole or fenbendazole. Oral fenbendazole may also be an option in large animals and some birds. Metronidazole (25 mg/

kg, PO, bid for 5-7 days) is ~65% effective in eliminating Giardia spp from infected dogs but may be associated with acute development of anorexia and vomiting, which may occasionally progress to pronounced generalized ataxia and vertical positional nystagmus. Metronidazole may be administered to cats at 10-25 mg/kg, PO, bid for 5 days. Furazolidone at 4 mg/kg, PO, bid for 7 days, is also effective in cats and small dogs, although diarrhea and vomiting are possible side effects; it is also suspected of teratogenicity. A killed vaccine, available for dogs and cats, reportedly reduces clinical signs and the number and duration of cysts shed into the environment.

Control: Giardia cysts are immediately infective when passed in the feces and survive in the environment. Cysts are a source of infection and reinfection for animals, particularly those in crowded conditions (eg, kennels and catteries). Prompt removal of feces from cages, runs, and yards limits environmental contamination.

Cysts are inactivated by most quaternary ammonium compounds, household bleach (1:32 or 1:16 dilution), steam, and boiling water. To increase the efficacy of disinfectants, solutions should be left for 5-20 min before being rinsed off kennel or run surfaces. Disinfection of grass yards or runs is impossible. These areas should be considered contaminated for at least a month after infected dogs last had access. Cysts are susceptible to desiccation, and areas should be allowed to dry thoroughly after cleaning. Cysts contaminating the hair of dogs and cats may be a source of reinfection. Shampooing and rinsing the animals well can help remove cysts from hair. The killed vaccines that are available for dogs and cats aid in disease prevention by decreasing or preventing cyst shedding.

Colic in Horses: Introduction

In its strictest definition, the term "colic" means abdominal pain. Over the years, it has become a broad term for a variety of conditions that cause the horse to exhibit clinical signs of abdominal pain. Consequently, it is used to refer to conditions of widely varying etiologies and severity. To understand these etiologies, make a diagnosis, and initiate appropriate treatments, veterinarians must first appreciate the clinically relevant aspects of equine GI anatomy, the physiologic processes involved in movement of ingesta and fluid along the GI tract, and the extreme sensitivity of the horse to the deleterious effects of bacterial endotoxin that normally exists within the lumen of the intestine.

GI Anatomy: The horse is a monogastric animal, with a relatively small stomach (capacity 8-10 L) that is located on the left side of the abdomen beneath the rib cage. The junction of the distal esophagus and the cardia is a functional 1-way valve, permitting gas and fluid to move into the stomach but not out. Consequently, conditions that impede the normal aboral movement of gas and fluid through the small intestine may result in severe dilation and rupture of the stomach.

Because of its position, the stomach is difficult to visualize with radiography or ultrasonography in large adult horses. The smaller size of the foal, however, permits assessment of gastric emptying by contrast radiography. The small intestine comprises the duodenum, jejunum, and ileum, with the latter joining the cecum at a distinct ileocecal junction.

The duodenum is positioned primarily dorsally on the horse's right side, where it is suspended from the dorsal body wall by a small mesentery of 3-5 cm. Consequently, the duodenum is not involved in small-intestinal displacements involving the mesentery (volvulus). At the base of the cecum in the right paralumbar fossa region, the duodenum turns toward the midline.

It is at this point that the duodenum, if distended with gas or fluid (eg, in horses with proximal enteritis), can be felt on rectal examination. As the small intestine reaches the dorsal midline, it becomes the jejunum. The characteristic long mesentery allows loops of the jejunum to rest on the contents of the ventral portion of the abdomen.

The jejunum is ~65 ft (19.5 m) long; its length, coupled with its long mesentery, allow it to be involved in small intestinal volvulus and incarcerations. At the end of the jejunum, the wall of the intestine becomes more muscular, the lumen is narrowed, and an additional mesenteric attachment becomes apparent. The last 18 in. (45 cm) of the small intestine, the ileum, joins the cecum at its dorsal medial aspect. This junction is identified by the attachment of the ileocecal fold from the ileum to the dorsal band of the cecum. This ileocecal fold is used as a landmark to locate the ileum at surgery. From the ileum, the ingesta enters the cecum, a large, blind-ended fermentation vat that is situated primarily on the horse's right side, extending from the region of the paralumbar fossa to the xiphoid cartilage on ventral midline. The cecum is 4-5 ft (1.2-1.5 m) long and can hold 27-30 L of feed and fluid. Under the influence of the cecal musculature, the ingesta in the cecum is massaged, mixed with microorganisms capable of digesting cellulose, and eventually passed through the cecocolic opening into the right ventral colon. The attachment of the cecum to the dorsal body wall is wide, thus minimizing the likelihood that the cecum can become displaced or twisted on its own.

The right ventral colon is divided into sacculations that help mix and retain plant fibres until they are digested. It is located on the ventral aspect of the abdomen from the flank region to the rib cage. The ventral colon then turns toward the left, becoming the sternal flexure and then the left ventral colon. The left ventral colon, which also is large and sacculated, passes caudally to the left flank area.

Near the pelvic region, the diametre of the colon decreases markedly, and the colon folds back on itself. This region, which is called the pelvic flexure, is the initial portion of the unsacculated left dorsal colon. Presumably due to the abrupt decrease in diametre, the junction between the left ventral colon and pelvic flexure is the most common location for impactions.

The diametre of the dorsal colon is maximal either at its diaphragmatic flexure or at the right dorsal colon. There are no sacculations in either the left or right portion of the dorsal colon. The right dorsal colon is closely attached to the right ventral colon by a short intercolic fold and to the body wall by a tough common mesenteric attachment with the base of the cecum. In contrast, neither the left ventral nor the left dorsal colons are attached directly to the body wall, allowing these portions of the colon to become displaced or twisted. Ingesta moves from the large right dorsal colon into the short transverse colon, which has a diametre of ~10 cm and is fixed firmly to the most dorsal aspect of the abdominal cavity by a strong, short, fibrous mesentery. The transverse colon is located cranial to the cranial mesenteric artery. Finally, the ingesta enters the sacculated descending colon, which is 10-12 ft (3-3.6 m) long.

Blood Supply to the GI Tract: The celiac and cranial mesenteric arteries (branches of the abdominal aorta) supply blood to the GI tract. The celiac artery supplies arterial blood to the stomach, pancreas, liver, spleen, and the first portion of the duodenum.

The cranial mesenteric artery supplies arterial blood to the remaining portion of the duodenum; to all of the jejunum, ileum, cecum, large colon, and transverse colon; and to the first portion of the descending colon. Because the large colon is attached to the body wall only in the region near the cranial mesenteric artery, the blood supplying all portions of the colon must traverse the entire length of the colon.

The pelvic flexure receives its blood supply from 2 branches of the cranial mesenteric artery; one branch supplies the right dorsal and left dorsal colons before reaching the pelvic flexure, and the other branch supplies the right and left ventral colons before reaching the pelvic flexure. Thus, volvulus of the large colon near the junction of the colon and cecum may impede the flow of blood to the entire left colon. The major branches of the cranial mesenteric artery can be damaged by the migrating forms of Strongylus vulgaris.

Natural Openings in the Abdomen: There are several natural openings or spaces within the abdominal cavity that can be important in conditions causing colic. The inguinal canal provides an opening through which intestine might pass and become trapped.

Although inguinal hernias are common in young foals, they rarely cause clinical problems; the situation is considerably different in stallions. Similarly, if the ventral abdominal wall fails to form properly around the umbilicus, an opening remains and the potential exists for intestinal problems to develop secondary to an umbilical hernia. The epiploic foramen, a natural opening between the portal vein, the caudal vena cava, and the caudate lobe of the liver, can be the site of intestinal incarcerations. Finally, there is a natural space between the dorsal aspect of the spleen and the left kidney. This space is bounded by the renosplenic ligament, a strong band of tissue that connects the dorsomedial aspect of the spleen with the fibrous capsule of the left kidney. This ligament provides a "shelf" over which large colon can be displaced.

Colonic Motility Patterns: Normograde peristalsis in the left ventral colon moves ingesta toward the left dorsal colon, and the muscles in the wall of the left dorsal colon contract to move the ingesta toward the diaphragmatic flexure. There is evidence, however, that the muscles in the left ventral colon contract in a retrograde fashion, from the pelvic flexure region toward the sternal flexure. Furthermore, these contractions originate from a pacemaker region in the pelvic flexure. It has been hypothesized that this pacemaker senses either the size or the consistency of the feed particles in the ingesta and then initiates the appropriate motility pattern. If the ingesta has been digested sufficiently, it is moved in a normograde direction; if additional digestion is necessary, the ingesta is moved in a retrograde direction to retain it in the ventral colon. This theory has been proposed to account for the common clinical occurrence of obstruction at or near the pelvic flexure.

Diagnosis: A diagnosis can be made and appropriate treatment begun only after thoroughly examining the horse, considering the history of any previous problems or treatments, determining which part of the intestinal tract is involved, and identifying the cause of the particular episode of colic. In most instances, colic develops for one of 4 reasons: 1) The wall of the intestine is stretched excessively by either gas, fluid, or ingesta. This stimulates the stretch-sensitive nerve endings located within the intestinal wall, and pain impulses are transmitted to the brain. 2) Pain develops due to excessive tension on the mesentery. 3) Ischemia develops, most often as a result of incarceration or severe twisting of the intestine. 4) Inflammation develops and may involve either the entire intestinal wall (enteritis) or the covering of the intestine (peritonitis). Under such circumstances, proinflammatory mediators in the wall of the intestine decrease the threshold for painful stimuli. The list of possible conditions that cause colic is long, and it is reasonable first to determine the most likely type of disease and begin appropriate treatments and then to make a more specific diagnosis, if possible. The general types of disease that cause colic include excessive gas in the intestinal lumen (flatulent colic), simple obstruction of the intestinal lumen, obstruction of both the intestinal lumen and the blood supply to the intestine (strangulating obstruction), interruption of the blood supply to the intestine alone (nonstrangulating infarction), inflammation of the intestine (enteritis), inflammation of the lining of the abdominal cavity (peritonitis), erosion of the intestinal lining (ulceration), and "unexplained colic."

In general, horses with strangulating obstructions and complete obstructions require emergency abdominal surgery, whereas horses with the other types of disease can be treated medically. The history of the present colic episode and previous episodes, if any, must be ascertained to determine if the horse has had repeated or similar problems, or if this episode is an isolated event.

The duration of the episode, the rate of deterioration of cardiovascular status, the severity of pain, whether feces have been passed, and the response to treatment are important information. It is also critical to determine the horse's deworming history (schedule, treatment dates, drugs used), when the teeth were floated last, if any changes in feed or water supply or amount have occurred, and whether the horse was at rest or exercising when the colic episode started.The physical examination should include assessment of the cardiopulmonary and GI systems.

The oral mucous membranes should be evaluated for colour, moistness, and capillary refill time. The mucous membranes may become cyanotic or pale in acute cardiovascular compromise and eventually hyperemic or muddy as peripheral vasodilation develops later in shock.

The capillary refill time (normal ~1.5 sec) may be shortened early but usually becomes prolonged as vascular stasis (venous pooling) develops. The membranes become dry as the horse becomes dehydrated. The heart rate increases due to pain, hemoconcentration, and hypotension; therefore, higher heart rates have been associated with more severe intestinal problems (strangulating obstruction). However, not all conditions requiring surgery are accompanied by a high heart rate. An important aspect of the physical examination is passing a nasogastric tube. Because horses can neither regurgitate nor vomit, adynamic ileus, obstructions involving the small intestine, or distention of the stomach with gas or fluid may result in gastric rupture. Passing a stomach tube may, therefore, save the horse's life and assist in diagnosis of these conditions. If fluid reflux occurs, the volume and colour of the fluid should be noted. The abdomen and thorax should be auscultated, and the abdomen percussed.

The abdomen should be auscultated over several areas (cecum on the right, small intestine high on the left, colon lower on the left). Intestinal sounds associated with episodes of pain may indicate an intraluminal obstruction (eg, impaction, enterolith). Gas sounds may indicate ileus or distention of a viscus. Fluid sounds may indicate impending diarrhea associated with colitis. A complete lack of sounds is usually associated with adynamic ileus or ischemia. Percussion will assist in identifying a grossly distended segment of intestine (cecum on right, colon on left) that may need to be trocarized. The respiratory rate may be increased due to fever, pain, acidosis, or an underlying respiratory problem. Diaphragmatic hernia is also a possible cause of colic. The most definitive part of the examination is the rectal examination.

The Veterinarian should Develop a Consistent Method of Palpating for the following: aorta, cranial mesenteric artery, cecal base and ventral cecal band, duodenum, bladder, peritoneal surface, inguinal rings in stallions and geldings or the ovaries and uterus in mares, pelvic flexure, spleen, and left kidney. The intestine should be palpated for size, consistency of contents (gas, fluid, or impacted ingesta), distention, edematous walls, and pain on palpation. A sample of peritoneal fluid (obtained via paracentesis performed aseptically on midline) often reflects the degree of intestinal damage. The colour, cell count and differential, and total protein concentration should be evaluated. Normal peritoneal fluid is clear to yellow, contains <5,000 WBC/μL, most of which are mononuclear cells, and <2.5 g of protein/dL. The age of the horse is important because a number of age-related conditions cause colic.

The More Common of these include the Following: in foals—atresia coli, meconium retention, uroperitoneum, and gastroduodenal ulcers; in yearlings—ascarid impaction; in the young—small-intestinal intussusception, nonstrangulating infarction, and foreign body obstruction; in the middle-aged—cecal impaction, enteroliths, and large-colon volvulus; and in the aged—pedunculated lipoma and mesocolic rupture. Ultrasonographic evaluation of the abdomen may help clinicians differentiate between diseases that can be treated medically and those that require surgery.

The technique also can be applied transrectally to clarify findings noted on rectal palpation. In foals, echoes from the large colon and small intestine are commonly identified from the ventral abdominal wall, whereas only large colon echoes are usually seen in adult horses. The large colon can be identified by its sacculated appearance.

The duodenum can be identified in the tenth intercostal space and traced around the caudal aspect of the right kidney. The jejunum is rarely identified during transabdominal ultrasonographic examination of normal adult horses, whereas the thick-walled ileum can be identified by transrectal examination.

The most common abnormalities identified by ultrasonography include inguinal hernia, renosplenic entrapment of the large colon, sand colic, intussusception, enterocolitis, right dorsal colitis, and peritonitis. Stallions with inguinal hernia have incarcerated intestine on the affected side; it is possible to identify the intestine, and to obtain information concerning the thickness of its wall and presence or lack of peristalsis can be obtained.

In horses with renosplenic entrapment of the large colon, the tail of the spleen or the left kidney cannot be imaged, or the gas-filled large colon is present in the caudodorsal aspect of the abdomen in the region of the renosplenic space. Horses with sand colic have granular hyperechoic echoes originating from the affected portion of the colon. The characteristic finding in horses with intussusception is the "bull's eye" appearance of the affected portion of the small intestine. Very often the intestine proximal to the intussusception is distended and the strangulated portion is thickened. Horses with enterocolitis frequently have evidence of hyperperistalsis, thickened areas of the bowel wall, and fluid distention of the intestine.

In contrast, horses with right dorsal colitis commonly have marked thickening of the wall of the right dorsal colon. In horses with peritonitis, the peritoneal fluid may be anechoic or there may be evidence of flocculent material and fibrin between serosal surfaces of the viscera.

Treatment: Horses with colic may need either medical or surgical treatments. Almost all require some form of medical treatment, but only those with certain mechanical obstructions of the intestine need surgery. The type of medical treatment is determined by the cause of colic and the severity of the disease. In some instances, the horse may be treated medically first and the response evaluated; this is particularly appropriate if the horse is mildly painful and the cardiovascular system is functioning normally.

Ultrasonography can be used to evaluate the effectiveness of nonsurgical treatment. If necessary, surgery can be used for a diagnosis as well as a treatment. If evidence of intestinal obstruction with dry ingesta is found on rectal examination, a primary aim of treatment is to hydrate and evacuate the intestinal contents.

If the horse is severely painful and has clinical signs indicating loss of fluid from the bloodstream (high heart rate, prolonged capillary refill time, and discolouration of the mucous membranes), the initial aims of treatment are to relieve pain, restore tissue perfusion, and correct any abnormalities in the composition of the blood and body fluids. If damage to the intestinal wall (as a result of either severe inflammation or a displacement or strangulating obstruction) is suspected, steps should be taken to prevent or counteract the ill effects of bacterial endotoxin that leaves the intestine and enters the bloodstream. Finally, if there is evidence that the colic episode is caused by parasites, one aim of treatment is to eliminate the parasites.

Pain Relief: In most cases of colic, pain is mild, and analgesia is all that is needed. In these instances, the cause of colic is presumed to be spasm of intestinal muscle or excessive gas in a portion of the intestine. If, however, the pain is due to an intestinal twist or displacement, some of the stronger analgesics may mask the clinical signs that would be useful in making a diagnosis. For these reasons, a thorough physical examination should be completed before any medications are given. However, because horses with severe colic or pain may hurt themselves and become dangerous to people nearby, analgesics often must be given first. Additionally, many horses with less severe problems may need pain relief until the other treatments have time to be effective.

An analgesic that has the fewest side effects and causes the least alteration in the horse's attitude should be selected. Medications used commonly for abdominal pain are NSAID that reduce the production of prostaglandins. When these drugs are used as recommended, their toxic effects on the kidneys and GI tract occur infrequently. Clinical experience suggests that flunixin meglumine may mask the early signs of conditions that require surgery and, therefore, must be used carefully in horses with colic.

The most commonly used sedative for colic is xylazine, an α_2-agonist. Within a few minutes after administration, the horse stands quietly and is less responsive to pain. Unfortunately, the effects of xylazine are short-lived, and it inhibits the intestinal muscles; it also decreases cardiac output and thus reduces blood flow to the tissues. Detomidine, a more potent α_2-agonist that is much longer-acting, is used successfully under similar circumstances. Of the narcotic analgesics, but orphanol is used most often in horses with colic. Butorphanol has few adverse effects on the GI tract or heart. However, when given in large doses, narcotics can cause excitement, and the horse may become unstable. Butorphanol is frequently combined with an α_2-agonist to produce a more prolonged period of analgesia. Although pain relief usually is provided by analgesics, there are other important ways to reduce the degree of pain. For example, passing a nasogastric tube (also an important part of the diagnostic workup) may remove any fluid that has accumulated in the stomach because of an obstruction of the small intestine. The removal of this fluid not only relieves pain from gastric distention but also prevents rupture of the stomach.

Fluid Therapy: Many horses with colic benefit from fluid therapy to prevent dehydration and maintain blood supply to the kidneys and other vital organs. The fluids may be given either through the nasogastric tube or IV, depending on the particular intestinal problem. Horses with strangulating obstruction or enteritis must be given fluids IV because absorption of fluids from the diseased intestine is reduced and fluid may be secreted into the lumen of the intestine. The latter mechanism causes a buildup of fluid in the intestine, which must be removed from the stomach through a nasogastric tube. This abnormal movement of body fluids into the intestine contributes to the development of circulatory shock, which is often the ultimate cause of death.

Horses with colic may need either medical or surgical treatments. Almost all require some form of medical treatment, but only those with certain mechanical obstructions of the intestine need surgery. The type of medical treatment is determined by the cause of colic and the severity of the disease. In some instances, the horse may be treated medically first and the response evaluated; this is particularly appropriate if the horse is mildly painful and the cardiovascular system is functioning normally. Ultrasonography can be used to evaluate the effectiveness of nonsurgical treatment. If necessary, surgery can be used for a diagnosis as well as a treatment.

If evidence of intestinal obstruction with dry ingesta is found on rectal examination, a primary aim of treatment is to hydrate and evacuate the intestinal contents. If the horse is severely painful and has clinical signs indicating loss of fluid from the bloodstream (high heart rate, prolonged capillary refill time, and discolouration of the mucous membranes), the initial aims of treatment are to relieve pain, restore tissue perfusion, and correct any abnormalities in the composition of the blood and body fluids. If damage to the intestinal wall (as a result of either severe inflammation or a displacement or strangulating obstruction) is suspected, steps should be taken to prevent or counteract the ill effects of bacterial endotoxin that leaves the intestine and enters the bloodstream. Finally, if there is evidence that the colic episode is caused by parasites, one aim of treatment is to eliminate the parasites.

Pain Relief: In most cases of colic, pain is mild, and analgesia is all that is needed. In these instances, the cause of colic is presumed to be spasm of intestinal muscle or excessive gas in a portion of the intestine. If, however, the pain is due to an intestinal twist or displacement, some of the stronger analgesics may mask the clinical signs that would be useful in making a diagnosis. For these reasons, a thorough physical examination should be completed before any medications are given.

However, because horses with severe colic or pain may hurt themselves and become dangerous to people nearby, analgesics often must be given first. Additionally, many horses with less severe problems may need pain relief until the other treatments have time to be effective. An analgesic that has the fewest side effects and causes the least alteration in the horse's attitude should be selected.

Medications used commonly for abdominal pain are NSAID that reduce the production of prostaglandins. When these drugs are used as recommended, their toxic effects on the kidneys and GI tract occur infrequently. Clinical experience suggests that flunixin meglumine may mask the early signs of conditions that require surgery and, therefore, must be used carefully in horses with colic.

The most commonly used sedative for colic is xylazine, an α_2-agonist. Within a few minutes after administration, the horse stands quietly and is less responsive to pain. Unfortunately, the effects of xylazine are short-lived, and it inhibits the intestinal muscles; it also decreases cardiac output and thus reduces blood flow to the tissues. Detomidine, a more potent α_2-agonist that is much longer-acting, is used successfully under similar circumstances. Of the narcotic analgesics, butorphanol is used most often in horses with colic. Butorphanol has few adverse effects on the GI tract or heart. However, when given in large doses, narcotics can cause excitement, and the horse may become unstable. Butorphanol is frequently combined with an α_2-agonist to produce a more prolonged period of analgesia.

Although pain relief usually is provided by analgesics, there are other important ways to reduce the degree of pain. For example, passing a nasogastric tube (also an important part of the diagnostic workup) may remove any fluid that has accumulated in the stomach because of an obstruction of the small intestine. The removal of this fluid not only relieves pain from gastric distention but also prevents rupture of the stomach.

Fluid Therapy: Many horses with colic benefit from fluid therapy to prevent dehydration and maintain blood supply to the kidneys and other vital organs. The fluids may be given either through the nasogastric tube or IV, depending on the particular intestinal problem.

Horses with strangulating obstruction or enteritis must be given fluids IV because absorption of fluids from the diseased intestine is reduced and fluid may be secreted into the lumen of the intestine. The latter mechanism causes a buildup of fluid in the intestine, which must be removed from the stomach through a nasogastric tube. This abnormal movement of body fluids into the intestine contributes to the development of circulatory shock, which is often the ultimate cause of death.

Most of the fluid is reabsorbed from the ingesta in the cecum and colons. In fact, ~95% of the fluid that normally enters the lumen of the large intestine is returned to the bloodstream.

Therefore, horses with intestinal obstructions near the pelvic flexure usually require relatively small amounts of IV fluids, whereas horses with small-intestinal obstructions need extremely large amounts. The volume and type of fluid to be given are determined by the severity and cause of the problem. Laboratory tests to determine the degree of hemoconcentration and whether concentrations of electrolytes are abnormal are critical for accurate treatment of a horse with severe colic. The balance of body fluids can be reestablished by administering IV fluids formulated to replenish the deficient electrolyte(s).

In most instances, however, fluid therapy must be started before laboratory results are available, particularly when the horse is showing clinical signs of circulatory shock. When IV fluids are needed but the clinical signs are mild to moderate, the horse is usually given 8-10 L of a sterile replacement fluid that contains electrolytes in concentrations that normally exist in the blood. This volume is administered over 1-2 hr, and the horse is reevaluated to determine if additional fluids are needed. Horses in circulatory shock require much larger volumes of IV fluids, given as rapidly as possible; up to 20 L in 1 hr may be needed to reestablish tissue perfusion. In severe cases, hypertonic saline (7% NaCl) may be given to rapidly increase plasma volume. Depending on the cause of colic, IV fluids may be needed for several days until intestinal function has returned, electrolyte concentrations are balanced, and the horse can maintain its fluid needs by drinking.

Under such circumstances, the daily IV fluid requirements may range from 30 to 100 L.Fluids are sometimes given through the nasogastric tube as part of the treatment of impactions of the colon.

Many clinicians believe that the same result can be accomplished by giving large volumes of fluids IV. If the horse will not drink voluntarily and there is no obstruction in the small intestine, hydration may be maintained by administering fluids through the tube. Fluids or medications should not be given through the nasogastric tube if fluid reflux is being removed from the stomach, as this indicates either the stomach or the small intestine is not emptying properly.

Protection Against Bacterial Endotoxin: Endotoxin, a part of the outer coating of enteric gram-negative bacteria, is released when the bacteria die or multiply rapidly. Normally, endotoxin is restricted to the intestinal lumen, but if the intestinal mucosal lining is damaged due to ischemia, endotoxin moves into the peritoneal cavity or the bloodstream.

It then interacts with mononuclear phagocytes and triggers an inflammatory response that can include fever, depression, hypotension, coagulation abnormalities, and eventually death. Minimizing the inflammatory responses to endotoxemia is a vital part of colic therapy.

Prostaglandins are involved in causing many of endotoxin's early ill effects. Flunixin meglumine reduces the cellular production of prostaglandins and can help prevent some of their effects.

Because flunixin can help prevent some of the early effects of endotoxemia at dosages less than the recommended dosage (1.1 mg/kg), smaller dosages (0.25 mg/kg) can be administered without masking clinical signs associated with conditions that require surgery. There is considerable controversy regarding the efficacy of plasma or serum that contains antibodies designed to neutralize endotoxin. These antibodies are directed against the components of endotoxins that are consistent among different gram-negative bacteria. The results of clinical studies using such antibodies have been conflicting, with evidence of protection being seen in some studies and no positive effects identified in others.

Because endotoxin itself stimulates the generation of a wide array of inflammatory substances that ultimately produce the pathophysiologic effects, neutralizing antibodies should be used as early in the course of the disease as possible. As an alternative approach, polymyxin B has been used to prevent endotoxin from interacting with the horse's inflammatory cells. Polymyxin B has well documented nephrotoxicity; however, concentrations of polymyxin B that bind endotoxin are far less than those that cause toxic effects.

Polymyxin B has been evaluated in several recent experimental studies of endotoxemia and currently is being used in clinical cases at 1,000-5,000 U/kg, bid-tid. This form of therapy should be initiated as early as possible in the clinical course of the disease. In addition, fluid replacement therapy should be maintained in hypovolemic animals, and serum creatinine concentration should be closely monitored. This latter concern is especially relevant to azotemic neonatal foals, as they appear to be more susceptible to the nephrotoxic side effects of polymyxin B.

Intestinal Lubricants and Laxatives: A common cause of colic in horses is simple obstruction of the large intestine by dried ingesta, sometimes mixed with sand. These impactions of the large intestine generally develop near the pelvic flexure or in the right dorsal colon but may involve any portion of the large colon, descending colon, or cecum.

In most instances, lubricants or fecal-softening agents given through a nasogastric tube soften the impacted ingesta, allowing it to be passed. This form of therapy can be aided by the simultaneous administration of IV fluids. Keeping the horse muzzled is advised to prevent further impaction of feed material while the obstruction is softening. Mineral oil is the most commonly used medication in the treatment of a large colon impaction. It coats the inside of the intestine and aids the normal movement of ingesta along the GI tract. It is administered through a nasogastric tube, up to 4 L, sid-bid, until the impaction is resolved. Although mineral oil is safe, it is not highly effective in treating severe impactions or sand impactions because it may simply pass by the obstruction without softening it. Dioctyl sodium sulfosuccinate (DSS) is a soap-like compound that acts by drawing water into the dry ingesta. It is more effective than mineral oil in softening impactions; however, it may interfere with the normal fluid absorptive functions of the colon and can be toxic.

Thus, DSS can be given safely only in small quantities 2 times 48 hr apart. A safe and useful compound for treating impactions, especially those containing sand, is psyllium hydrophilic mucilloid.

When mixed with water, it forms a gelatinous mass that carries ingesta along the GI tract. Although usually given through a nasogastric tube to horses with impactions, psyllium also may be used as a preventive by mixing the dry powder into the feed. Horses that live in a sandy environment or that persistently develop impactions may be given psyllium powder, 400 g/500 kg, sid in their feed for 7 days.

This treatment is repeated 2-3 times each year in an effort to prevent the development of sand impactions. Strong laxatives that stimulate intestinal contractions are not commonly used to treat impactions and, in fact, may worsen the problem. Occasionally, horses with extremely hard impactions are treated with magnesium sulfate, which draws body fluids into the GI tract. Side effects include dehydration and an increased risk of diarrhea. Fluid therapy, whether the fluids are administered through a nasogastric tube or IV, is an important and effective part of treating horses with colonic or cecal impactions. If an impaction does not start to break down within 3-5 days, surgery may be necessary to evacuate the intestine and aid in restoring normal motility.

Larvicidal Deworming: The normal migratory routes of the larvae of large bloodworms, particularly Strongylus vulgaris, have been implicated in many cases of colic. In response to the migratory and maturation processes of the larvae in the cranial mesenteric artery, the wall of the artery becomes thickened and forms loose plaques of inflammatory tissue. It has been hypothesized that these plaques activate coagulation, resulting in thromboembolism. The blood supply to the intestine may be reduced, resulting in altered intestinal motility, a change in the absorption of nutrients from the intestine, or death of the intestine. Thus, thromboembolism has been presumed to be a cause of recurrent episodes of colic and weight loss.

Modern deworming medications, such as ivermectin and moxidectin, have activity against migrating S vulgaris larvae. Fenbendazole kills migrating strongyles if given at twice the recommended dosage daily for 5 days or at 10 times the recommended dosage daily for 3 days.

As a result of common use of these anthelmintics, chronic intermittent colic once thought to be caused by thromboembolism or parasite larval migration has largely been eliminated from equine practice. There is considerable evidence that damage caused by cyathostomes causes colic, diarrhea, and loss of condition, particularly in young horses. These signs are seen on a seasonal basis and are synchronous with the emergence of large numbers of encysted larvae into the lumen of the large colon. In temperate areas of the Northern hemisphere, the larvae encyst during the winter months and emerge in the late winter and spring causing ulceration, edema, and inflammation of the mucosa of the large colon. This may result in diarrhea, protein loss, weight loss, and mild intermittent colic and fever. Horses with cyathostomiasis require treatment with larvacidal dosages of anthelmintics such as ivermectin, moxidectin, and fenbendazole. Some horses require analgesics, supportive care, and proper nutritional support.

Surgery: Surgery usually is necessary if there is a mechanical obstruction to the normal flow of ingesta that cannot be corrected medically or if the obstruction also interferes with the intestinal blood supply. The latter conditions cause death of the horse unless surgery is performed quickly. Occasionally, surgery is indicated as an exploratory diagnostic procedure for horses with chronic colic that have not responded to routine medical therapy. Under most circumstances, horses exhibiting signs of severe abdominal pain nonresponsive to analgesic therapy require emergency abdominal surgery. Generally, the lumen of the intestine is completely obstructed, such as is caused by strangulating obstruction or severe displacement. Similarly, horses with an abnormally distended intestine on rectal examination and peritoneal fluid with an increased total protein concentration and number of RBC probably have a strangulating lesion that requires surgical correction. These classic findings that characterize horses requiring emergency surgery often are the exception rather than the rule. Some horses with mild or moderate pain may also require surgery, and a judgment must be based on a thorough physical examination and other methods of evaluation.

Some of the more commonly used indications for surgery in horses with colic include uncontrollable pain; >4 L of fluid reflux from the stomach; no borborygmi on auscultation; peritoneal fluid with increased protein, erythrocytes, and toxic neutrophils; and a tightly distended intestine, displaced colon, or enterolith or foreign body identified on rectal examination. Performing surgery (if indicated) early is critical to success and improves the prognosis for survival.

Therefore, it is more important to decide if the horse should be referred to a clinic where surgery could be performed if needed, rather than trying to determine if emergency surgery is definitively required. It is generally prudent to refer the following types of cases: 1) a horse that responds initially to an analgesic but requires additional analgesic therapy a few hours later, 2) a horse that continues to exhibit signs of pain despite administration of analgesics, 3) a horse that remains painful but has normal peritoneal fluid, 4) a horse with distended small intestine on rectal examination but lacking fluid reflux, or 5) a horse with large quantities of fluid removed from the stomach but no distended small intestine palpable on rectal examination.

When surgery is required, in most instances, the horse is anesthetized and positioned on its back, and the surgical incision is made on the ventral midline. Once the peritoneal cavity is entered, portions of the intestine should be examined to determine the definitive cause of the colic.

Correction may involve repositioning a displaced portion of intestine, removing an obstruction, or resecting devitalized intestine. When devitalized segments of intestine must be removed or an enterotomy performed, postoperative care may include antibiotics, IV fluids, polymyxin B, antibodies directed against endotoxin, and NSAID to combat endotoxemia. When a displaced segment of intestine is simply returned to its normal location, the postoperative care is much less intense. Each horse must be handled individually, and its treatment needs are based on its response to surgery and the development of complications.

Prognosis: A large retrospective study in the USA documented an overall survival rate of 60% for horses with colic, and a survival rate of 50% for those horses undergoing abdominal surgery, including those euthanized on the surgery table for inoperative conditions. Survival rates for horses with strangulating obstruction and inflammatory diseases were only 24% and 42%, respectively.

In contrast, horses with an undefined cause for the colic episode had a survival rate of 94%. When the segment of the GI tract was considered, the survival rates for conditions affecting the small intestine and stomach were poorer than for those affecting the large colon.

In addition, conditions that interfered with both the passage of ingesta and the intestinal blood supply dramatically decreased the chances of survival. The results of more recent studies are far more promising, with survival rates for horses undergoing emergency abdominal surgery often >80%.

Furthermore, there have been reports documenting survival rates of 70% for horses requiring resection of strangulated small intestine or correction of large colon volvulus. In earlier retrospective studies, these conditions were associated with survival rates d"30%.

Although data on longterm survival (ie, the horse returning to its intended use) are more difficult to obtain, recent findings indicate that most horses that die or are euthanized because of serious problems do so within 3 mo after surgery. Values obtained from several variables are often combined to predict survival in horses with colic. Prognostic indicators include pain assessment, intestinal distention, mucous membrane colour, and cardiovascular system function. Survival rates are highest for horses with mild abdominal pain and are lowest for horses with severe pain. Horses with palpable intestinal distention have lower survival rates than horses lacking evidence of intestinal distention, and survival rates are even lower if no intestinal sounds are audible on auscultation of the abdomen.

Red mucous membranes are frequently associated with bacterial endotoxemia, which decreases the survival rate. Cardiovascular system function reflects the degree of shock and, therefore, correlates with the prognosis for survival. For instance, horses with low systolic blood pressure or a high heart rate have a decreased chance of survival.

Of the laboratory analyses used to predict survival, blood lactate concentration and the anion gap are used most often. Measurement of blood lactate has been used as an indicator of tissue perfusion, with increasing concentrations of lactic acid corresponding with poor tissue perfusion. Similarly, the anion gap (the calculated difference between the measured cations and the measured anions) reflects the generation of organic anions, most notably lactic acid, due to reduced tissue perfusion. The concentration of protein in the peritoneal fluid also has been used to predict survival, with higher concentrations associated with a poorer prognosis.

Chapter 5

Growth Disturbances

Several diseases involve abnormalities of tissue growth. These vary from congenital defects in organ development, to neoplasia. Throughout the embryonic and postnatal development of an individual, tissues grow mainly due to the process of cell proliferation. Admittedly, tissue mass also can be increased by an increase in cell size, but as a component of growth, this mechanism is unimportant. Many tissues retain the capacity for cellular proliferation throughout the life of the individual. In some, there is continual mitotic division to replace cells that are lost. In the skin, for instance, there is continual loss of keratinised epithelial cells requiring replacement by proliferation of basal cells. Similarly in the bone marrow there is continual cell proliferation to replace cells of the peripheral blood whose lifetime is limited. Other cells, such as those of the renal tubular epithelium or of the liver, are not continually proliferating. However, they retain the capacity for mitotic division as a mechanism for repair. Most of the daughter cells that result from cell proliferation undergo differentiation, adopting the structural and functional characteristics of the tissue they are destined to become. Thus, cells committed to be epidermal cells only reproduce epidermal cells, liver cells produce liver cells, and so on. Usually, fully differentiated cells lose the capacity to divide so that loss of this capacity may be regarded as one feature of the process of differentiation.

The Cell Cycle

Most tissues can be regarded as containing a mixture of cells. Some cells are continually dividing, while others are not dividing but can return to the mitotic pool. Still, some component cells are terminally differentiated and no longer able to undergo mitosis. The sequence of events comprising mitosis is called the CELL CYCLE.

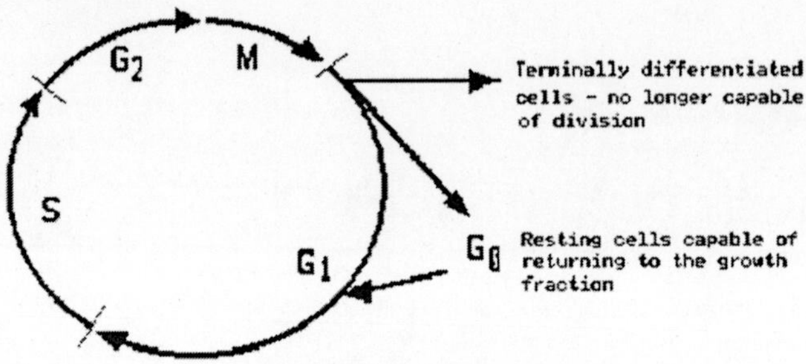

Figure: *The Cell Cycle.*

The cycle consists of four stages. Cell division occurs during the M phase. In the S phase, synthesis of DNA occurs. Daughter cells may undergo differentiation and no longer capable of division, or they may enter G0. Cells in G0 are mitotically inactive but may be recalled to the growth fraction under appropriate conditions. G1 is the most variable phase. The time taken to go through G1 largely decides the length of the cycle and therefore the rate of cell proliferation. During the S phase of the mitotic cycle, DNA and chromosomal proteins are synthesised. Proliferating cells must synthesize all their other components to avoid a progressive reduction in size during mitotic division.

It is also important to realise that the rate of proliferation of cells is not the only determinant of the rate of tissue growth. The rate of tissue growth depends on three factors:

- The rate of cell proliferation
- The fraction of cells in the mitotic pool (the growth fraction)
- The rate of cell loss .

In growth, as in all biological phenomena, there is variation between normal individuals. However, when outside the normal range, these variations may be regarded as pathologic and may result in functional abnormalities that we recognise as disease. Disturbances of growth may result in an excess or a deficit of tissue, or may produce an abnormal pattern of development.

Developmental Anomalies

Malformations may occur during the growth and development of a tissue or organ and are present at birth as congenital lesions. Although they may be due to genetic defects, they may also be caused by a variety of factors (toxic, infectious, etc.). Isolated cases of developmental anomalies therefore cannot be assumed to be inherited. The congenital anomalies reported in domestic animal species may be too many to be listed here, and will be dealt with later in the course. Their effect on the animal varies from negligible to lethal. Certain types of developmental abnormalities can be conceptualised more easily as abnormalities of growth, and these include AGENESIS, APLASIA, and HYPOPLASIA.

Agenesis of an organ or tissue suggests a complete failure of that tissue to develop. Aplasia suggests a failure to grow and therefore implies the presence of a rudimentary organ. The clinical significance depends on the organ involved. Example, aplasia of one kidney would be expected to be clinically not apparent, whereas bilateral aplasia of kidneys would be lethal. The term aplasia also is used to refer to failure of a tissue to renew itself (e.g., the term aplastic anaemia).

Hypoplasia refers to the failure of an organ to reach normal size. It is therefore a developmental defect occupying the spectrum between aplasia and normal development. Examples regularly seen are renal hypoplasia and testicular hypoplasia. Hypoplasia of an organ may cause clinical disease, and its severity depends on the organ affected, and the degree to which function is reduced.

Acquired Lesions

Some lesions included under growth abnormalities may be regarded as adaptive responses of cells to changes in the demand made upon them. These include the following:

- Atrophy
- Hypertrophy
- Hyperplasia
- Metaplasia
- Dysplasia..

Atrophy

Atrophy implies an acquired change in a previously normal tissue and is the subsequent decrease in the size of an organ or tissue. The reduction in size may be due to a decrease in the number of cells (numerical atrophy) or the size of the individual cells (quantitative atrophy), or both. The loss of cell is by apoptosis. This type of lesion must be differentiated from agenesis and hypoplasia. Atrophy can occur under physiological or pathological conditions.

Physiological atrophy occurs in many tissues as a normal manifestation (e.g., atrophy of the thymus, mammary gland in males, involution of the uterus post-partum, and involution of fetal structures after birth like the ductus arteriosus, and umbilical vessels). Pathological atrophy includes the following types:

- *Nutritional atrophy* - due to inadequate dietary intake, or in events of starvation;
- *Vascular atrophy* - due to ischaemia;
- *Disuse atrophy* - due to reduced functional activity (e.g., paralysed limb)
- *Pressure atrophy* - probably mediates through vascular insufficiency due to long standing pressure (e.g., by tumour growth, surgical cast)
- *Endocrine atrophy* - due to loss of stimulation from trophic hormones (e.g., pituitary cyst leading to generalised somatic atrophy)
- Atrophy due to:
    - o Metabolic diseases
    - o Infections
    - o Neoplasms.

The differing types listed above are based on clinical varieties, but the basic aetiology is a deprivation of blood supply or nutritional requirements to the tissue with resultant atrophy. Grossly, the tissues or organs are smaller than normal but usually retain their normal shape. Microscopically, there are fewer cells than normal and these cells are smaller than normal. The tissue, however, appears more cellular due to the diminished amount of cytoplasm surrounding the remaining nuclei.

Hypertrophy and Hyperplasia

Hypertrophy is the increase in the size of the tissues or organ due to an increase in the size of individual cells. In pure form, hypertrophy occurs only in muscle and is usually a response to an increased demand for work.

Hyperplasia is an increase in tissue mass or organ size due to an increase in the number of constituent cells. Frequently, these two changes occur simultaneously in the tissues, but hypertrophy occurs alone in those tissues that are incapable of regeneration (e.g., cardiac muscle: See lecture notes on Inflammation and Healing). Both processes may be physiological or pathological, and the main factors are work load or endocrine stimulation. Types include the following:

- *Endocrine* - e.g., mammary gland during lactation
- *Compensatory* - e.g., when one kidney is hypoplastic or surgically removed
- *Functional* - e.g., muscles in response to heavy exercise; left ventricular myocardium following narrowing of aortic valve (aortic stenosis)
- *Replacement* - as part of the repair process (e.g., healing of fractured bone, healing of liver defect by regeneration)
- *Reactive* - e.g., reactive hyperplasia of lymphoid tissues and bone marrow in response to infection or anaemia; Also in response to chronic irritation e.g., thickening of the skin in mange mite infestation.
- *Neoplastic* - tumours are formed because of localised areas of increase in cell number

Usually, there is no well-defined cut off between physiologic and pathologic response. A response that at one level may be considered physiologic may be considered pathologic when it exceeds some arbitrarily selected limits.

Patterns of Hyperplasia include the following:

- *Nodular hyperplasia* - where the added tissue masses assume nodules e.g., in liver tissue remodelling
- *Cystic hyperplasia* - form spaces lined with epithelia e.g., cystic prostatic hyperplasia

- *Papillary hyperplasia* - form frond like projections e.g., hyperplasia of lining epithelia of tubular organs
- *Adenomatous hyperplasia* - form gland-like mass resembling neoplasm .

Metaplasia

Metaplasia is an adaptive response in which a different but related type replaces one type of mature differentiated cell. It is usually reversible and is most commonly seen from more specialised to less specialised but more resistant cell type (e.g., columnar or transitional cell type to squamous epithelia).

Epithelial metaplasia occurs following prolonged irritation or chronic infection (e.g., stones in urinary bladder), and in nutritional deficiencies (e.g., Vitamin A deficiency cause squamous cell metaplasia of prostate gland). Connective tissue metaplasia on the one hand, occur in association with repair processes (e.g., Fibroblast retains their mesenchymal ability to change into other connective tissue cells - may form bone, cartilage, or fibrocartilage).

Metaplasia does not occur because of alterations in existing mature cells. Rather it depends on proliferation of germinal cells whose progenies undergo modified differentiation. The change often is associated with hyperplasia and is usually orderly. Loss of orderly arrangements leads to dysplasia.

Dysplasia

Dysplasia literally means “abnormal growth”. However, it is used in a more restricted sense to describe a proliferative response accompanied by loss of regular differentiation and by cellular atypia and disorderliness.

Thus, it may be thought of as disorderly or atypical hyperplasia. These changes most frequently are observed in epithelia subjected to chronic irritation or inflammation. Cellular atypia is characterised by PLEOMORPHISM (variation in size and shape) and HYPERCHROMICITY (increased staining). There is a loss of the normal regular progression from germinal to fully differentiated cells and mitosis is found in abnormal positions. Dysplasia is however reversible if the cause is removed. Yet, when left alone, dysplasia may progress to become neoplasms.

Disorders of Micturition

Disorders of micturition result from a dysfunction in the storage or voiding of urine and may be neurogenic or non-neurogenic in origin. Urinary incontinence is the failure of voluntarily control micturition, with constant or intermittent unconscious passage of urine. Incontinent animals may leave a pool of urine where they have been lying or may dribble urine while walking. The coat around the vulva or prepuce may be wet, and perivulvar or peripreputial dermatitis can result from urine scalding.

Failure of urine storage is characterized by inappropriate leakage of urine due to failure of bladder relaxation, urethral incompetence, anatomic defects, or overflow of stored urine. Urge incontinence is seen with detrusor irritability, usually associated with cystitis.

The most common non-neurogenic incontinence is attributed to deficiency of sex hormones in neutered animals, particularly female dogs, and is referred to as hormonal-responsive urethral incompetence. Idiopathic urethral sphincter incompetence also is seen. Urinary incontinence associated with anatomic defects may be detected in animals at an early age. For example, an animal with a unilateral congenital ectopic ureter may void normally but "dribble" urine intermittently, whereas animals with bilateral ectopic ureters are less likely to void normally. Paradoxical urinary incontinence may develop when there is a partial obstruction of the urethra leading to bladder distention and overflow incontinence.

Failure of normal voiding is characterized by frequent attempts to urinate with stranguria, and passage of only small amounts of urine. Inability to urinate can be due to mechanical obstruction of the urethra by calculi, neoplasms, or strictures; detrusor atony from overdistention of the bladder; or neurologic disease. Animals with abnormalities of the voiding phase may develop overflow incontinence due to dribbling of urine associated with bladder overdistention.

Neurologic causes of micturition disorders can be categorized as upper (UMN) or lower motor neuron (LMN) lesions. Lesions in the sacral spinal cord, pelvic nerve, and detrusor atony lead to LMN signs, which are often characterized by a distended, easily expressed bladder. Dysautonomia in cats is a multisystemic disease characterized by widespread disruption of autonomic system functions, including urinary incontinence of LMN origin.

Damage to the thoracolumbar spinal cord or disease of the cerebrum, cerebellum, or brain stem can lead to UMN signs, which are characterized by a distended bladder that is difficult to express. Another neurologic cause of inability to urinate is functional obstruction (detrusor-sphincter reflex dyssynergia), which occurs when there is incoordination of the normal micturition reflex; this is believed to result from overdischarge of sympathetic nerve impulses to the urethral sphincter, resulting in a failure of urethral relaxation during detrusor contraction.

Animals with neurogenic incontinence may leak urine (LMN) and/or develop overflow incontinence due to dribbling of urine associated with bladder overdistension (any neurogenic cause).

Diagnosis: Clinical signs are usually suggestive of a micturition disorder. The history should include age of onset, sexual status of the animal, age at neutering, current medication, and history of previous urinary tract disorders.

A thorough physical and neurologic examination is indicated, and the act of voiding should be observed, including estimation of initial and final bladder volume. Animals with LMN lesions or an atonic bladder have a large, distended bladder that can be expressed with minimal pressure.

Animals with mechanical or functional obstruction or with spinal lesions causing UMN also have a large distended bladder, but urine cannot be readily expressed. Caution must be exercised when attempting to express urine from these animals to avoid rupturing the bladder. Plain or contrast radiography, cystoscopy, or ultrasonography are necessary to determine the type and location of mechanical obstruction. Animals with functional obstruction (reflex dyssynergia) generally exhibit pollakiuria with interrupted urine stream, distended urinary bladder, no identifiable structural cause of obstruction, and overflow incontinence, and generally have an abnormal neurologic examination. A catheter can easily be passed into the bladder in animals with functional obstruction but will not pass in animals with mechanical obstruction.

Animals with functional obstruction (reflex dyssynergia) generally exhibit pollakiuria with interrupted urine stream, distended urinary bladder, no identifiable structural cause of obstruction, and overflow incontinence, and generally have an abnormal neurologic examination. A catheter can easily be passed into the bladder in animals with functional obstruction but will not pass in animals with mechanical obstruction.

Treatment: Accurate diagnosis or localisation of the lesion is essential for appropriate pharmacologic management. Animals with hormonal incontinence were formerly treated with the appropriate sex hormone—diethylstilbestrol in females and testosterone in males. The dose should be adjusted to the minimum required to maintain continence. Diethylstilbestrol may be unavailable or difficult to obtain. Alternatively, an α-adrenergic agonist drug (eg, phenylpropanolamine, 2-4 mg/kg/day in divided doses) can be given to animals with urethral incompetence. Urge incontinence (detrusor instability) is treated with anticholinergic drugs such as oxybutin chloride (0.5 mg/kg, PO, sid) or propantheline (dogs <20 kg, 7.5 mg/day; dogs >20 kg, 15 mg/day; cats, 7.5 mg every 72 hr). Cholinergic drugs such as bethanechol are used in animals with detrusor atony. Functional obstruction is treated with sympatholytic drugs (eg, phenoxybenzamine, 2.5-10 mg, sid-tid); cholinergic drugs may also be necessary.

Complete mechanical obstruction of the urethra is a medical emergency and should be relieved by catheterization and retropulsion of the obstructing material into the bladder or by surgery. Animals with detrusor atony from overdistention but without neurologic lesions benefit from decompression of the bladder by placement of an indwelling urinary catheter for 3-7 days. This may be done continuously or intermittently. Those with neurogenic atony, which usually does not respond to medical management, may require manual expression of the bladder or catheterization several times daily.

Immunopathologic Mechanisms

The primary role of the immune system is the discrimination of self and non-self. The fundamental purpose of recognition of non-self is to protect against invading microorganisms, chemical agents, or other foreign substances.

To eliminate non-self agents, the immune system has developed a variety of mechanisms, including inactivation of biologic agents, lysis of foreign cells, agglutination or precipitation of molecules or cells, or phagocytosis of foreign materials. Generating the right class of immune response is under the control of dendritic cells (DC).

DC can be considered immunologic sensors—they are scattered throughout the body, sense environmental stimuli, and convey this information to naïve lymphocytes to tune the relevant immune response. For example, in response to intracellular microbes such as viruses or certain bacteria, DC secrete interleukin-12 (IL_{12}), inducing T-helper cells (T_H) to differentiate into T_H1. T_H1 cells promote cell-mediated immunity through production of ã-interferon (IFNã) and IL_2.

In contrast, extracellular pathogens such as helminths lead DC to secrete IL_4 and to trigger the naïve T_H cells toward T_H 2 differentiation. T_H2 cells promote antibody production through the secretion of IL_4, IL_5, IL_{10}, and IL_{13}, which increase IgE production, eosinophils and mast cells. The protective immune response against a non-self agent is a complex program including the nature of the stimuli, DC subsets, T_H subsets, and polarized cytokine profiles.

However, under certain circumstances, these normally protective responses can result in significant tissue damage; these immunopathologic mechanisms are called immune-mediated diseases. There are 4 general classical classifications of these diseases, which are mediated either through antibodies (Types I, II, and III) or by cells (Type IV). Many theories exist to explain immune-mediated diseases including external environmental factors, genetic predisposition, and hormonal influences. Recently immune-mediated diseases have been categorized in light of T_H1 and T_H 2 polarization. T_H1 cells are associated with autoimmune diseases (Type II) and T_H 2 cells with allergic diseases, immune complex disorders, and delayed-type hypersensitivity (Types I, III, and IV).

Corticosteroids, with or without other immunosuppressive drugs, are currently the mainstay of immune-mediated disease treatment. The primary challenge in this area is to find specific agents that precisely correct the dysregulation of T_H1/T_H 2 homeostasis.

Type I Reactions (Anaphylaxis)

Anaphylaxis is an acute systemic manifestation of the interaction of an antigen (allergen) binding to IgE antibodies, which are bound to mast cells and basophils.

This binding of antigens to cell-bound IgE antibodies triggers the release of chemical substances from the mast cells and basophils. The major biologically active mediators produced by mast cells and basophils include histamine, leukotrienes, eosinophilic chemotactic factor, platelet activating factor, kinins, serotonins, and proteolytic enzymes.

These chemicals directly affect both the vascular system, causing vasodilation and increased vascular permeability, and smooth muscles, causing contraction.

Additionally, they result in the migration of eosinophils to the triggering site. The severity of the reaction depends on the type of antigen, the amount of IgE antibodies produced, and the amount of antigen and route of exposure. Agents that can cause anaphylactic and allergic reactions are numerous and include the venom of stinging and biting insects, vaccines, drugs of any kind, foods, and blood products.

Clinical signs can be localised or generalized and include restlessness and excitement, pruritis around the head or site of exposure, facial edema, salivation, lacrimation, vomiting, abdominal pain, diarrhea, dyspnea, cyanosis, shock, incoordination, collapse, convulsions, and death.

Dogs differ from other domestic animals in that the major organ affected by anaphylactic shock is the liver, rather than the lungs. Signs in dogs are associated with constriction of hepatic veins, which results in portal hypertension and visceral pooling of blood.

Therefore, GI signs rather than respiratory signs are more apt to be seen in dogs.

Supportive therapy, in addition to treating respiratory distress, consists of the administration of epinephrine (both locally and systemically as needed), IV fluids for the treatment of shock, antihistamines (systemically for severe acute anaphylaxis or orally as a means to control chronic signs of allergy or milder allergic signs), and corticosteroids if needed.

Type II Reactions (Antibody-Mediated Cytotoxic Reactions)

Type II reactions occur when an antibody binds to an antigen present on the surface of the cell. This antibody-antigen complex then can activate the complement pathway, resulting in cell lysis or, through an antibody-mediated or complement-fragment-mediated receptor binding of a phagocytic cell, an antibody-mediated cytotoxicity.

It is unclear what triggers this antibody-mediated cytotoxicity but, as with all immune-mediated pathologic events, the combination of external factors and an infectious process in a genetically predisposed animal can lead to the development of immunopathologic disorders.

It has been hypothesized that acute viral infections can lead to changes in immune regulatory pathways that result in an overreaction of the immune system or to conversion of the protective immune response into a pathologic process. Also, cross-reactive antibodies can develop during an infectious process.

These cross-reactive antibodies directed toward an infectious agent will bind to normal tissue and result in antibody-mediated cytotoxicity. For example, in streptococcal infection in horses a cross-reaction between streptococcal antigen and vascular basement membranes can occur, leading to an immunopathologic disease. Lastly, certain pathogens such as Babesia or Haemobartonella may parasitize tissues, causing an immune response that destroys those tissues as part of the protective mechanism.

Clinical signs of a Type II hypersensitivity are variable and depend on the organ in which the reaction is occurring. They can include fever, cutaneous signs, polyarthritis, pain or joint swelling, and CNS signs. Glomerular nephritis is recognised by proteinuria or acute renal failure. Hematologic abnormalities such as hemolytic anemia, thrombocytopenia, neutropenia, or lymphopenia may be seen. Vague signs such as vomiting, diarrhea, or abdominal pain may also be seen. The diagnosis is primarily made by elimination of more obvious causes for the signs mentioned above and by histopathologic and immunohistopathologic analysis of organ biopsies. Supportive treatment consists of elimination of the offending infectious agent (if determined) and anti-inflammatory or immunosuppressive drug therapy.

Type III Reactions (Immune Complex Disease)

Type III reactions occur when antigen-antibody complexes are deposited along the endothelium. These complexes stimulate, both directly and via the complement pathway, a neutrophilic inflammatory response and vascular damage. The result is a multisystemic vasculitis. The most commonly affected sites include the joints, skin, kidneys, lungs, and brain.

The prerequisite for the development of such disease is continued presence of soluble antigen and continuous production of antibody. When there is slightly more antigen than antibody, the soluble complexes become deposited along endothelial cells. The reason for their deposition is not entirely clear; however, it is presumed that large complexes are removed by phagocytosis and very small complexes can easily pass through the cellular membrane, whereas complexes of intermediate size become trapped on the basement membrane of endothelial cells.

These deposited immune complexes then activate the complement cascade. Complement fragments cleaved from precursor molecules in this cascade incite inflammatory cells and are also directly vasoactive. The end result is a vasculitis. There are a number of reasons for the continuous presence of antigen, including chronic persistent infections (due to viruses, bacteria, fungi, protozoa, or parasites) and certain neoplastic conditions, particularly lymphoreticular neoplasms. Drug administration can result in an animal mounting an antibody response to the drug. Chronic antigen exposure is possible with repository medications or if the drug is continually administered. Lastly, some animals respond to self antigens, which represent a source of chronic antigen. In many cases, the origin of the antigen cannot be determined and, therefore, the cause of the disease is unidentifiable.

Clinical signs are variable but include fever, cutaneous signs (such as erythema multiforme), and polyarthritis (demonstrated by the presence of a shifting-leg lameness or painful, swollen joints). Other signs include ataxia, behaviour change, proteinuria, isosthenuria, polydipsia, polyuria, or vague signs such as vomiting, diarrhea, or abdominal pain. Diagnosis is based on the elimination of more common causes of clinical signs. Supporting evidence to confirm the diagnosis includes establishing a temporal relationship if a drug is suspected as the cause, identifying chronic infections or malignancies, and performing various laboratory tests (such as a Coombs' test or an antinuclear antibody test) as well as histopathology and immunohistochemistry analyses to identify immune-mediated vasculitides or nephritis.

Therapy should include supportive treatment associated with the affected organ and removal of the causative agent or treatment of the underlying disorder (eg, appropriate antibiotic therapy for bacterial infections, surgical drainage of abscesses or infected tissue, therapy for heartworm disease, the withdrawal of drugs, etc).

Immunosuppression and anti-inflammatory therapy may be needed to stop the continued formation of immune complexes and to lessen some of the inflammation associated with deposition of immune complexes.

Type IV Reactions (Cell-mediated Immune Reactions)

Cell-mediated immune reactions occur when T_H cells respond to foreign antigen or small molecules bound to cell tissue to form a complete antigen. T cells elaborate a variety of cytokines. IL_1 and other cytokines attract mononuclear phagocytes to the site of antigen. The infiltration of mononuclear cells and the elaboration of a variety of substances from these cells result in the pathologic processes of cell-mediated immune reactions.

The antigens usually responsible for the development of Type IV reactions include intercellular bacteria or parasites, some viruses, chemicals, and (in certain situations) cell antigen. This type of reaction can occur in any organ and, therefore, the clinical signs will vary. The diagnosis is based on ruling out other causes for organ-specific diseases and by a classic histologic description of delayed-type hypersensitivity reaction in tissue. The goals of treatment are to provide supportive therapy based on the organ-specific disease process, to identify (if possible) and eliminate the source of antigen that is responsible for the reaction, and to provide anti-inflammatory or immunosuppressive therapy if needed.

Immunopathologic Diseases: Introduction

Specific disease entities with an immune basis have been best characterized in companion and laboratory animal species. The clinical manifestations and treatment usually are similar among species, except for the relative frequencies of these various disorders.

Diseases Involving Anaphylactic Reactions: Overview (Type I Reactions, Atopic Disease)

Type I reactions are either systemic or localised. If the animal has been previously exposed to an allergen (antigen) and produces IgE antibodies, then injection of the sensitizing antigens directly into the bloodstream can result in anaphylactic shock or more focal reactions (eg, hives, urticaria, facial-conjunctival edema). If the sensitizing allergen enters through the mucous membranes or the skin, more localised reactions usually occur.

Systemic Anaphylaxis (Generalized Anaphylactic Reactions)

Anaphylactic shock occurs in sensitized animals after parenteral injection of vaccines or drugs, ingestion of foods, or insect bites. Clinical signs occur within seconds to minutes after exposure to the allergen. This latent period is the time required for the allergen to bind to sensitized mast cells and for vasoactive mediators to be released. In people and most domestic animals, lungs are the primary target organ and the portal-mesenteric vasculature is secondary; this is reversed in dogs. Mast cell degranulation in the pulmonary vasculature causes constriction of bronchial airways or pulmonary veins and pooling of blood in the pulmonary vascular bed, which results in severe respiratory distress. Mast cell degranulation in the portosystemic vasculature causes venous dilatation and pooling of blood in the intestines and liver, with resultant shock, agitation, colic, nausea, vomiting and diarrhea, hypersalivation, dyspnea, cyanosis, and in severe cases, death.

Anaphylactic shock is treated with an IV injection of epinephrine to counteract bronchial constriction and portal-mesenteric vasodilation. Ancillary support of blood pressure and respiration may be necessary. Because of the peracute onset of signs, antihistamines are of little therapeutic benefit. Antihistamines are more effective in treating urticarial reactions and facial-conjunctival edema, but even in those cases, antihistamines are more effective when used to prevent attacks in animals with a known allergic predisposition.

Urticarial reactions (hives or angioedematous plaques) of the skin and subcutaneous tissue and acute edema of the lips, conjunctiva, and skin of the face (facial-conjunctival angioedema) are less severe manifestations of a systemic allergic reaction. Hives are the least severe reaction and are seldom associated with other clinical abnormalities.

Facial-conjunctival edema is more severe and can be associated with mild to moderately severe systemic anaphylaxis. These reactions usually follow administration of vaccines or drugs, ingestion of certain foods, or insect bites. Urticarial reactions and facial-conjunctival edema occur in most species and usually resolve spontaneously within 24 hr. Not all urticarial reactions are mediated by IgE antibody.

Milk allergy occurs occasionally in cows and less frequently in mares. This can happen when intramammary pressure increases enough that normally sequestered milk components, notably casein, gain access to the circulation; these "foreign" proteins induce a Type I hypersensitivity. The reaction can be localised or systemic. Recovery usually is prompt once the gland is emptied.

Localised Anaphylactic Reactions

Allergic rhinitis is manifest by serous nasal discharge and sneezing. It is less common in other animals than in people. Often, it is seasonal, correlating with pollen exposure.

Nonseasonal rhinitis may be associated with exposure to ubiquitous allergens, such as molds, danders, bedding, and feeds. Recurrent airway obstruction in horses (*Recurrent Airway Obstruction*) may be a sequela of low-grade respiratory allergies. Summer snuffles is a seasonal allergic rhinitis occurring commonly in Guernsey or Jersey cattle placed on certain types of flowering pastures in late summer and early autumn. Allergic rhinitis can be diagnosed tentatively by the following: 1) identification of eosinophils in the nasal exudate, 2) demonstration of a favourable response to antihistamines, 3) disappearance of signs when the offending allergen is removed, or 4) occasionally, its seasonal nature. Unlike in people, skin testing is not an accurate means to diagnose nasal allergies in animals.

Chronic allergic bronchitis has been best characterized in dogs. A dry, harsh, hacking cough that is easily precipitated by exertion or by pressure on the trachea is a characteristic clinical sign. The disease may be seasonal or occur year-round. Usually, it is not associated with other signs of illness. The bronchial exudate is rich in eosinophils and free of bacteria. Chest radiographs are normal, and there may or may not be a low-grade peripheral eosinophilia. The condition is treated with bronchial dilators and expectorants (aminophylline and potassium iodide or guaifenesin), which aid in the removal of thick, tenacious mucus. Glucocorticoids dramatically alleviate clinical signs, especially when their use can be limited to certain seasons or to low-dose, alternate-day therapy. Avoidance of the offending allergen(s) usually is not possible because only rarely is it identifiable.

Allergic bronchiolitis is most common in cats. It is manifest by a low-grade cough, wheezing, some dyspnea, and increased peribronchiolar density on radiographs, and it may be mistaken for other conditions (allergic asthma or lungworm disease). Early in the course of the disease, clinical signs can be modified by antihistamine therapy, but if the disease increases in severity, moderate to high dosages of corticosteroids may be necessary. The offending allergen usually is not identified.

Diseases Involving Cytotoxic Antibodies

Autoimmune Hemolytic Anemia and Thrombocytopenia. These are the most common Type II reactions. Antibody and complement attach to RBC either directly or indirectly via an absorbed antigen and mediate RBC destruction, resulting in a severe, life-threatening anemia. Concurrent thrombocytopenia is found in 60% of cases. Type II reactions can be associated with systemic lupus erythematosus (SLE [more common in dogs]) or with lymphoreticular malignancies (more common in horses and cats). Drugs, vaccines, or infections also can precipitate attacks of hemolytic anemia or thrombocytopenia in most species. More often than not, the triggering cause is unknown. However, as more information becomes available about rickettsia, these intracellular pathogens may be found responsible for many of the idiopathic immune-mediated disorders.

Autoimmune hemolytic anemia (AIHA) has 4 basic forms: peracute, acute or subacute, chronic, and pure red cell aplasia. Most forms are treatable, and relapses are uncommon.

Peracute AIHA is seen mainly in middle-aged, larger breeds of dogs. Affected dogs are acutely depressed and within 24-48 hr have a fulminant decrease in PCV with bilirubinemia, variable icterus, and sometimes hemoglobinuria. Initially, the anemia is nonresponsive, but it becomes responsive within 3-5 days. Thrombocytopenia and thrombotic phenomena may be accompanying features. The Coombs' test is often negative, and spherocytes may or may not be present, but in-tube or slide agglutination of RBC is marked. The autoagglutination is not dispersed by saline dilution, hence the term hemolytic anemia with in-saline agglutinins. The serum usually contains autoantibodies that cause agglutination of most donor RBC (including heterospecies). The prognosis of peracute AIHA is poor even with prompt and vigorous therapy. The most effective therapy involves immediate use of high dosages of glucocorticoids plus cyclophosphamide. Incompatible blood transfusions should be avoided if possible, because they will provide more foreign material to provoke the failing immune system. If incompatible blood must be used, the animal should first be heparinized and maintained on heparin for the first 10 days. Even without transfusion, heparinization may be beneficial for the first 2 wk or more. Bovine hemoglobin blood substitute and human immunoglobulin can be used to support the patient until immunosuppressive treatment reduces the destruction of RBC.

Acute AIHA is the most common form of the disease, with a breed predilection in Cocker Spaniels. Initial signs are pallor, fatigue, and less commonly, icterus. Hepatosplenomegaly is a prominent sign. The WBC count often is increased due to bone marrow hyperplasia. Autoagglutination of RBC is uncommon, and the Coombs' test is generally positive. These animals usually respond well to glucocorticoid therapy. If a favourable response is not seen within 7-10 days, cytotoxic drugs (cyclophosphamide or azathioprine) should be added to the regimen.

Chronic AIHA differs from the acute form in that the PCV falls to a constant level and remains there for weeks or months. The bone marrow is either normal or hyperresponsive, and the Coombs' test is often negative. Chronic AIHA is relatively more common in cats than in dogs. Usually, the anemia is responsive early in the course of disease but responds minimally or not at all by the time it becomes severe. Initial treatment is with glucocorticoids; if there is no response within 2 wk, cytotoxic drugs are added to the regimen.

Pure red cell aplasia (*Primary Bone Marrow Diseases*) is a variant of the above disorders and is most common in dogs. It occurs in 2 forms, one in postweanling to adolescent puppies and the other in adults. Unlike AIHA, the bone marrow shows a selective depression of erythroid elements; granulocytes and platelets are unaffected. Therefore, the peripheral anemia is unresponsive. The immune attack apparently is directed at RBC precursors, and the Coombs' test is usually negative. However, there is often some difficulty in identifying compatible donors. Treatment is usually as for chronic AIHA.

Autoimmune thrombocytopenia is common, especially in dogs. It occurs more often in females than males. The most frequent clinical signs are hemorrhages of the skin and mucous membranes. Melena, epistaxis, and hematuria may be accompanying features and can cause profound anemia. Hemolytic anemia and thrombocytopenia sometimes occur together. Autoimmune thrombocytopenia usually is diagnosed on the basis of low peripheral platelet counts despite a pronounced megakaryocytosis in the marrow. Occasionally, megakaryocytes may be selectively absent from the marrow—a condition analogous to pure red cell aplasia. Tests for antiplatelet antibodies are difficult to conduct and may be positive in £70% of cases. The diagnosis is usually made on clinical appearance and response to therapy, rather than on antiplatelet antibody tests.

Animals with autoimmune thrombocytopenia that show only petechial and ecchymotic hemorrhages, with no significant blood loss and megakaryocytes in the marrow, are usually treated initially with glucocorticoids alone. The clinical signs should abate and the platelet count begin to rise after 5-7 days. If the platelet count has not increased significantly by days 7-

10, either cyclophosphamide, azathioprine, or vincristine can be added to the glucocorticoid regimen. In animals with megakaryocytes in the marrow and severe blood loss, a more rapid response to therapy is desirable. Such animals are treated with a single injection of vincristine combined with daily glucocorticoids; a favourable response usually occurs after 3-5 days. If the blood loss is life-threatening, platelet-rich whole blood should be administered.

If the platelet count has risen by day 7, remission is maintained on glucocorticoids alone. If there is no response after 7 days, a second dose of vincristine is given. If the platelet count is still low after 2 wk, vincristine is discontinued and either cyclophosphamide or azathioprine is added. Animals with thrombocytopenia and no megakaryocytes respond much more slowly to glucocorticoids, or to glucocorticoids and vincristine.

Preferred treatment for these animals is with prednisolone and cyclophosphamide, and a response should not be expected much earlier than 1-2 wk after beginning therapy. Therapy can be discontinued in most animals with autoimmune thrombocytopenia 1-3 mo after the platelet count returns to normal.

Some animals have more or less persistent thrombocytopenia despite drug therapy, or they can be maintained in remission only with chronic high-dose treatment. The alternatives are to allow the animal to live with the thrombocytopenia if signs are minimal or to use longterm combination drug therapy with glucocorticoids and either vincristine, azathioprine, or cyclophosphamide. Splenectomy may be helpful; it is seldom curative by itself but may allow use of lower and safer dosages of immunosuppressive drugs.

Cold agglutinin (hemolytic) disease is an AIHA that has been recognised most often in dogs and horses. It is often idiopathic but can be secondary to a chronic infection, other autoimmune diseases, or a neoplastic process. The IgM autoantibodies can be agglutinating or nonagglutinating. Complete agglutination is not seen at body temperature but rather at some lower temperature, thus it is more frequent in colder climates and seasons. Initial signs may be of a hemolytic disease; in the agglutinating type, there also may be microcapillary stasis with subsequent acrocyanosis and necrosis of the nose, tips of the ears and tail, digits, scrotum, and prepuce. Diagnosis is based on a reversible autoagglutination that occurs only at a cool temperature.

The direct Coombs' reaction is usually negative for IgG, frequently positive for C3, and usually positive for IgM if the reaction is performed in the cold. Mortality is high. In the absence of precipitating disorders, eg, infection or neoplasia, the disease is best controlled with high doses of glucocorticoids used in combination with cyclophosphamide. Cyclophosphamide is withdrawn when the anemia disappears and cold agglutinins are no longer detected.

Autoimmune Skin Disorders

In these immunologic skin disorders, antibodies are directed against intracellular cement substances at the basal cell layer, which results in separation of the epidermal cells (acantholysis). Pemphigus foliaceus is more common in dogs than in cats and horses but is still an uncommon disease. It is characterized clinically by erosions, ulcerations, and thick encrustations of the skin and mucocutaneous junctions.

The absence of lesions in the mouth, and the widespread thick, crusty nature of the skin lesions, tend to differentiate pemphigus foliaceus from pemphigus vulgaris. Autoantibodies are present in the skin and react with intracellular cement substance.

These autoantibodies cause a separation of the cornified from uncornified cell layers. High doses of glucocorticoids are used initially, but low-dose, alternate-day therapy is used once the disease is under control. More potent immunosuppressive drugs such as cyclophosphamide or azathioprine are used with glucocorticoids in cases unresponsive to steroids. Gold salts, in conjunction with low doses of glucocorticoids, are sometimes helpful in maintaining remission in animals in which steroids alone are ineffective. Animals that respond poorly to initial therapy, or require high dosages of drugs to control lesions, have a poor longterm prognosis.

Pemphigus vulgaris is rarer than pemphigus foliaceus. It is characterized by bullous lesions along the mucocutaneous junctions of the mouth, anus, prepuce, and vulva, and in the oral cavity. Other areas of the skin are only mildly involved. Because the epidermis of animals is relatively thin (compared with human skin), the bullae rupture rapidly and form erosions; consequently, characteristic bullae are seldom seen. The bullae occur as a result of suprabasilar acantholysis. Secondary bacterial infection often complicates the lesions, and if untreated, the disorder is often fatal. It is treated with high doses of glucocorticoids alone or in combination with other drugs such as cyclophosphamide, azathioprine, or gold salts. The disease is difficult to maintain in remission, and the longterm prognosis is fair to poor.

Bullous pemphigoid has been recognised in dogs, most often in Collies and Doberman Pinschers. Lesions are often widespread but tend to be concentrated in the groin. The involved skin resembles a severe scald. Bullae also may be seen; they are subepidermal and may be full of eosinophils. Autoantibodies to the basal lamina proteins are seen in immunohistopathologic sections. The treatment of choice is prednisolone and azathioprine used in combination; remission is frequent, but continuous drug therapy at relatively high dosages may be required to keep the disease under control. The longterm prognosis is poor.

Myasthenia Gravis

The acquired form of myasthenia gravis occurs in dogs and rarely in goats and cats. Affected animals produce autoantibodies to acetylcholine receptors, which bind to the receptor and reduce acetylcholine. The clinical manifestations mimic those produced by curare. Extreme generalized muscle weakness, accentuated by mild exercise, is common. Megaesophagus is a frequent primary or accompanying complaint in dogs. Thymomas are often associated with myasthenia gravis in humans, but this is uncommon in other animals. Administration of a short-acting anticholinesterase (edrophonium chloride) produces a dramatic increase in muscle strength. Treatment is with a long-acting anticholinesterase. Chronic immunosuppressive drug therapy for this disease is logical and should be investigated. Autoantibodies to the acetylcholine receptors can be detected in the serum of affected animals by an indirect immunohistopathologic analysis using normal muscle as a substrate.

Diseases Involving Immune Complexes (Type III Reactions)

Immune complex disorders are among the most common of the immunologic diseases. They may be idiopathic or of secondary origin. The site of deposition of the immune complexes determines the nature of the disease. Glomerulonephritis (*Glomerular Disease*) is caused by deposition of antigen-antibody complexes in the subendothelial or subepithelial surface of the glomerular basement membrane.

Secondary glomerulonephritis occurs as a side effect of chronic infectious, neoplastic, or immunologic disorders. Animals with idiopathic glomerulonephritis (>50% of cases) usually have signs of renal disease, whereas secondary glomerulonephritis is often a relatively minor part of a more serious disease.

Hypersensitivity pneumonitis is caused by deposition of immune complexes in the alveoli; it is most common in large animals that are exposed to antigenic dusts. The most potent antigens of this type are those contained in the spores of thermophilic actinomycetes from moldy hay.

Inhalation of these spores causes farmer's lung disease in humans and a similar condition in cattle (*Hypersensitivity Pneumonitis*). Hypersensitivity pneumonitis is characterized by the onset of respiratory distress 4-6 hr after exposure to moldy hay. The most effective treatment is removal of the source of the antigen; otherwise, corticosteroid therapy may help.

Systemic lupus erythematosus (SLE) occurs in dogs, is rare in cats, and has been reported in large animals.

It has 2 Immunologic Features: immune complex disease and a heightened antibody responsiveness with a tendency to produce autoantibodies. Therefore, it is a combination of Type II and III diseases. Antibodies to nucleic acid are the diagnostic hallmark of SLE, but in some individuals, antibodies to RBC, platelets, lymphocytes, clotting factors, immunoglobulin (rheumatoid factors), and thyroglobulin also may be present. These autoantibodies, in particular those to nucleic acids, are not always pathogenic by themselves. Rather, they should be considered markers of the disease. Although combinations of autoantibodies and self-antigens may contribute to the total pool of immune complexes, they are not the sole source of immune complexes. Usually, either the immune complex or the autoantibody aspect of the disease predominates in a given animal. Immune complex deposition around small blood vessels leads to synovitis, dermal reactions, oral erosions and ulcers, myositis, neuritis, meningitis, arteritis, myelopathy, glomerulonephritis, and pleuritis. Glomerulonephritis is one of the major life-threatening complications of SLE in cats but not in dogs. Psychosis, a major sign of SLE in people, is also seen in animals with SLE. Autoimmune hemolytic anemia or thrombocytopenia, or both, are the most common autoantibody manifestations of SLE in animals.

SLE is characterized by the presence of antinuclear antibodies (ANA), and tests for these or the associated LE cells may help in diagnosis. However, some healthy animals may have ANA, and not all animals with SLE have detectable ANA in their blood. Diagnosis of SLE should be based on the entire clinical syndrome—not just on the presence or absence of ANA.

SLE usually can be treated with glucocorticoids. Initially, they are used in high daily doses, and when remission occurs, alternate-day, low-dose therapy is used. Drug treatment should be continued for ≥2-3 mo after all clinical signs have disappeared. Cyclophosphamide or azathioprine, or both, are used in combination with glucocorticoids in animals with SLE that is difficult to control with glucocorticoids alone.

Vasculitis mediated by immune complexes occurs in animals, especially dogs and horses. Lesions are most prevalent in the dermis of the distal limbs and mucous membranes of the mouth, particularly the palate and tongue (dogs) and lips (horses). Involvement of the nose, ears, eyelids, cornea, and anus is less common. Early lesions are seen as reddened areas that rapidly form shallow erosions. A scab quickly forms over dermal erosions. Edema of the limbs is common in horses and a less frequent but equally striking sign in dogs. Vasculitis is a feature of SLE in some animals but most often is idiopathic. Drug-induced vasculitis has been well recognised in dogs. The vasculitis is detected on histopathologic and immunohistopathologic examination of superficial and deep biopsies taken from the margins of lesions.

Vasculitis is treated by withdrawal of offending drugs (if implicated in the cause) or by immunosuppressive drug therapy.

Glucocorticoids used alone or in combination with other agents such as azathioprine or cyclophosphamide are usually used to treat non-drug-induced cases.

Purpura hemorrhagica of horses is a form of nonthrombocytopenic purpura (*Congenital Thrombocytopenia*) that often is a sequela of an earlier Streptococcus equi respiratory infection; it is mediated by immune complexes of antibody and streptococcal antigen in vascular basement membranes.

Anterior uveitis (*Anterior Uvea*) often involves immune-complex-mediated reactions; it frequently occurs in the recovery stage of infectious canine hepatitis (*Infectious Canine Hepatitis: Introduction*) due to the reaction of serum antibodies with uveal endothelial cells that contain canine adenovirus 1. Similarly, equine recurrent uveitis (*Equine Recurrent Uveitis: Introduction*) or anterior uveitis of horses may be associated with immunologic reactions to Leptospira or Onchocerca spp . Uveitis caused by Toxoplasma and feline infectious peritonitis virus infections of cats also has an immunologic basis.

Canine rheumatoid arthritis manifests initially as a shifting lameness with soft-tissue swelling around involved joints. Within weeks or months, the disease localises in individual joints, and characteristic radiographic changes develop. The earliest radiographic changes consist of soft-tissue swelling and a loss of trabecular bone density in the area of the joint. Lucent, cyst-like areas frequently are seen in the subchondral bone. The prominent lesion is a progressive erosion of cartilage and subchondral bone in the area of synovial attachments, which results in loss of articular cartilage and collapse of the joint space. Angular deformities often occur, and luxation of the joint is a frequent sequela. Deformities are most frequent in the carpal, tarsal, and phalangeal joints, and less frequent in the elbow and stifle. Synovial fluid changes indicate a sterile, inflammatory synovitis, with increased total cell count and a high proportion of neutrophils in the synovial fluid cell population. The condition is believed to be due to deposition of immune complexes in the synovia.

A rheumatoid arthritis also has been recognised in cats. It tends to occur in older male cats and frequently is associated with feline leukemia virus infection. The development of disease in cats is much more insidious than in dogs.

Plasmacytic-lymphocytic synovitis, possibly a variant of rheumatoid arthritis, occurs in medium and large breeds of dogs. Although multiple joints often are involved, the disease has a predisposition for the stifles. The most common clinical sign is hindlimb lameness and anterior drawer motion of the stifles. Lymphocytes and polymorphonuclear neutrophils predominate in the synovial fluid, although in some cases the fluid is essentially normal. Gross inspection of the joint reveals a yellowish proliferation of the synovial membrane and stretching or rupture of the cruciate ligaments.

Canine rheumatoid arthritis and plasmacytic-lymphocytic synovitis respond poorly to systemic glucocorticoids alone. Cyclophosphamide and azathioprine frequently are used with glucocorticoids to treat these disorders; NSAID (eg, aspirin, carprofen, etodolac, meloxicam) may help bring relief.

Idiopathic polyarthritis is most common in large dogs, particularly German Shepherds, Doberman Pinschers, retrievers, spaniels, and pointers. In toy breeds, it is most frequent in Toy Poodles, Yorkshire Terriers, and Chihuahuas, or mixes of these breeds. There is no evidence of a primary chronic infectious disease process or systemic lupus erythematosus; joint disease is often the sole manifestation. Diagnosis is based on the history of cyclic antibiotic-unresponsive fever, malaise, and anorexia, with stiffness or lameness. Bony changes are not seen on radiographs until the disease is well established. Even then, radiographic changes are mild and can mimic degenerative joint disease. Synovial fluid is inflammatory in nature but sterile. The disease may be controlled with daily high-dose glucocorticoids followed by low-dose, alternate-day therapy. Treatment usually can be discontinued after 3-5 mo. Dogs that do not respond well to such therapy (>50%) are treated with more potent immunosuppressive drugs such as azathioprine or cyclophosphamide in addition to glucocorticoids. Gold salts may be helpful in augmenting glucocorticoid therapy in some animals.

Periarteritis nodosa (polyarteritis nodosa, necrotizing polyarteritis) is a rare, idiopathic disease of domestic animals that usually occurs as a secondary immunologic manifestation caused by deposition of immune complexes and inflammation in walls of small and medium-sized arteries. Among farm animals, it is most common in pigs, usually associated with erysipelas and streptococcal infections, and is attributed to a hypertensive arterial reaction to these bacteria or to their vaccines. It has been reported in cats, although it is often mistaken for the noneffusive form of feline infectious peritonitis.

Immune-mediated meningitis is believed to occur in dogs. The condition also has been called periarteritis nodosa, although its relationship to the human syndrome is uncertain. A steroid-responsive meningitis has been seen in adolescent or young adult Beagles, Boxers, German Shorthaired Pointers, and Akitas, but is very rare in other pure and mixed breeds. The clinical signs in Beagles, Boxers, and German Shorthaired Pointers consist of cyclic bouts of fever, severe neck pain and rigidity, reluctance to move, and depression. Each attack lasts 5-10 days, with intervening periods of complete or partial normalcy lasting ≥1 wk. During attacks, protein and neutrophils in the CSF are increased. The lesion is an arteritis, primarily of the meningeal vessels, but occasionally of other organs as well. The disease is often self-limiting over several months; attacks become milder and less frequent. Glucocorticoid therapy reduces the severity of attacks. In some animals, the disease becomes chronic and only partially amenable to therapy.

A more severe form of this meningitis has been reported in a litter of young Bernese Mountain Dogs. The disease in this litter was somewhat cyclical, but the resolution in intervening periods was less than in the disorder of Beagles, German Shorthaired Pointers, and Boxers. CSF abnormalities resembled those of the disease in other breeds. The condition was less self-limiting and required longterm, high-dose glucocorticoid therapy to keep the animals comfortable.

A syndrome of meningitis, often associated with polyarthritis, is seen in Akitas as young as 12 wk old. The dogs show severe (but somewhat cyclical) bouts of fever, depression, cervical pain and rigidity, and generalized stiffness. Affected dogs grow at a slower rate and often appear unthrifty. The condition responds poorly to glucocorticoid and combination immunosuppressive therapy, and most dogs are euthanized as young adults. In older Akitas, a milder and more drug-responsive form of the disease is seen, which may be associated with pemphigus foliaceus, uveitis, and plasmacytic-lymphocytic thyroiditis.

Diseases Involving Cell-Mediated Immunity (Type IV Reactions)

Granulomatous reactions to microorganisms such as mycobacteria, Coccidioides, Blastomyces, and Histoplasma spp, and possibly feline infectious peritonitis virus, may be due to chronic cell-mediated immune reactions. Although cell-mediated immunity effectively controls these types of infection in most individuals, for poorly understood reasons, these same mechanisms are only partially effective in others. A granulomatous reaction occurs, characterized by a fibrous stroma and an infiltration of macrophages, giant cells, and lymphocytes.

Lymphocytic choriomeningitis is a viral infection of mice (*Generalized Diseases*) in which CNS damage is due to the destruction of virus-infected cells by thymus-derived lymphocytes. Old-dog encephalitis (*Canine Distemper: Introduction*) also may result from cell-mediated immune mechanisms directed against cells persistently infected with canine distemper virus. The initiating canine distemper virus infection is usually clinically inapparent and may precede the encephalitis by years.

Contact hypersensitivity results from chemicals reacting with dermal proteins, which modify self-proteins. These modified proteins are antigenic, and the host's cell-mediated immune response against these chemically altered dermal proteins damages the skin, eg, poison oak and poison ivy reactions in humans. This reaction has been described in both dogs and horses and usually occurs as a result of contact with sensitizing chemicals incorporated in plastic food dishes, plastic collars, and drugs placed on the skin.

Autoimmune thyroiditis has been recognised in dogs and is characterized by destruction of the thyroid gland by an autoimmune process that has both humoral (Type II) and cell-mediated (Type IV) components. The disease is particularly prevalent in Doberman Pinschers, Beagles, Golden Retrievers, and Akitas. Hypothyroidism (*Hypothyroidism*) may be the sole manifestation of the disease or may be a clinical or subclinical component of a broader autoimmune disorder such as systemic lupus erythematosus, idiopathic polyarthritis, immune-mediated meningitis (periarteritis nodosa), panendocrinopathy, and rheumatoid arthritis.

Autoimmune adrenalitis has been reported in dogs. The adrenal glands are slowly destroyed by a plasmacytic-lymphocytic infiltrate. When sufficient glandular tissue is destroyed, the dogs develop Addison's syndrome (adrenocortical insufficiency, *Hypoadrenocorticism*). The condition is sometimes associated with a similar immune attack against other endocrine glands, in particular the thyroid.

Keratitis sicca occurs in dogs, with a genetic predisposition in Cocker Spaniels. It can occur in either a primary form or secondary to chronic use of sulfonamides. It is associated with an immune-mediated destruction of the lacrimal glands and is somewhat analogous to Sjögren's syndrome of humans, which is caused by disease of the salivary glands and a lack of saliva. Of affected dogs, ≥50% respond favourably to eyedrops that contain cyclosporine, which selectively inhibits disorders mediated by T lymphocytes.

Immune-deficiency Diseases: Overview

Deficiencies in Phagocytosis

Phagocytosis is an essential feature of the immune system. Phagocytes are found underlying the mucous membranes and skin and in the bloodstream, spleen, lymph nodes, meninges, synovial membrane, bone marrow, and around blood vessels throughout the body. Phagocytes are either in the tissue (histiocytes, synovial macrophages, Kupffer cells, etc) or in the blood (polymorphonuclear leukocytes, monocytes). Phagocytes have immunoglobulin and complement receptors on their surfaces that assist in the engulfment (opsonization) of foreign material coated with specific antibody (opsonins) or complement, or both. Phagocytosis involves chemotaxis of the phagocyte to foreign, noxious, or damaged material; adherence of the material to the plasma membrane of the phagocyte; incorporation of the material into a pinocytotic vesicle; formation of a phagosome; and activation of the respiratory burst and lysosomal enzymes in the phagosome.

Deficiencies in phagocytosis can involve acquired or congenital defects in any of these steps, or can be due to the available number of phagocytes. They often manifest as an increased susceptibility to bacterial infections of the skin, respiratory system, and GI tract. These infections respond poorly to antibiotics.

Acquired phagocytic deficiencies include disorders that lead to profound and chronic depressions of WBC. Feline leukemia virus infection, feline panleukopenia virus infection, feline immunodeficiency virus infection, tropical canine pancytopenia, idiopathic granulocytopenias, drug-induced granulocytopenias (anticancer drugs, estrogens, anticonvulsants, sulfonamides, etc), and myeloproliferative disorders are a few conditions in which secondary infections can develop as life-threatening complications.

A cyclic decrease of all cellular elements, most notably neutrophils, occurs in the peripheral blood and lowers the resistance to infection of gray Collies and Collie crosses.

Congenital abnormalities that lead to impaired phagocytosis are well documented in humans. Deficiencies of opsonins, complement factors, chemotactic abilities, myeloperoxidase, and lysosomal enzyme activation have been recognised in humans but not in other animals. Chronic granulomatous disease has been recognised as an X-linked defect in some Irish Setters (canine granulocytopathy syndrome). Some lines of Weimaraners develop bacterial septicemias (usually manifested by bone and joint infections) as puppies. The underlying cause for this phenomenon is unknown; some of the affected dogs have lower than normal levels of IgM and IgG, and preliminary research indicates that WBC have a bactericidal defect.

Leukocyte Adhesion Deficiency

Leukocyte adhesion deficiency (canine granulocytopathy syndrome) is a primary immunodeficiency disorder inherited as an autosomal recessive trait. It has been described in humans, Irish Setters, and Holstein cows. This deficiency is the result of a deficient expression of leukocyte surface glycoproteins. Clinically, it is characterized by recurrent, severe bacterial infections; impaired pus formation; and delayed wound healing. Infected animals usually have severe pyrexia, anorexia, and weight loss; response to antibiotic therapy is usually poor. Extreme, persistent leukocytosis may occur (>100,000 WBC/μL) and consists predominantly of mature neutrophils.

Deficiencies in Immunoglobulins

These may be acquired or congenital. Acquired deficiencies occur in neonates that do not receive adequate maternal antibodies (failure of passive transfer) or in older animals due to conditions that decrease active immunoglobulin synthesis. Failure of passive transfer of immunoglobulin occurs occasionally in all species that have colostrum as the major source of maternal antibodies. It is commonly associated with clinical problems in calves, lambs, and foals.

Failure of passive transfer can occur when the young animal fails to nurse properly during the first several days of life or when the dam's colostrum contains low levels of specific antibodies.

Theoretically, problems with the intestinal absorption of immunoglobulin in the milk also can occur. Immunoglobulin levels <400 mg/dL in a postnursing serum sample indicate a failure of passive transfer in foals. Removing calves from their dams too soon is a frequent problem in dairy herds and is a leading cause of failure of passive transfer in dairy calves. Newborn animals that do not obtain adequate maternal antibodies often succumb to fatal bacterial or viral infections of the GI and respiratory tracts.

Idiopathic (essential) hypogammaglobulinemia has not been described in animals other than humans, but undoubtedly it occurs. It is associated with excessive regulatory cell activity that depresses antigen-stimulated immunoglobulin synthesis to B lymphocytes.

Hypogammaglobulinemia of clinical significance can be associated with any disorder that interferes with immunoglobulin synthesis. Tumors, such as plasma cell myelomas or lymphosarcomas that occasionally secrete large amounts of monoclonal antibody, can be associated with profound deficiencies of normal beneficial antibodies.

This may be because the tumor cells are competing for necessary substrate substances with normal immunoglobulin-producing cells, or because thymus-derived regulatory lymphocytes in the blood nonselectively inhibit the abnormal immunoglobulin production. Animals with tumors that produce monoclonal antibodies can have severe secondary infections.

Some viral infections, eg, canine distemper and canine parvovirus, may damage the lymphoreticular system so severely that normal antibody production is virtually stopped.

Congenital hypogammaglobulinemia (common variable immunodeficiency) has been recognised either by itself or in combination with deficiencies in cell-mediated immunity (combined immunodeficiency, *see* below). Deficiencies in IgG subclass synthesis have been seen in some breeds of cattle; IgM deficiency has been described in horses; and IgA deficiencies have been described in Beagles, German Shepherds, and Shar-Peis. Cattle with IgG subclass deficiency are usually asymptomatic. Older foals with IgM deficiencies develop respiratory infections. Dogs with IgA deficiency, like their human counterparts, suffer mainly from chronic skin infections, chronic respiratory infections, and possibly allergies. The IgA deficiency of Beagles appears to be due to a defect in the secretion of IgA, because IgA-positive cells are present in normal numbers. Some German Shepherds seem to have lower IgA levels than other breeds and a higher incidence of GI allergies. IgA deficiency in Shar-Peis is highly variable; some have negligible serum and secretory levels, and some have normal serum levels and low or negligible secretory levels. Like the German Shepherds, affected Shar-Peis have more problems than expected with allergies. Patients with common variable immunodeficiency have a higher than usual incidence of autoimmune disorders and autoantibodies (eg, autoimmune hemolytic anemia, thrombocytopenia, systemic lupus erythematosis). Longterm treatment with broad-spectrum antibiotics is required and IV human g-globulin is usually needed.

Transient hypogammaglobulinemia has been recognised most frequently in foals and puppies. It may be more common in Spitz-type puppies than in other breeds. It is congenital and manifest by a delay in development of active immunity associated with a maturational defect of both T_H function and the B cell response to foreign antigens. Puppies with this condition develop recurrent respiratory infections at 1-6 mo of age but recover and are essentially normal by 8 mo of age. Affected foals frequently develop clinical signs of hypogammaglobulinemia (usually respiratory infections) at ~6 mo of age when their maternal antibody reaches a very low level. After another 3-5 mo, they begin to produce immunoglobulin. Appropriate antibiotic treatment is often sufficient.

Deficiencies in Cell-mediated Immunity

Pure deficiencies in cell-mediated immunity are rare in humans and have not yet been described in other animals. In general, deficiencies in cell-mediated immune responses are associated with thymic aplasia, an absent or very small thymus. This is seen in some inbred lines of dogs and cattle; these animals were deficient in cell-mediated immune functions, such as lymphocyte blastogenesis, as well as having pituitary dysfunction.

Combined Immunodeficiency Disease

An autosomal recessive type of this disease has been identified in Arabian foals and Basset Hounds. Sporadic cases of combined immunodeficiency, probably heritable, have also been seen in Toy Poodle, Rottweiler, and mixed-breed puppies. Affected dogs are frequently asymptomatic during the first several months of life but become progressively more susceptible to microbial infections as maternal antibody wanes. Puppies with combined immunodeficiency disease generally are normal until 6-12 wk old. The most common cause of death from this condition is canine distemper as a consequence of routine immunization with modified live virus distemper vaccine. Arabian foals with the disorder frequently succumb to adenovirus pneumonia or other infections when ~2 mo old. The foals are persistently lymphopenic. Precolostral serum samples have no detectable IgM antibody. Immunoglobulin levels are normal after nursing but progressively decrease after that time compared with levels in normal foals. At necropsy, the thymus gland is difficult to identify and is architecturally abnormal. Lymphoid elements are markedly depleted in the lymph nodes, Peyer's patches, and spleen.

Complement Deficiencies

A congenital deficiency of C3 has been described in an inbred line of Brittany Spaniels. These dogs developed recurrent bacterial infections, especially skin diseases and pneumonias. Although complement is necessary for opsonization and neutrophil chemotaxis, bacterial infections do not always develop in people or laboratory animals with these deficiencies. This is mainly because the existence of 2 pathways provides a way of activating the system even if one pathway is blocked.

Congenital deficiency in the C1 inhibitor has been recognised in humans and occurs rarely in dogs. Affected animals suffer from recurrent bouts of facial edema. Diagnosis is based on a blood test showing <30% of the normal C3 level. There is no specific treatment for complement deficiencies. Vaccination and antibiotics are used to prevent and treat infection.

Selective Immunodeficiencies

Rottweiler puppies have a breed predilection for severe and often fatal canine parvovirus infections (*Canine Parvovirus*). Their resistance to other diseases is essentially normal, and the basis of this selective immunodeficiency is unknown. Persian cats have a predilection toward severe, and sometimes protracted, dermatophyte infections (*Dermatophytosis: Introduction*). In some Persian cats, the fungal infections invade the dermis and cause granulomatous disease (mycetomas). Mink with the Aleutian coat colour mutation are susceptible to chronic parvovirus infection and develop a disorder called Aleutian disease (*Viral Diseases*). Other strains of mink are susceptible to infection with this virus but do not develop clinical disease. Focal and systemic aspergillosis (*Aspergillosis: Introduction*), and mycoses due to related fungi, affect certain types of dogs. Long-nosed breeds, in particular German Shepherds and shepherd-crosses, are prone to develop focal aspergillosis in the nasal passages. Systemic aspergillosis is seen almost exclusively in German Shepherds, and more commonly in western Australia than elsewhere. It is characterized by fungal pyelonephritis, osteomyelitis, and discospondylitis. The organism can be isolated readily from blood and urine.

Viral-Induced Immunodeficiencies

These have been caused by a number of agents in animals. Canine distemper virus causes a profound combined immunodeficiency in affected puppies. The infection is associated with a progressive decline in levels of antibody globulin and increased susceptibility to agents normally contained by cellular immunity, eg, Toxoplasma, Nocardia .

Parvoviral infection in both dogs and cats causes a profound and transient depression in the number of neutrophils and in lymphocyte responsiveness. This has led to an increased incidence of fungal infections (aspergillosis, mucormycosis, candidiasis) in the immediate post-recovery period. A severe immunodeficiency syndrome induced by parvovirus has also been seen in mice.

Retroviral-induced immunodeficiency has received increased scrutiny since the appearance of acquired immunodeficiency syndrome (AIDS) in humans. Feline leukemia virus (FeLV) infection is associated with acquired immunodeficiency and increased incidence of secondary and opportunistic infections. Acquired immunodeficiency in FeLV infection is multifactorial and broad in nature. Infected cats can have deficiencies of neutrophils, decreased synthesis of antibodies (especially to bacterial antigens), decreased cellular immunity, and variable levels of complement. Immune responses to FeLV infection also appear to inhibit ongoing feline infectious peritonitis (FIP) virus immunity specifically, which leads to reactivation of quiescent FIP.

Simian type D retrovirus (types 1-5 and Mason-Pfizer monkey virus) infection of macaques has a similar pathogenesis to that of FeLV infection of cats but can induce even more severe immunodeficiency. Each serotype tends to be found in specific species of macaques in the wild and within defined geographic areas. Type D retrovirus infection of macaques can cause severe disease in adolescent animals from zoos and in primate centres with large breeding groups. Although the infection rate in the wild may be high, these viruses cause a less severe syndrome in wild than in captive populations. Affected macaques either die within several months with fever, lymphadenopathy, and opportunistic infections of the CNS, respiratory tract, and intestines; become lifelong asymptomatic carriers; or recover fully. A progressive retroperitoneal fibrosis is a feature with some serotypes. Healthy monkeys can be antibody positive and have virus in their blood and saliva (asymptomatic carriers) or can be antibody positive without isolatable virus (immune). Animals with clinical signs are always viremic but may or may not have serum antibodies, depending on disease severity.

Simian immunodeficiency virus (SIV) is a lentivirus with considerable genetic homology to human immunodeficiency virus (HIV). Many strains of SIV exist in nature. The common hosts are African primates such as African green monkeys, sooty mangabeys, mandrills, baboons, and other guenons. Transmission between infected and noninfected monkeys is probably by bites and in utero exposure. SIV is not present in native populations of Asian primates. It rarely causes disease in the host African species. If infected animals are under heavy stress, as in captivity, some may develop AIDS-like disease. SIV, especially of sooty mangabey origin, causes severe disease in macaques (rhesus, stump-tail, pig-tail, bonnet, etc). Most affected macaques have come from zoos and primate centres where contact is allowed between African and Asian species, and tissues and body fluids are often exchanged between animals for research purposes. The immunosuppression associated with SIV can last for weeks or years. Encephalitis (usually asymptomatic except for wasting) and lymphomas are frequent sequelae of SIV infection in macaques. Infected animals, whether healthy or diseased, carry the infection for life. Monkeys that are infected with SIV usually make serum antibodies that are detectable by a number of procedures. Because the infection is lifelong, the presence of serum antibodies to SIV indicates the presence of virus in the body.

Feline immunodeficiency virus (FIV, originally feline T-lymphotropic lentivirus) is a related lentivirus that has been identified in domestic cats and cheetahs. The infection is endemic in cats throughout the world. Virus is shed mainly in the saliva, and the principal mode of transmission is through bites. Free-roaming (feral and pet), male, and aged cats are at the greatest risk of infection. FIV infection is uncommon in closed purebred catteries. After infection, there is a transient period of fever, lymphadenopathy, and neutropenia. Most cats recover from this stage and appear normal for months or years before immunodeficiency occurs. The percentage of infected cats that enter the terminal phase of the illness is unknown. Cats with acquired immunodeficiency induced by FIV develop chronic secondary and opportunistic infections of the respiratory, GI (including mouth), and urinary tracts, as well as the skin. FIV-infected cats have a higher than expected incidence of FeLV-negative lymphomas, usually of the B-cell type, and myeloproliferative disorders (neoplasias and dysplasias). Of affected cats, ~5% have neurologic signs referable to cerebral cortex disease (behavioural abnormalities, psychomotor disturbances, dementia, convulsions). Cats remain infected for life; the presence of serum antibodies is directly correlated with the ability to isolate virus from blood cells and saliva.

Bovine immunodeficiency-like virus is a lentivirus that was originally isolated from bovine leukemia virus (BLV)-negative cattle with persistent lymphocytosis and hemolymphadenopathy. It also has been isolated from cattle with BLV-negative lymphosarcomas. The overall incidence in cattle appears to be ~1% although in some herds it may be ≥15%. Preliminary evidence indicates that the virus is not a cause of immunodeficiency in cattle. Some infected cattle can be detected by serologic tests for viral antibodies. Virus isolation from blood appears to be the most accurate way to detect infected animals.

Tumors of the Immune System

Studies of the immunologic response to tumors conducted in the past 15 years have changed the definition of cancer, which is now perceived as a chronic immune disease. In response to genotoxic stress, carcinogens, or viruses, the targeted cells induce expression of stress proteins and tumor-associated antigens. These mark the abnormal cells for the immune system, which eliminates them through cell-mediated cytoxicity. In cancer patients, tumor cells escape from the immune attack by relying on both immunoparalysis and tumor cell modification. The demonstration that even bulky, invasive tumors can undergo complete remission under appropriate stimulation (eg, IL_2) has shown that it is indeed possible to treat cancer successfully by immune manipulation.

Cancer is the number one cause of death in dogs; 45% of dogs ≥10 yr old die of cancer. Lymphoma is one of the most prevalent tumors in dogs and cats. Boxers, Basset Hounds, and Rottweilers are predisposed to developing lymphomas. The normal immune response requires a burst of rapid proliferation of lymphocytes. On occasion however, this proliferation may be uncontrolled, and lymphoid neoplasms result. Because lymphocytes are present in all organs, tumor development can occur in any organ. Lymphomas can be multicentric, mediastinal, gastrointestinal, renal, nervous, or leukemic. Less commonly, they occur in the eyes, skin, or nose. To determine the stage of the disease, CBC, serum chemistry profiles, abdominal ultrasound, abdominal radiographs, and bone marrow analyses are useful. Immunofluorescent staining can be performed in dogs and cats to characterize lymphomas. They may be either T cell or B cell in origin.

Most cases of canine lymphosarcoma, Marek's disease, calf leukosis, and feline leukemia are of T-cell origin, as are thymomas. Thymomas, which are relatively uncommon in domestic animals, generally cause loss of condition and respiratory distress. They are commonly confirmed by radiography. In humans, thymomas may be associated with signs of myasthenia gravis. While this association has been reported in dogs, it is uncommon. Many T-cell lymphomas are associated with a simultaneous immunosuppression manifest by a predisposition to recurrent infections.

Adult bovine and ovine leukosis, alimentary feline leukemia, and avian leukosis are usually of B-cell origin. Under some circumstances, neoplastic B cells may develop into plasma cells. Plasma-cell tumors are known as myelomas. Because neoplastic plasma cells can secrete immunoglobulins, they give rise to gammopathies.

Combination chemotherapy (eg, vincristine, l-asparaginase, cyclophosphamide, doxorubicin, prednisone) is recommended for lymphoma treatment. Side effects include vomiting, diarrhea, lack of appetite, and fever. Hair loss is not observed in dogs and cats. Lymphomas are rarely cured, but remission of up to 1 yr is common after combination chemotherapy.

Gammopathies

Gammopathies are conditions in which serum immunoglobulin levels are greatly increased. Using electrophonetic patterns, they can be classified either as polyclonal (increases in all major immunoglobulin classes) or monoclonal (increases in a single homogeneous immunoglobulin). Polyclonal gammopathies in animals are seen in chronic pyodermas; chronic viral, bacterial, or fungal infections; granulomatous diseases; abscessation; chronic parasitic infections; chronic rickettsial diseases, such as tropical canine pancytopenia; chronic immunologic diseases, such as systemic lupus erythematosus, rheumatoid arthritis, and myositis; or with neoplasia. They also may be idiopathic. In some animals, the gammopathy may appear initially to be monoclonal because of a predominance of 1 immunoglobulin class (usually IgG). Examples of this phenomenon have been seen in cats with noneffusive feline infectious peritonitis and in dogs with chronic tropical canine pancytopenia.

Monoclonal gammopathies are characterized by the presence of a homogeneous serum immunoglobulin protein. Uninvolved immunoglobulin classes are usually depressed. Monoclonal gammopathies are either benign (ie, associated with no underlying disease), or potentially associated with immunoglobulin-secreting tumors. In humans, benign gammopathies may become malignant at a later date; in other animals, they are rare and are not associated with a demonstrable tumor or clinical illness.

Tumors that secrete monoclonal antibodies originate either from plasma cells (myeloma) or lymphoblasts (lymphosarcoma). Plasma-cell myelomas can secrete intact proteins of any immunoglobulin class or immunoglobulin subunits (light chains or heavy chains). Myeloma proteins in dogs are commonly IgG or IgA types and less commonly IgM. Myelomas of the IgA type are particularly common in Doberman Pinschers. Monoclonal immunoglobulin produced by lymphosarcoma are often of the IgM class, regardless of species. Myeloma proteins in cats and horses usually are IgG and, uncommonly, IgM, IgG (T) (horses), or IgA.

Clinical signs depend on the location and severity of the primary neoplasm and on the amount and type of immunoglobulin secreted. Plasma-cell myelomas frequently develop in marrow cavities of flat bones of the skull, ribs, and pelvis, and in the vertebrae. Pathologic fractures of diseased bone can lead to CNS or spinal disorders or to pain and lameness. Lymphosarcomas frequently involve parenchymatous organs; therefore, clinical signs are more diverse.

Clinically evident illness can result from the presence of the monoclonal protein itself. Amyloidosis (*Amyloidosis: Introduction*) can be due to increased immunoglobulin catabolism. Hyperviscosity syndrome appears in 20% of dogs with monoclonal gammopathy, especially with IgM or IgA monoclonal proteins, and can occur if the protein levels in blood are high. In this syndrome, plasma viscosity can be many times normal, which leads to profound vascular disturbances, thrombosis, and bleeding diathesis. Depression, blindness, and neurologic manifestations can be due to hemorrhage in the nervous system and retina. Some IgM monoclonal proteins act as cryoglobulins and aggregate in vitro and in vivo when the plasma is cooled. Animals with cryoglobulinemia often develop gangrenous sloughs of the ear tips, eyelids, digits, and tip of the tail, especially during cold weather. Myelomas that produce autoantibodies to various tissues have been identified in humans, but not in other animals. Finally, animals with monoclonal gammopathies may have greatly depressed levels of normal immunoglobulins and, therefore, may develop serious secondary infections.

Immunoglobulin-secreting tumors usually are treated with glucocorticoids and alkylating drugs. The prognosis for remission after therapy is much better in dogs than cats. Even in dogs, however, the longterm prognosis is poor and relapse is common after 6-12 mo. Plasmapheresis may be needed to lower serum viscosity in animals with clinical signs of hyperviscosity syndrome. Antibiotics and globulin injections may help prevent secondary infections.

Urinary System, Introduction: Introduction

Primary functions of the urinary system include: 1) excretion of waste products of metabolism; 2) maintenance of a constant extracellular environment through conservation and excretion of water and electrolytes; 3) production of the hormones erythropoietin and renin, which regulate hematopoiesis, blood pressure, and sodium reabsorption; and 4) metabolism of vitamin D to its active form (1,25-dihydroxycholecalciferol). Many abnormalities of the urinary system can be diagnosed from the signalment of the patient, history and physical examination findings, serum chemistry profile, urinalysis, and aerobic bacterial urine culture. The history should include information regarding changes in water consumption, frequency of urination, volume of urine produced, appearance of urine, and behaviour of the patient. It is also important to obtain information about historical and current drug administration, appetite, diet, changes in body weight, and previous illnesses or injuries. The physical examination should include palpation of the bladder and examination of external genitalia. In dogs, rectal examination should be performed to evaluate the urethra in both sexes and for evaluation of the prostate in male dogs. Rectal examination in cats may not be feasible due to their small size; however, the kidneys are generally easier to palpate in cats than in dogs. A full neurologic examination should be performed on all animals with micturition disorders. Additional diagnostic tests, such as CBC, blood gas analysis for acid-base status, blood pressure, urine protein:creatinine ratio, iohexol clearance test, survey abdominal radiography, abdominal ultrasonography, contrast studies of the upper and lower urinary tract, cystoscopic examination of the urinary bladder, and renal biopsy may also provide valuable information.

Urinalysis: One of the most important diagnostic tests for evaluation of urinary tract disorders is a urinalysis. Urine may be collected by one of 4 methods: spontaneous micturition, manual compression of the urinary bladder, catheterization, and cystocentesis. Each method has advantages and disadvantages. A urinalysis should include method of collection, urine specific gravity, colour, turbidity, pH, glucose, ketones, bilirubin ictotest, occult blood, protein, and leukocytes (urine dipstick leukocyte tests are unreliable in cats). Microscopic examination of urine sediment should include RBC, WBC, epithelial cells, renal casts, bacteria, yeast, parasitic ova, fat, sperm, and crystals. Delay in analyzing urine samples can result in artifacts (eg, changes in urine pH, formation of crystals, etc), so it is important to note the time when the sample was collected and the time when it was analyzed. If a sample will not be analyzed immediately, it should be refrigerated.

Protein in urine should be evaluated in light of the urine specific gravity. Protein in a concentrated urine sample may not be significant, whereas the same amount in a dilute sample may be significant. Urine dipsticks provide a semiquantitative assessment of protein and can be influenced by urine pH. Therefore, they should be used only as a screening test for protein, not as a definitive diagnosis of proteinuria.

A Urine Protein: creatinine ratio from a single urine sample or from a 24-hr urine sample is required to quantitate the amount of protein in urine. In dogs, the following guidelines should be used for interpretation of urine protein:creatinine ratios: 0.0-0.3 = normal; 0.3-1.0 = questionable; and >1.0 = abnormal. In cats, a urine protein:creatinine ratio <0.7 is considered normal. Urine protein:creatinine ratios must be interpreted in the context of other information from the urinalysis. Inflammation and hematuria can falsely elevate urine protein:creatinine ratios.

Bacterial Culture of Urine: A urinalysis is unreliable for ruling out a urinary tract infection (UTI). Not all UTI are associated with an inflammatory response. In addition, >10,000 bacterial rods/mL and >100,000 bacterial cocci/mL of urine are required to consistently find bacteria in a urine sample using light microscopy. About 25-30% of all dogs with UTI have urine bacterial counts below these figures at the time of specimen collection, so urine culture is important to rule out a UTI.

Urine samples for bacterial culture may be obtained by the same methods used for obtaining samples for urinalysis; however, the preferred method is cystocentesis. Urine obtained by cystocentesis should be sterile. If urine samples are collected by methods other than cystocentesis, a quantitative urine culture should be requested. If the sample is collected by spontaneous micturition or manual compression, significant numbers of bacteria are present if ≥100,000 colony forming units (CFU)/mL of urine in dogs or ≥10,000 CFU/mL of urine in cats are detected. Samples with >10,000-90,000 CFU/mL in dogs and >1,000-10,000 CFU/mL in cats are suspicious for a UTI. If the sample is collected by catheterization, ≥10,000 CFU/mL in dogs and ≥1,000 CFU/mL in cats is significant, while samples containing 1,000-10,000 CFU/mL in dogs and 100-1,000 CFU/mL in cats are suspicious for a UTI.

Serum Chemistry Profile: Evaluation of serum chemistries, including BUN, creatinine, calcium, phosphorus, and serum electrolytes, is useful in many urinary tract disorders and can provide a crude indication of glomerular filtration rate (GFR). Although elevations in BUN and creatinine are supportive of renal dysfunction, these tests are influenced by nonrenal factors as well. For example, dehydration can cause increases in BUN and serum creatinine not associated with renal failure. BUN can also be influenced by diet and GI bleeding and is considered inferior to creatinine for evaluating GFR. Serum creatinine levels can be falsely lowered in patients with severe muscle wasting and falsely elevated in patients with severe muscle damage. Although BUN and serum creatinine increase as GFR declines, this relationship is not linear. Large changes in GFR early in renal disease cause only small increases in BUN and serum creatinine, while small changes in GFR in advanced renal disease may be associated with large changes in BUN and serum creatinine.

Additional Diagnostic Tests: More sensitive methods for detecting renal dysfunction include plasma clearance tests (eg, inulin clearance), radionuclide techniques, endogenous creatinine clearance, and exogenous creatinine clearance. However, these tests are impractical to perform routinely in clinical practice. The iohexol clearance test is a recently developed alternative for detecting renal dysfunction. It entails recording an accurate body weight, administering a precise amount of iohexol IV, and accurately timing collection of blood samples as directed following administration. This test does not require timed collection of urine samples or special equipment.

Depending on the cause of the urinary tract disorder, radiographic procedures, sonographic examination, and cystoscopic examination of the bladder may provide additional valuable information. The kidneys have a limited range of responses to disease; therefore, renal biopsies are rarely useful when evaluating renal dysfunction. An exception to this is in animals with significant proteinuria.

Blood gas analysis or serum bicarbonate levels provide useful information on acid-base status, especially in animals with renal dysfunction. Metabolic acidosis is a common problem in chronic renal failure and can result in protein catabolism.

Principles of Therapy

Diseases of the urinary system can result from a variety of pathologic processes, and appropriate therapy (as discussed in the following chapters) depends on the location, severity, and etiology of the problem. *See also* systemic pharmacotherapeutics of the urinary system, *Systemic Pharmacotherapeutics of the Urinary System: Introduction* . If the condition is not life threatening, appropriate diagnostic samples should be collected before initiating therapy. It is important to remember that some diagnostic tests and treatments have the potential to cause significant harm. If the specific cause cannot be determined, nonspecific and supportive therapy (eg, monitoring fluids, treating acidosis) should be instituted.

Congenital and Inherited Anomalies of the Urinary System

Congenital and inherited anomalies of the urinary system comprise a group of anatomic defects that may have functional consequences. They are uncommon but remain important components of basic medical knowledge for veterinarians.

Renal Anomalies

Renal Dysplasia and Hypoplasia: These defects are most common in dogs and have been reported in many breeds, including Alaskan Malamutes, Bedlington Terriers, Chow Chows, Cocker Spaniels, Doberman Pinschers, Keeshonden, Lhasa Apsos, Miniature Schnauzers, Norwegian Elkhounds, Samoyeds, Shih Tzus, Soft-coated Wheaten Terriers, and Standard Poodles. Renal dysplasia may be unilateral or bilateral. The kidneys are usually small, firm, and pale; they may have a uniformly diminished renal cortex. Histologic examination reveals immature glomeruli, primitive tubules, and secondary inflammatory lesions, especially interstitial fibrous connective tissue.

Affected animals usually have polydipsia and polyuria that precede signs of uremia. Dwarfing may be noticed if the onset of renal failure occurs within the first few months of life. Urinalysis, hemogram, and blood chemistry changes are the same as in other chronic, progressive renal diseases. Uremia is usually identified between 6 mo and 2 yr of age. The diagnosis is suspected based on the breed and age of disease onset and is confirmed by renal biopsy. Treatment is aimed at managing the associated chronic renal failure.

Renal Agenesis: Renal agenesis is always accompanied by ureteral aplasia and may be associated with aplastic reproductive tissues on the same side. The condition is typically an incidental finding so long as the other kidney is functioning normally. Bilateral agenesis results in early perinatal death.

Polycystic Kidneys: Multiple cysts form within the renal parenchyma, and such kidneys are usually grossly enlarged on palpation. This condition may be associated with hepatic biliary cysts. Polycystic kidneys may cause no clinical signs or may lead to progressive renal failure. This condition is familial in Beagles, Cairn Terriers, Persian cats, and domestic long-haired cats. Diagnosis is based on physical and radiographic findings, ultrasonic examination, or exploratory laparotomy. Pyelonephritis may be seen concurrently and precipitate renal insufficiency.

Simple Renal Cysts: These solitary, unilocular cysts generally do not communicate with the renal collecting system; the rest of the kidney is normal. The origin of these cysts is uncertain. They are usually an incidental finding.

Perirenal Pseudocysts: Perirenal pseudocysts are accumulations of fluid that develop external to the renal parenchyma; they have been identified in cats. Their origin is unknown.

The accumulated fluid may be located between the renal parenchyma and the renal capsule or between the renal capsule and a thin-walled fibrous sac attached to the capsule. They are termed pseudocysts rather than cysts because they are not lined by epithelium. Because only a limited number have been examined histologically, it is unknown whether all perirenal fluid-filled structures are pseudocysts.

The fluid contained within these structures is not urine or lymph but is described as a transudate. Clinical signs are characterized by progressive abdominal enlargement. Abdominal palpation reveals a large, firm, nonpainful mass located in the area of the kidneys. Renal function tests and urinalysis are typically normal; however, a mild azotemia may occur. Diagnosis is made by excretory urography or ultrasono-graphy. Treatment involves exploratory surgery to confirm the diagnosis, drainage of the pseudocyst fluid, and resection of as much of the pseudocyst wall as possible. The prognosis appears to be good; however, only a limited number of cases have been evaluated.

Miscellaneous Renal Anomalies: Double or multiple renal arteries are seen in ~5% of dogs. Other congenital defects include renal malpositioning, renal fusion, and nephroblastoma. Nephroblastoma is an embryonal tumor and is rare in domestic animals except pigs. It may cause no problems but may be very large and cause abdominal distention.

Ureteral Anomalies

This defect is most commonly reported in 3- to 6-mo-old dogs, with females affected 8 times more frequently than males. Other anomalies frequently associated with ectopic ureter include hydroureter, hydronephrosis, renal hypoplasia, bladder hypoplasia, and urethral sphincter incompetence. Continual dripping of urine is the classic sign, although animals with unilateral ectopic ureter may void normally; the inability to void normally suggests bilateral ectopic ureters.

A low-grade vaginitis or vulvitis may also be present due to urine scalding. Involved ureters may open into the urethra, the uterus, or the vagina. Unilateral ectopic ureter is seen with equal frequency on right and left sides, and involvement is bilateral in ~25% of cases. Ectopic ureters generally result from disruption of development of the mesonephric and metanephric duct systems.

A genetic component is suspected on the basis of identifying high-risk breeds (West Highland White Terriers, Fox Terriers, and Miniature and Toy Poodles) and a familial occurrence in Siberian Huskies and Labrador Retrievers. Diagnosis is confirmed by IV urography that traces the course of the ureter. Successful surgical treatments usually involve transplantation of affected ureters into the bladder, or ureteronephrectomy. Indications for ureteronephrectomy may include severe ipsilateral renal disease such as hypoplasia, hydronephrosis, or pyelonephritis in the presence of a normally functioning contralateral kidney. Important postoperative complications are persistent incontinence, hydronephrosis, and dysuria. Incontinence occurs most often in cases of bilateral ectopic ureters and may be due to abnormal development of the bladder neck and urethra. An adrenergic agent such as phenylpropanolamine (0.5-1.5 mg/kg, PO, every 8-12 hr) may help minimize the incontinence.

Miscellaneous Ureteral Anomalies: Less frequently recognised ureteral anomalies include aplasia, duplication, and ureterocele. Ureteroceles are characterized by dilation of the submucosal ureter segment within the bladder. Diagnosis is by excretory urography. Appropriate therapy is ureteronephrectomy if the lesion is unilateral with secondary hydronephrosis and hydroureter. If the proximal ureter and kidney are normal, excision or incision of the ureterocele, in addition to ligation of any ectopic distal channel, has been successful.

Bladder Anomalies

Urachal Remnants: Congenital anomalies resulting from incomplete urachal closure include patent urachus, urachal diverticulum, umbilical urachal sinus, and intra-abdominal urachal cyst. Clinical signs and appropriate therapy depend on the type of anomaly. Patent urachus is typically associated with continuous urinary incontinence, urine scalding of the ventral abdomen, and development of bacterial urinary tract infections. Urachal diverticula also predispose to urinary tract infection by serving as a nidus for bacteria. Definitive diagnosis of both disorders is by positive contrast cystography. Treatment consists of surgical resection and 2-4 wk of appropriate antibiotic therapy when indicated. Surgical resection is the standard treatment for umbilical urachal sinuses and intra-abdominal urachal cysts.

Miscellaneous Bladder Anomalies: Bladder duplication, dysplasia, hypoplasia, agenesis, and exstrophy have been reported and are often associated with other urinary tract defects. Diagnosis is by physical examination, observation of micturition, and contrast radiography. Clinical signs and therapy depend on the type of anomaly.

Urethral Anomalies

Congenital or hereditary urethral anomalies are uncommon; they include urethral agenesis, imperforate urethra, hypospadias, epispadias in combination with bladder exstrophy, urethral duplication, urethral diverticula, urethrorectal fistula, and urethral stenosis.

Hypospadias: This developmental defect results from failure of the urethral grooves to fuse during phallus elongation. The urethral opening is ventral and caudal to the tip of the penis and is classified on the basis of anatomic localisation as glandular, penile, scrotal, perineal, or anal. The penis or scrotum may be underdeveloped as well. Clinical signs depend on the site of the urethral meatus and include urine scalding and complications of increased susceptibility to urinary tract infection. Although surgical correction also depends on the site of the urethral meatus, a modification of the prescrotal urethrostomy is generally useful.

Urethrorectal Fistulas: These appear to be more prevalent in English Bulldogs, possibly as a congenital defect due to abnormal separation of the embryonal cloaca into the urethra and rectum. Clinical signs include hematuria and dysuria secondary to urinary tract infection. Simultaneous passage of urine from the anus and urethra during micturition may be noted. Appropriate therapy consists of surgical correction and concurrent management of urinary tract infection.

Urolithiasis

Urethral Obstruction

Some mineral solutes precipitate to form crystals in urine; these crystals may aggregate and grow to macroscopic size, at which time they are known as uroliths (calculi or stones). Uroliths generally contain an organic matrix that is believed to vary minimally among uroliths and that constitutes ~2-10% of the stone's chemical composition. The remaining 90-98% of the urolith is composed of minerals that vary depending on the type of urolith. Urolithiasis is a general term referring to stones located anywhere within the urinary tract. Uroliths can develop in the kidney, ureter, bladder, or urethra and are referred to as nephroliths, ureteroliths, urocystoliths, and urethroliths, respectively.

Uroliths in all animal species are composed of ~10 different minerals. Identification of the minerals in uroliths by quantitative analysis is unreliable. The type of minerals in uroliths can be readily identified by optical crystallography, infrared spectroscopy, and/or x-ray diffraction. Minerals found in uroliths have a chemical name and often a mineral or crystal name (*Table: Urolith Names*). Variation in urine characteristics over time can result in more than one crystal type within a single urolith. In such instances, the urolith core corresponds to conditions that were present when the urolith initially formed, and the outer layers correspond to more recent conditions that favoured continued growth.

Mechanisms involved in stone formation have not been completely defined. However, three main contributing factors are: 1) matrix—the inorganic protein core may facilitate initial urolith formation, 2) crystallization inhibitors—organic and inorganic crystallization inhibitors may be lacking or dysfunctional in animals with uroliths, and 3) precipitation crystallization factors—a complex relationship among urine solutes and other chemical factors in the urine can lead to conditions favouring crystallization.

Regardless of the underlying mechanism(s), uroliths are not produced unless sufficiently high urine concentrations of urolith-forming constituents exist, and transit time of crystals within the urinary tract is prolonged. For selected stones (eg, struvite, cystine, urate), other favourable conditions (eg, proper pH) for crystallization must also exist. These criteria can be affected by urinary tract infection, diet, intestinal absorption, urine volume, frequency of urination, therapeutic agents, and genetics.

Clinical signs associated with urolithiasis are seldom caused by microscopic crystals. However, formation of macroscopic uroliths in the lower urinary tract that interfere with the flow of urine and/or irritate the mucosal surface often results in dysuria, hematuria, and stranguria. Nephroliths often are asymptomatic unless pyelonephritis exists concurrently or they pass into the ureter.

Ureteral obstruction may produce signs of vomiting, lethargy, and/or flank and renal pain, particularly if there is acute total obstruction with distention of the renal capsule. The only clinical sign associated with unilateral urethroliths may be pain, which can be difficult to detect in dogs and cats. If these initial signs of ureteral obstruction do not lead to a diagnosis, unilateral ureteral obstruction may result in hydronephrosis with loss of function of the ipsilateral kidney. Ureteroliths may also precipitate a uremic crisis in cats with previously compensated chronic renal failure. Because clinical signs of renal dysfunction are generally not apparent until two-thirds or more of total functional renal parenchyma is lost, clinical signs may not be observed unless both ureters are obstructed, there is contralateral chronic kidney disease, or a renal infection develops. Unilateral ureteroliths may be identified serendipitously during abdominal imaging studies or surgery.

Abdominal palpation is helpful in detecting urocystoliths; the bladder wall may be thickened and a grating sensation may be felt when the bladder is palpated. Although palpation may reveal a single large urolith or multiple uroliths by their crepitation, it cannot dependably identify all animals with uroliths; urethral calculi may be detected by rectal palpation or located by passing a catheter.

Because multiple uroliths may be present throughout the urinary tract, a complete radiographic examination of the tract is indicated; radiodense calculi >3 mm in diametre are usually visible on radiographs. Urate, and occasionally cystine, uroliths may be radiolucent, requiring contrast radiography or ultrasonography to confirm their presence. Urinalysis, including identification of crystals on microscopic examination of fresh, warm urine and bacterial culture and sensitivity testing, is a critical part of the evaluation and may be helpful in determining the type of urolith present. Ultrasonography and cystoscopy may also be useful.

Urethral Obstruction: Urethral obstruction is common in male dogs and cats. It may occur suddenly or may develop over days or weeks. Initially, the animal may exhibit frequent attempts to urinate and produce only a fine stream, a few drops, or nothing. Animals may also exhibit extreme pain manifested by crying out when attempting to urinate. Complete obstruction causes uremia within 36-48 hr, which leads to depression, anorexia, vomiting, diarrhea, dehydration, coma, and death within ~72 hr. Urethral obstruction is an emergency condition, and treatment should begin immediately.

If the bladder is intact, it is distended, hard, and painful; care should be used when palpating the bladder to avoid iatrogenic rupture. If the bladder has ruptured, it cannot be palpated and urine can sometimes, but not always, be obtained from the abdominal cavity by paracentesis. Animals with spontaneous bladder rupture may appear temporarily improved because the pain associated with bladder distention has been relieved; however, peritonitis and absorption of uremic toxins and potassium occur rapidly and lead to depression, abdominal distention, cardiac arrhythmias, and death.

Hyperkalemia and metabolic acidosis are life-threatening complications of urethral obstruction. An ECG (to record cardiac rhythm and rate) and a serum potassium are indicated. Initial emergency care involves immediate relief of obstruction by catheterization and fluid therapy with normal saline. Occasionally, an obstruction at the external urethral orifice can be dislodged by gentle massage.

Sometimes, when a portion of the urethra is dilated with fluid under pressure and then suddenly released, urethral calculi can be flushed out. The urolith nearly always can be flushed back into the bladder by using the largest catheter that can be easily passed to the calculus, occluding the distal end of the urethral lumen around the catheter, and infusing a sterile mixture of equal parts of isotonic saline solution and an aqueous lubricant.

If the urethrolith cannot be flushed back into the bladder, a urethrotomy should be performed to remove the obstructing stone(s). Depending on the clinical circumstances, the urethrotomy site may be sutured or a permanent urethrostomy created. Calculi that are flushed back into the bladder should be removed by cystotomy to prevent recurrence, although in some cases they can be dissolved. The stone should be sent for quantitative analysis, and the animal managed medically to prevent stone recurrence based on the results.

Urolithiasis in Ruminants

Uroliths in cattle, sheep, and goats are common. Although uroliths can be found anywhere within the urinary tract, urethroliths are responsible for most clinical problems. Obstruction induced by urethroliths causes urine retention and leads to bladder distention, abdominal pain, and eventual urethral perforation or bladder rupture, with death from uremia or septicemia. It is an important disease of feeder animals but is also seen in mature breeding animals. Urolithiasis is seen most often during winter in steers and wethers on full feed, or on range during severe weather conditions with limited water intake, especially when the water has a high mineral content. Urolithiasis has no specific geographic distribution, and the different urolith types reflect the mineral distribution of the feed. Uroliths occur in either sex, but obstructive urolithiasis develops primarily in males because of anatomic differences.

Etiology and Pathogenesis: Ruminant urolithiasis is considered primarily a nutritional disease. The prevalence of urolithiasis in the USA is highest in calves, lambs, and kids castrated at an early age and fed high-grain diets with roughly a 1:1 calcium to phosphorus ratio or a diet high in magnesium. Ruminants fed high-grain diets with a low calcium to phosphorus ratio are at increased risk of developing struvite uroliths, while ruminants grazing on silica-rich soil are predisposed to form silica uroliths. Diets high in calcium (eg, subterranean clover) may result in calcium carbonate uroliths, while plants such as halogeton or tops from the common sugar beet may be a factor in calcium oxalate formation. The mineral composition of water, in concert with dietary mineral imbalances, probably contributes more to initiating urolith formation than does the lack of water itself. A definitive diagnosis of urolithiasis in a single animal suggests that all males in the population are at risk for the disease.

The distal aspect of the sigmoid flexure of cattle and the sigmoid flexure and urethral process of sheep and goats are the most common sites for uroliths to lodge. Irritation at the site of lodging causes inflammation and swelling that contributes to urethral occlusion. Castration of young males also predisposes to urolith-induced urethral obstruction by removing hormonal influences necessary for mature development of the penis and urethra.

Clinical Findings: Clinical signs may be associated with partial or complete urethral occlusion. Animals with partial obstruction dribble blood-tinged urine after prolonged, painful (stranguria) attempts at urination; before complete occlusion occurs, urine may dry on the preputial hairs and leave detectable mineral deposits. Animals with complete urethral obstruction exhibit tenesmus, tail twitching, weight shifting, and signs consistent with colic. Inappetence, bloat, depression, and rectal prolapse may also be seen. Affected steers may elevate the tail and show urethral pulsations just ventral to the rectum. Goats may vocalize.

Common sequelae of complete urethral obstruction include urethral perforation or urinary bladder rupture. Bladder rupture often results in death from uremia. The disease course may be 5-7 days. Although urethral perforation may also cause uremia and death, it is not uncommon for the ventral abdominal skin to necrose and slough, allowing the development of a pseudourethra.

Diagnosis: Diagnosis based on the history, clinical signs, and physical examination is usually straightforward. Hypersensitivity in the region of the sigmoid flexure may be evident. Palpation may identify abnormal pulsations of the urethra and tissue swelling associated with the obstruction. Rectal palpation may reveal an enlarged, distended bladder, or the bladder may be nonpalpable, consistent with bladder rupture.

Examination of the urethral process in sheep and goats may reveal the occluding urolith. If early clinical signs of obstructive uropathy are missed, the animal may show only inappetence, depression, subcutaneous swelling along the penis, or uroperitoneum; abdominal distention due to uroperitoneum must be differentiated from ruminal tympany, peritonitis, peritoneal tumors, and GI tract obstructions.

Ballottement allows detection of the fluid, and when viewing the animal from behind, the abdomen appears symmetrically enlarged and pear-shaped. Ultrasound examination of the abdomen reveals a large amount of hypoechoic fluid. Confirmation is obtained by examining fluid collected by abdominocentesis and finding that the creatinine in peritoneal fluid is 2 times or more that in plasma. Subcutaneous swellings along the prepuce and ventral abdomen due to a perforated urethra must be differentiated from traumatic injury, subcutaneous abscesses, and umbilical or ventral hernias. In breeding animals, preputial lacerations with prolapse and sheath infection, and hematoma of the penis must also be differentiated. In animals with clinical signs of acute colic, other causes of abdominal pain must be eliminated; these diseases include indigestion, stasis or obstruction of the GI tract, primary enteritis, abomasal ulcers, and coccidiosis.

Treatment and Control: Treatment of obstructive urolithiasis generally involves establishing a patent urethra and correcting fluid and electrolyte imbalances. In many instances, surgical management of the obstruction is all that is necessary; however, severely uremic and depressed animals require rehydration and correction of acid-base and electrolyte abnormalities. If a rupture of the urinary tract has occurred, hyponatremia, hypochloremia, hyperphosphatemia, and metabolic alkalosis with variable potassium concentrations are found. Treatment with IV normal saline is indicated. The volume of fluid administered should be calculated to correct clinical dehydration. Once the animal is rehydrated, fluid therapy may be continued to encourage diuresis.

Animals with an intact urethra and bladder, with early clinical signs of obstructive urethral disease, may benefit from conservative therapy using antispasmodics and tranquilizers. This is believed to relax the retractor penis muscles with straightening of the sigmoid flexure. However, conservative therapy is only rarely beneficial in small ruminants, and is warranted only in cases of acute or partial obstruction without evidence of urethral or bladder damage; it should not be used in complicated or advanced cases. Uroliths trapped within the urethral process of sheep and goats may be removed by gentle manipulation or by amputation of the urethral process. Proper restraint, tranquilization, and a regional anesthetic are necessary. The techniques may vary, but the typical procedure requires exteriorization of the penis. Although amputation may be effective, relief is typically temporary (<2 days) in most animals, in which obstruction recurs due to the presence of multiple uroliths.

Perineal urethrostomy has also been recommended as an effective surgical technique in castrated males. Short-term complications associated with perineal urethrostomy may include postoperative hemorrhage, surgical wound dehiscence, and subcutaneous urine accumulation. Urethral stricture is a common longterm complication. In addition, perineal urethrostomy is associated with loss of breeding ability in intact males. In more complicated cases, such as those with urethral perforation, amputation of the penis proximal to the sigmoid flexure or near the perineal area may be necessary as a salvage procedure. Animals that develop urethral perforation also require drainage of accumulated subcutaneous urine; this is accomplished by lancing the skin overlying the area of accumulated urine. Topical antiseptics and fly repellents may be applied to these ventral lacerations, and parenteral antibiotics are recommended to prevent infection.

Cystotomy followed by dietary management is believed to be a more effective longterm solution to urolithiasis in sheep and goats than is perineal urethrostomy. Cystotomy allows removal of multiple urocystoliths, permits bidirectional urethral flushing, and poses less risk for urethral stricture. Tube cystotomy is generally considered the treatment of choice, allowing time for the calculi to be expelled spontaneously.

If the bladder is ruptured, the ability to urinate must be restored and uremia corrected. In animals with substantial uroperitoneum, the peritoneal cavity should be slowly drained using a teat tube or trocar. Urine removal may also reduce the severity of peritonitis and make the animal more comfortable. Fluid, electrolyte, and acid-base homeostasis normally returns within 24 hr after restoration of a patent urinary system. Persistent uremia indicates the possibility of hydronephrosis or ascending pyelonephritis, or both. A urethrostomy should be performed to provide unobstructed passage of urine. Attempts to surgically repair the ruptured bladder have been largely unsuccessful due to the chronic distention prior to rupture. The bladder may heal spontaneously after urethrostomy and removal of abdominal fluid; however, these animals are best salvaged within 3-4 mo to avoid further complications. Despite treatment, some animals fail to pass urine effectively and the uroperitoneum recurs. These animals may be treated by performing tube cystotomy, followed by appropriate antibiotic and fluid therapy.

Several measures to prevent the formation of urethral calculi have been recommended. The most important is to provide a calcium: phosphorus ratio of 2:1 in the complete ration. Intensive concentrate feeding, such as in many finishing programs, frequently leads to urolith formation and urethral obstruction. Thus, any feeding program incorporating concentrate feeding must include appropriate calcium supplementation. Adjunct measures to minimize the formation of urethral calculi include adding sodium chloride up to 4% of the total ration. This promotes increased sodium and chloride concentration in the urine, water intake, and urine dilution, which increases the mineral solubility. Ammonium chloride can be used as a urinary acidifying agent (7-10 g/head/day for a 30-kg lamb or kid; 50-80 g/head/day for a 240-kg steer). Urine acidification antagonizes magnesium-ammonium-phosphate crystal formation and has been shown empirically to be a useful preventive measure. These adjunct measures should not be used in lieu of a properly balanced ration. In operations with a significant problem of urolith formation, evaluation of the ration is the most important measure that can be taken to reduce the incidence.

Urolithiasis in Horses

Urolithiasis is a less common condition in horses than in small ruminants or steers. The disease can affect immature horses but is seen most frequently in adults. There is no breed predilection. Urolithiasis is seen more frequently in males than females, which has been attributed to anatomic differences between the male and female urethra.

Equine uroliths have a diametre of 0.5-21 cm, weigh as much as 6.5 kg, and are found most often within the bladder. Most equine uroliths are composed of calcium carbonate, in various hydrated forms, with struvite uroliths occasionally noted. Calcium carbonate uroliths have 2 separate clinical forms. The first form is a concretion of salts and mucoproteins that varies in consistency from friable to firm. These uroliths are usually yellow and oval or irregularly shaped; they frequently have a rough or spiculated surface and are generally soft enough to be fragmented during surgery. The second calcium carbonate form is a firm concretion that is hard and resistant to fragmentation and is typically smooth and white. There appears to be no difference in chemical composition between these forms.

Etiology: The mechanism of urolith formation in horses is unknown, although the alkaline pH and high mineral content of normal equine urine may favour crystal formation and precipitation. Normal equine urine also contains large amounts of mucoproteins, which may serve as a cementing substance to adhere crystals. Consumption of feed and water high in mineral content may increase urinary solute concentrations and thereby promote crystallization and precipitation. Multiple nephroliths may develop in horses with renal papillary necrosis (associated with NSAID administration while dehydrated) and mineralization of the papillae.

Clinical Findings: Clinical signs depend on the urolith location. Most uroliths are located in the bladder and cause dysuria, pollakiuria, and hematuria. Hematuria is most evident after exercise and toward the end of a voided urine stream. Affected horses frequently stretch out to urinate and may maintain this posture for variable periods before and after micturition. Additional signs may include scalding of the perineum in females or of the medial aspect of the hindlimbs in males. Geldings and stallions may protrude the penis flaccidly for prolonged periods while intermittently dribbling urine. Affected horses may occasionally exhibit recurrent bouts of colic or an altered hindlimb gait. Urethral obstruction may also develop as the result of a trapped urolith and is typically accompanied by restlessness, sweating, varying degrees of colic, and frequent attempts to urinate. The bladder is distended on rectal examination. In most fatal cases, a single large urolith, occasionally accompanied by smaller ones, is found in the bladder; less frequently, the urolith may be found lodged at the bladder neck or the ischial arch. Nephroliths are occasionally found via ultrasonography in horses with cystic calculi; owners of such horses should be informed that obstruction may recur.

Bilateral nephroliths are not uncommon in adult horses that have been used for performance. Intermittent chronic obstruction of ureters will eventually cause renal failure, resulting in weight loss and anorexia.

Diagnosis: Tentative diagnosis of urolithiasis is usually based on the history and clinical signs and confirmed most easily by rectal palpation of a firm, ovoid, intravesicular mass at or near the neck of the bladder. In most cases, urolith palpation is not difficult because clinical signs are rarely evident until the stone is several centimetres in diametre. Transrectal ultrasonography with a 7.5 mHz linear probe allows visualization of the stone. If ultrasound examination cannot be performed, the distended bladder should be catheterized to facilitate palpation and eliminate the possibility of urethroliths, urethral stricture, or smegma impaction of the urethral sinus. Urinalysis frequently reveals RBC, neutrophils, calcium carbonate crystals, and proteinuria.

Cystoscopy, ultrasonography, and radiology are not essential for detection of urocystoliths in horses but may provide additional diagnostic or prognostic information. Ultrasonography is necessary to identify nephroliths.

Treatment: Several surgical procedures have been described for urocystolith removal. The surgical options include midline or paramedian laparotomy and cystotomy, pararectal cystotomy, subischial urethrostomy, urethral sphincterotomy, and laser lithotripsy. The selection of a procedure is dictated by the size, location, and number of uroliths; the sex and physiologic status of the horse; and the availability of surgical facilities.

Uroperitoneum in Foals

Uroperitoneum is defined as urine leakage into the peritoneal space. In foals, this most commonly results from tearing of the bladder during parturition or rupture of the urachus secondary to umbilical abscessation. Ureteral or urethral tears are rare. Some studies indicate a higher incidence of bladder rupture in males than in females, possibly because the narrower pelvis and the longer, narrower urethra of colts is a predisposing factor. Urachal rupture occurs in both males and females. Traumatic bladder rupture is thought to be caused by uterine contractions on a full bladder as the foal passes through the birth canal. Although most ruptured bladders at birth are thought to be traumatic, the presence of smooth edges and absence of hemorrhage around the tear in some foals suggest a congenital origin (developmental defect of the bladder wall). Most bladder tears are located on the dorsum of the bladder. In the case of a ruptured urachus, infection in the umbilical stump can weaken the urachal wall and result in leakage of urine into the abdomen. Prematurity, cystitis, ascending infection, abdominal trauma, failure of passive transfer, and sepsis may predispose the foal to bladder rupture.

Clinical Findings: Foals generally appear normal at birth but progressively become lethargic, tachycardic, and tachypneic over 24-48 hr. Signs may not appear for a longer period in foals with a ruptured urachus. As the condition progresses, the abdomen becomes noticeably distended, and ballottement may produce a fluid wave. Most foals attempt to urinate often, with small amounts of urine being produced. This stranguria is often misinterpreted as straining to defecate. Other foals may be anuric or urinate normally.

Diagnosis: Blood and peritoneal fluid analysis can be helpful in diagnosis. Foals usually have a neutrophilic leukocytosis. Serum hyperkalemia combined with hyponatremia and hypochloremia are seen due to the high concentration of potassium and low levels of sodium and chloride in the urine, which rapidly equilibrate across the peritoneum. An ECG may show broad QRS complexes and very tall T waves due to hyperkalemia. The increased serum potassium predisposes the foal to bradycardia and cardiac arrhythmias (AV block, atrial standstill, and cardiac arrest) if not corrected. Serum BUN and creatinine values can be normal or increased. Blood gas analysis may also be normal or reveal a metabolic acidosis. Abdominal fluid is pale yellow and copious and can be easily detected on ultrasonographic evaluation. The creatinine level in the peritoneal fluid is at least double that in the serum. This test is the most accurate in diagnosing the problem. If laboratory testing is not available, then 10 mL of methylene blue can be injected into the bladder via a urinary catheter. If the bladder is patent to the peritoneal space, then dye should be seen in the peritoneal fluid within 15 min.

The clinical signs of progressive depression and stranguria can confuse the diagnosis. Differential diagnoses include septicemia (*Septicemia in Foals: Introduction*), hypoxic ischemic encephalopathy (*Hypoxic Ischemic Encephalopathy: Introduction*), persistent meconium impaction, or colic for other reasons.

In the case of a urachal rupture, abdominal ultrasonography may be helpful to establish an etiologic diagnosis. Ultrasonography of the umbilical remnants may suggest the presence of infection or abscessation. A large amount of fluid in the abdomen is also seen.

Treatment: Surgery is necessary to correct the defect and, in uncomplicated cases, is very successful. The foal should be stabilized before surgery. Potassium >5 mEq/L should be lowered preoperatively by administration of insulin at 0.1 mg/kg, IV, in 500 mL of normal saline plus 5% dextrose, over 30-40 min. Sodium bicarbonate administration is also helpful in driving potassium into cells. Peritoneal dialysis can be considered if the above treatment is unsuccessful.

The bladder should be repaired using absorbable sutures. Because surgical staples have migrated into the bladder and become the nidus for stone formation at a later date, they should not be used. If the umbilical structures are enlarged (indicating infection), they should be removed at the time of surgery and cultured. After surgical correction of the bladder, an indwelling urinary catheter may be placed for 48 hr to decrease bladder distention and leakage of urine at the repair site.

If a bladder rupture is recognised early in an otherwise healthy foal and the foal is stabilized appropriately prior to surgery, the prognosis for recovery is good to excellent, with success rates as high as 95%. In septic or premature foals, in which complications such as peritonitis, incisional complications, adhesions, and anesthetic death are encountered more frequently, the prognosis is fair.

Chapter 6

Infectious Diseases of the Urinary System in Small Animals

Pyelonephritis

Kidney infection (pyelonephritis) is usually due to ascending bacteria, although hematogenous spread is possible. The organisms and predisposing causes are similar to those of bacterial cystitis. Renoliths and ureteroliths, which impede the normal flow of urine out of the renal pelvis, are a common cause. In young dogs or cats, congenital malformations (eg, ectopic ureters) are a predisposing cause. Animals at risk for pyelonephritis are the very young, the very old, the immunosuppressed, or those with inadequate urine-concentrating ability. In many instances, an underlying cause is not identified.

Animals with acute pyelonephritis exhibit kidney or flank pain, fever, malaise, and sometimes vomiting, polyuria, and polydipsia. Urinalysis shows proteinuria, pyuria, bacteriuria, and/or hematuria. WBC casts are often present in fresh urine sediment. The urine culture is usually positive; the CBC may show leukocytosis with a left shift. The biochemical profile may be normal or show azotemia (prerenal or renal) and/or hyperglobulinemia. The animal may be in renal failure. Chronic pyelonephritis is more difficult to recognise because clinical signs may be subtle or absent. Polyuria and polydipsia are frequent. In many cases, the disease goes unrecognised until renal failure occurs. Although abnormalities in the urinalysis are present, they are often less dramatic than with acute kidney infection. A single urine culture can be negative if bacterial numbers are low. Other useful diagnostic tests include renal ultrasonography and IV pyelograms. Both studies may show dilation of one or both renal pelvises secondary to inflammation and partial obstruction. Asymmetric renal size and architectural changes with renal pelvic dilatation is highly suggestive of chronic pyelonephritis. In some cases, nephropyelocentesis via ultrasonographic guidance is useful to obtain a sample of urine from the dilated renal pelvis for analysis and culture.

Pyelonephritis should be treated aggressively with broad-spectrum antibiotics, based on urine culture and antimicrobial susceptibility testing, for 4-6 wk. The infection may respond to the same antibiotics recommended for cystitis, but more frequent administration (eg, amoxicillin tid rather than bid) and/or higher dosages are indicated.

A fluoroquinolone or a combination of a fluoroquinolone with a α-lactam antibiotic is often effective. Dosages should be the same as for other soft-tissue infections. Animals that are febrile, anorectic, dehydrated, or azotemic should be hospitalized for IV antibiotics and fluid therapy.

Fluid therapy may prevent acute pyelonephritis from progressing to acute renal failure and will improve renal perfusion and uremic signs in animals already in renal failure. Animals with acute pyelonephritis may recover normal renal function, depending on the amount of damage that occurred prior to treatment. In selected cases of chronic pyelonephritis with a severely hydronephrotic, nonfunctional kidney, a nephrectomy may be the treatment of choice once the animal has been stabilized. This will remove the source of infection and hopefully save the opposite kidney. IV pyelography and/or renal scintigraphy are useful to assess the relative function of each kidney. If both kidneys are severely affected, medical management alone is the only alternative. Recovery to chronic, stable renal failure is possible in many cases.

The urine should be cultured after the first 5-7 days of therapy to assess antibiotic efficacy. A urinalysis and culture should be repeated 3-5 days following therapy, and then monthly for 3 consecutive months. If all of these cultures are negative, the interval between urine cultures may be gradually lengthened. Animals with pyelonephritis are at high risk for persistence or recurrence of kidney infection.

Interstitial Nephritis

Acute interstitial nephritis in dogs is caused most often by Leptospira *interrogans* (*Leptospirosis in Dogs*). Cats can develop leptospirosis, although signs are less severe than in dogs. Other infectious causes of interstitial nephritis in dogs include Leishmania *donovani* and Borrelia *burgdorferi*. Glomerulonephritis is the predominant renal pathology, so these diseases are considered immune complex diseases rather than true infections. Infectious diseases that cause vasculitis in dogs or cats (eg, feline infectious peritonitis, Rocky Mountain spotted fever, ehrlichiosis) may also cause renal failure.

Capillaria Plica *Infection*

Capillaria plica may infect the urinary bladder, and occasionally the ureters and renal pelvises, of dogs and cats. Distribution is worldwide, and wild animals appear to be the primary hosts. A similar but less common organism, C *felis cati*, is also found in cats.

Dogs and cats become infected with C *plica* by eating earthworms that contain the first-stage larvae. The worms are threadlike, yellowish, and 13-60 mm long. The eggs are colourless, operculated, have a slightly pitted shell, and are 63-68 × 24-27 μm in size.

Most dogs and cats are asymptomatic. Some animals show signs of pollakiuria, urinary incontinence, and urinating in abnormal places. The eggs are shed in the urine and may be found in the urine sediment. Microscopic hematuria and increased numbers of epithelial cells may also be present. Reported treatments include levamisole, fenbendazole, albendazole, and ivermectin. The treatment of choice is unknown, but a single dose of ivermectin at 0.2 mg/kg, SC, is likely to be effective. It is not FDA approved for this use and is contraindicated in Collie breeds. The parasite may be self-limiting in the absence of reinfection.

Giant Kidney Worm Infection in Mink and Dogs

Mink are the most common definitive host for Dioctophyma renale, the largest known nematode, which has a worldwide distribution. Many other species, including dogs and humans, can become infected. The definitive host contracts the parasite by ingesting encysted larvae in raw fish (eg, pike, bullhead) or frogs, or by ingesting an infected annelid worm. The larvae penetrate the bowel wall and migrate first to the liver and later to the kidneys. In dogs, the parasite often fails to reach the kidneys and may be found free in the abdominal cavity. Kidney worms grow larger in dogs than in mink, reaching up to 103 cm. Female worms are larger than male worms, and both are blood red. Both male and female worms must be present in the same kidney to complete the life cycle. Barrel-shaped, yellow-brown eggs with a thick pitted shell measuring 71-84 × 45-52 μm are shed into the urine.

In the kidneys, the worm(s) cause obstruction, hydronephrosis, and destruction of the renal parenchyma. The right kidney is most commonly affected in both mink and dogs. Kidney failure can result if both kidneys are parasitized. Chronic peritonitis, adhesions, and liver disease are also possible, especially in dogs.

Clinical signs are hematuria, pollakiuria, weight loss, and renal or abdominal pain. Urinalysis may reveal proteinuria, hematuria, and pyuria. IV pyelography or ultrasonography shows the enlarged hydronephrotic kidney.

The diagnosis is made by finding the eggs in the urine sediment if both sexes of the nematode are present in the kidney and the ureter is patent. Alternatively, exploratory laparotomy may reveal the diagnosis. Worms may be found in the peritoneal cavity, between the lobes of the liver, or within the affected kidney(s) via nephrotomy. Unilateral nephrectomy is the treatment of choice if the opposite kidney is unaffected. Preventing ingestion of raw fish or other aquatic organisms is recommended, especially in areas where the parasite is known to infect wild animals.

Bacterial Cystitis

Bacterial cystitis is infection and inflammation of the urinary bladder. Clinical signs are pollakiuria, hematuria, dysuria, and urinating in inappropriate places. Hematuria may be more noticeable at the end of the urine stream. An animal may exhibit pain on palpation of the caudal abdomen, and the bladder may feel thickened or irregular. Bacterial cystitis is occasionally diagnosed in an asymptomatic animal when a routine urinalysis is performed. Chronic glucocorticoid administration or hyperadrenocorticism are sometimes associated with asymptomatic urinary tract infections.

Urinalysis often shows increased protein and hemoglobin on the dipstick. The WBC part of the dipstick (ie, nitrate) is inaccurate in dogs and cats and should not be used. The urine pH may be alkaline (7.5-9.0) if the bacteria are urease positive (eg, Staphylococcus or Proteus). An alkaline urine pH by itself is not abnormal, however, as diet and other factors can affect urine pH. Urine sediment should be examined microscopically. Increased numbers of WBC, RBC, and/or bacteria are consistent with cystitis. Bacteria can be confused with stain precipitate; filtering the stain or evaluating the sediment without staining is advised. Lack of visible bacteria in the sediment does not rule out urinary tract infection.

If clinical signs and/or urinalysis are suggestive of infection, a urine culture and antimicrobial susceptibility should be performed. Cystocentesis is the preferred method for sample collection, followed by sterile urethral catheterization or a midstream free catch into a sterile collection cup. A quantitative culture is necessary to interpret the result, especially with samples not collected by cystocentesis. Ideally, the culture should be set up within 2 hr of collection. If the laboratory is off-site, the sample should be refrigerated and processed by the laboratory within 24 hr. If the specimen cannot be refrigerated, commercial collection kits that contain preservatives can be used to maintain a stable bacterial population at room temperature for 24 hr. Laboratories that can provide both quantitative culturing and a minimum inhibitory concentration-based method for antimicrobial susceptibility testing are preferred.

Simple bacterial cystitis is treated for 2 wk with a broad-spectrum antibiotic that achieves a high concentration in the urine. Appropriate initial choices include amoxicillin (10-20 mg/kg, PO, bid-tid), cefadroxil (22-30 mg/kg, PO, bid), or ometoprim-sulfadimethoxine (27 mg/kg, PO, day one, then 13.5 mg/kg, PO, sid). A repeat urine culture 3-5 days following therapy is recommended. If positive, another antibiotic based on the new susceptibility results is given for a longer treatment period (eg, 3-4 wk). Very resistant or recurrent infections should be treated for 4-6 wk. Every course of treatment should be followed by a urine culture, even if the signs have resolved. In animals that have a history of chronic or recurrent infections, a urine culture should be done every month for 3 mo following therapy. If all of these cultures are negative, then a urine culture every 2-4 mo for the next year is advisable. Because resistance to antibiotics can develop during therapy, antimicrobial susceptibility testing should be performed on every positive urine culture.

Animals with resistant or recurrent bacterial cystitis should be evaluated for an underlying cause. The history may reveal chronic glucocorticoid use. Survey abdominal radiographs are frequently diagnostic for cystic calculi. Negative survey films should be followed by double contrast cystourethrography, ultrasonography, and/or cystoscopy to rule out radiolucent urocystoliths, anatomic defects, and neoplasia. A serum biochemical profile and CBC are important to rule out predisposing systemic diseases. Other diagnostic considerations include feline immunodeficiency virus, feline leukemia virus, and hyperthyroidism in cats and hyperadrenocorticism in dogs.

In cases that respond to therapy but continue to have frequent bouts of cystitis without an identifiable cause, low-dose prophylactic antibiotics can be used to prevent ascending bacteria from establishing an infection according to the following protocol: 1) a therapeutic course of an antibiotic for the current infection is completed, 2) no antibiotics are given for 3 days, to allow collection of urine for a post-treatment culture, and 3) the prophylactic protocol is immediately started. Prophylaxis consists of using a broad-spectrum antibiotic (eg, amoxicillin, cefadroxil) at 1/3 of the total daily dose, given at bedtime, indefinitely. Every 6-8 wk, the antibiotic should be stopped for 3-5 days to obtain a sample for repeat urinalysis and culture. Every new infection should be treated with a therapeutic course of an antibiotic based on culture and susceptibility results. The treatment antibiotic will likely be different than the prophylactic antibiotic. The most valuable therapeutic antibiotics (eg, fluoroquinolones, second-generation cephalosporins) should be reserved for resistant infections. If the recurrent infection is resistant to the prophylactic antibiotic, this antibiotic can still be used for future prophylaxis after the infection is eradicated.

Encouraging frequent voiding during the daytime is helpful in preventing recurrent infections.

Noninfectious Diseases of the Urinary System in Small Animals

Renal Dysfunction: Overview

Failure of the filtration function of the kidneys leads to the development of azotemia (an excess of nitrogenous compounds in the blood), which may be classified as prerenal, renal, postrenal, or of mixed origin. Prerenal azotemia develops whenever mean systemic arterial blood pressure declines to values <60 mm Hg and/or when dehydration causes plasma protein concentration to increase. Conditions that may lead to the development of prerenal azotemia include dehydration, congestive heart failure, and shock. Prerenal azotemia generally resolves with appropriate treatment, because kidney structure has not been altered, which allows normal function to resume once renal perfusion has been restored. Renal azotemia refers to a reduction in glomerular filtration rate (GFR) of ~75% during acute or chronic primary renal (or intrarenal) diseases. Postrenal azotemia develops when the integrity of the urinary tract is disrupted (eg, bladder rupture) or urine outflow is obstructed (eg, urethral or bilateral ureteral obstruction). Once adequate urine flow is restored, postrenal azotemia will resolve.

Chronic Kidney Disease

This disease process involves a loss of functional renal tissue due to a prolonged (≥3 mo), usually progressive process. Dramatic changes in renal structure may be seen, although structural and functional changes in the kidney are only loosely correlated. Chronic kidney disease often smolders for many months or years before it becomes clinically apparent, and is invariably irreversible and progressive. Although congenital disease results in a transient increase in prevalence in animals <3 yr old, the prevalence increases with advancing age from 5-6 yr. In geriatric populations at referral institutions, chronic kidney disease affects up to 10% of dogs and 35% of cats. The prevalence in the general small animal population is likely to be lower. Several breeds of dogs and cats are afflicted with heritable chronic kidney disease. There is no apparent breed or sex predisposition for nonheritable chronic kidney disease in dogs or cats.

Chronic kidney disease is generally classified into various stages (*Table: International Renal Interest Society Classification of Stages of Kidney Disease*) based on laboratory tests and clinical signs. In Stage I, a process is damaging the kidneys but azotemia and clinical signs have not developed. Unfortunately, renal disease is uncommonly detected at this stage. In Stage II, the disease has progressed, GFR has fallen to <25% of normal, and azotemia is present, but clinical signs are not yet observed. However, this stage may be associated with impaired urine-concentrating ability and increased urine volume. Stage III occurs when GFR has declined further and both azotemia and clinical signs are often present. Stage IV reflects further progression and severe azotemia, with clinical signs present. This staging system applies to both chronic and acute kidney disease.

Etiology: Attempting to identify the primary process causing the kidney disease, especially in Stages I and II, is important to form a prognosis and treatment plan. Known causes of chronic kidney disease include diseases of the macrovascular compartment (eg, systemic hypertension, coagulopathies, chronic hypoperfusion), microvascular compartment (eg, systemic and glomerular hypertension, glomerulonephritis, developmental disorders, congenital collagen defects, amyloidosis), interstitial compartment (eg, pyelonephritis, neoplasia, obstructive uropathy, allergic and immune-mediated nephritis), and tubular compartment (eg, tubular reabsorptive defects, chronic low-grade nephrotoxicity, obstructive uropathy). Many causes of chronic, generalized renal disease are associated with progressive interstitial fibrosis. The severity of interstitial fibrosis is positively correlated to the magnitude of decline of GFR and negatively correlated with the prognosis. The glomerular, tubulointerstitial, and vascular lesions found in animals with generalized, chronic renal disease are often similar, regardless of the initiating cause. At this point, renal histology may show only marked interstitial fibrosis, which may be called chronic interstitial nephritis. This term describes the morphologic appearance of kidneys with end-stage chronic disease of any cause. Because acute kidney disease may progress to a chronic condition, any cause of acute kidney disease is also a possible cause of chronic kidney disease.

Clinical Findings: Generally, no clinical signs are observed as a direct result of disease until ≥75% of nephron function has been impaired (Stages III and IV). Exceptions are chronic kidney diseases that develop as part of a systemic disease with clinical signs referable to involvement of other body tissues (eg, systemic lupus erythematosus, systemic hypertension) or those associated with marked renal inflammation and capsular swelling leading to flank pain and occasionally to vomiting. Clinical evaluation may identify systemic hypertension and proteinuria with the nephrotic syndrome in any stage. Usually, the earliest clinical signs commonly attributable to renal dysfunction are polydipsia and polyuria, which are not observed until the function of approximately two-thirds of the nephrons has been impaired (late Stage II or early Stage III). Further destruction of renal tissue leads to azotemia without new clinical signs in Stage II, and finally to the clinically apparent uremic syndrome in Stage IV. Initially, uremia is associated with occasional vomiting and lethargy. As disease progresses within Stages III and IV over months (dogs) to years (cats), anorexia, weight loss, dehydration, oral ulceration, vomiting, and diarrhea become fully manifest. Loose teeth, deformable maxilla and mandible, or pathologic fractures may be seen with renal secondary osteodystrophy (*Renal Secondary Hyperparathyroidism*), but these are uncommon and generally observed only in young dogs with end-stage congenital renal disease. Physical examination and imaging studies of animals in Stages III and IV usually reveal small, irregular kidneys, although normal to large kidneys can be observed in animals with neoplasms, hydronephrosis, or glomerulonephritis. Mucous membranes are pale in late Stage III and Stage IV, due to the presence of a nonregenerative, normocytic, normochromic anemia.

Diagnosis: In Stages I and II, diagnosis is often missed or made incidentally during imaging studies or urinalyses conducted for other purposes. In Stages III and IV, the BUN, serum creatinine, and inorganic phosphorus concentrations are increased. Potassium depletion, due to renal potassium wasting combined with inadequate intake and the kaliuretic effects of acidosis, is frequently seen in cats and occasionally seen in dogs. Hyperkalemia associated with oliguria and anuria may be noted in terminal Stage IV or whenever marked prerenal azotemia is superimposed on chronic kidney disease. Systemic hypertension and associated complications develop in ~20% of affected cats and dogs and can occur at any stage. Osteoporosis may be seen radiographically, although this late finding is generally not helpful for diagnosis. In healthy dogs and cats, urine specific gravity generally ranges from 1.001-1.070, depending on body needs for water homeostasis; the normal range overlaps the abnormal or inappropriate range. In dogs and cats with dehydration and normal renal function, urine specific gravity should be >1.035. The inability to produce concentrated urine when challenged by dehydration is an early sign of chronic kidney disease; however, dogs with primary glomerular disease, and some cats, may become azotemic while retaining the ability to concentrate urine to a specific gravity >1.035. Even so, concentrated urine is rarely observed when the serum creatinine is >4 mg/dL in an animal with azotemia of renal origin.

The polydipsia and polyuria of chronic kidney disease must be differentiated from diseases that cause primary polydipsia (eg, psychogenic polydipsia, hyperthyroidism) or interfere directly with the urine-concentrating mechanism. This includes conditions that lead to retention of solute in tubular fluid (eg, diuretic administration, diabetes mellitus), central diabetes insipidus, and nephrogenic diabetes insipidus (eg, hyperadrenocorticism, hypercalcemia, pyometra, diseases causing septicemia). Adrenal insufficiency leads to a urine-concentrating defect and may thus be confused with Stage II and III oliguric renal disease because prerenal azotemia may be caused by the vomiting, diarrhea, and polydipsia associated with hypoadrenocorticism. Hyperkalemia, hyponatremia, and/or reduced plasma Na+/K+ ratio is most helpful in establishing a tentative diagnosis of adrenal insufficiency, which must be confirmed by hormonal assay(s). Also, animals with hypoadrenocorticism improve rapidly in response to proper therapy.

Combinations of survey radiography, abdominal ultrasonography, serial clinical pathology tests including urinalyses and urine cultures, and blood pressure measurements should be performed to evaluate the severity of disease, establish a prognosis, monitor the response to therapy, and identify complicating factors. Specific renal function tests and renal biopsy may be helpful to identify the exact cause in Stages I-III, but the presence of advanced pathologic changes in Stage IV is nonspecific and often precludes identification of an underlying cause by histologic studies. This condition in late Stage IV is often described as end-stage renal failure clinically and as chronic, generalized nephritis pathologically. Chronic kidney disease should be distinguished from the more readily reversible acute disease. Frequently, differentiation may be accomplished with an appropriate history, physical examination, and laboratory findings, although a renal biopsy may be required. However, therapy for chronic renal failure caused by a range of morphologic lesions is similar, so renal biopies may not be warranted.

Treatment: With appropriate therapy, animals can survive for long periods with only a small fraction of functional renal tissue, perhaps 5-8% in dogs and cats. Recommended treatment varies with the stage of the disease. In Stages I and II, animals usually have minimal clinical abnormalities. Efforts to identify and treat the primary cause of the disease should be thorough. The identification and supportive treatment of developing complications (eg, systemic hypertension, potassium homeostasis disorders, metabolic acidosis, bacterial urinary tract infection) should be aggressively pursued. The systemic hypertension seen in ~20% of animals with chronic kidney disease may be observed at any stage and is not effectively controlled by feeding a low-salt diet. The usual antihypertensive medications are a calcium-channel blocker such as amlodipine besylate (0.1-0.25 mg/kg, PO, sid) or an angiotensin-converting enzyme (ACE) inhibitor such as enalapril (0.5 mg/kg, sid-bid). While these may be administered together, a calcium-channel blocker is usually recommended as initial therapy in cats and an ACE inhibitor in dogs. In addition to providing a continual supply of fresh drinking water and encouraging (and documenting) adequate dietary intake, body condition scoring should be used routinely to assess adequacy of intake. Animals in this stage should be fed standard, commercially available maintenance diets, unless they are markedly proteinuric. All affected animals should be reevaluated every 3-6 mo, or sooner if problems develop.

In Stages II and III, the principles for management of complications are the same, except that the animal should be evaluated every 2-3 mo. These evaluations should include hematology, serum biochemistries, and urinalysis. Because dogs and cats with chronic kidney disease are prone to the development of bacterial urinary tract infections, urine culture should be performed twice annually or if urinalysis suggests infection. The progressive nature of this disease produces a vicious cycle of progressive renal destruction. Measures that may slow this progression include dietary phosphorus restriction (dogs and cats), dietary fish oil supplementation (dogs), antihypertensive agents (hypertensive dogs and cats), and administration of ACE inhibitors. Dietary restriction of phosphate and acid load is essential in this stage, and specialized diets for management of kidney disease should be fed. Potassium citrate or sodium bicarbonate, given PO, may be indicated if the animal is severely acidotic (plasma bicarbonate <15 mEq/L) or remains acidotic 2-3 wk after diet change. If dietary restriction of phosphorus is unsuccessful in maintaining a normal level of serum phosphorus within 2-3 mo, phosphate-binding gels containing calcium acetate, calcium carbonate, or aluminum hydroxide should be administered with meals to achieve the desired effect. In dogs only, there is a clear rationale for the inclusion of dietary n-3 polyunsaturated fatty acids in these stages.

In late Stage III and Stage IV, all of the principles of managing the preceding stages apply, except that the animal should be evaluated every 1-2 mo. Dietary restriction of protein may relieve some of the signs of uremia. High-quality protein (eg, egg protein) should be fed at a level of 2.0-2.8 g/kg/day for dogs and 2.8-3.8 g/kg/day for cats. Commercial diets formulated for cats and dogs with chronic kidney disease generally meet this recommendation. Administration of an H_2-receptor antagonist such as famotidine (5 mg/kg, PO, tid-qid) decreases gastric acidity and vomiting. Anabolic steroids, such as oxymethalone or nandrolone, have been administered to stimulate RBC production in anemic animals, but this is not effective. Recombinant erythropoietin is effective in stimulating RBC production, but antierythropoietin antibodies develop in ~50% of animals and may result in refractory anemia; until species-specific products become generally available, erythropoietin administration is now recommended only for animals showing clinically apparent signs of anemia (eg, weakness, marked lethargy not attributable to other factors), which generally occurs at a hematocrit <20%. Fluid therapy with polyionic solutions, given IV or SC in the hospital or SC by owners at home, is often beneficial in animals with intermittent signs of uremia. Although controversial, oral vitamin D administration may reduce uremic signs. However, vitamin D administration requires prior resolution of hyperphosphatemia and it may induce hypercalcemia. Feeding tubes may help manage chronic anorexia. Euthanasia or renal replacement therapy (renal transplantation and/or dialysis) should be carefully considered if therapy does not improve renal function and alleviate signs of uremia.

Acute Kidney Disease

Acute kidney disease is seen when a sudden, major insult damages the kidneys. The principal causes are toxins (eg, ethylene glycol, aminoglycoside antibiotics, hypercalcemia, hemoglobinuria) and ischemia (eg, embolic showers from disseminated intravascular coagulation or severe prolonged hypoperfusion).

Clinical Findings: Mild, acute kidney disease often goes unrecognised; severe initial or repeated bouts may lead to chronic kidney disease. The stages of acute and chronic kidney disease are the same. Most often, acute kidney disease is recognised in Stage IV and is characterized clinically by anorexia, depression, dehydration, oral ulceration, vomiting and/or diarrhea, or oliguria. Physical examination findings often reveal dehydration but otherwise are usually not remarkable, although pain is occasionally elicited on palpation of the kidneys, which may be normal-sized to slightly enlarged.

Diagnosis: A history of hypotension, shock, or recent exposure to known nephrotoxins in an animal with sudden-onset uremia (Stage IV) is the typical clinical picture of an animal with acute kidney disease. The presence of inappropriately concentrated urine (specific gravity 1.007-1.035) in the face of dehydration and/or azotemia suggests renal dysfunction. Differentiating between chronic and acute kidney disease (and establishing a specific cause in acute kidney disease) is important, as the prognosis and specific therapy may differ. Animals with acute kidney disease usually have a compatible history and other urinalysis abnormalities; marked cylindruria is a frequent and definitive finding. Other urinalysis findings may include the presence of a large number of renal epithelial cells and leukocytes in the urine sediment, glucosuria, crystalluria, and/or myoglobinuria/hemoglobinuria. Animals with Stage III or IV acute kidney disease have increased serum urea nitrogen, creatinine, and inorganic phosphorus concentrations and metabolic acidosis. Oliguria or anuria following rehydration, which is often associated with hyperkalemia, is a poor prognostic sign; in contrast, polyuric animals have a better prognosis, although they may become hypokalemic. Anemia is often, but not always, absent—a finding that may be helpful in differentiating acute from chronic kidney disease.

Following injury, the kidney has considerable potential for functional regeneration through the process of compensatory hypertrophy and adaptive hyperfunction. In animals with chronic kidney disease, it is likely that much of these processes has occurred prior to the initial diagnosis. In contrast, animals with acute kidney disease have considerably more potential for improvement of renal function, if they can be sustained through a uremic episode. The duration of the uremic episode may be substantial with some nephrotoxins (eg, 1-3 wk with aminoglycoside antibiotics and 4-8 wk with ethylene glycol). A renal biopsy may be of value in assessment of the severity, extent, cause, and potential reversibility of the disease.

Treatment: If the cause is known, specific therapy should be instituted, eg, 4-methyl-pyrazole or ethanol for ethylene glycol toxicity in dogs (*Ethylene Glycol Toxicity: Introduction*). Fluid therapy is indicated for all dehydrated and inappetant animals. A polyionic fluid such as lactated Ringer's solution is satisfactory unless hyperkalemia is present, in which case normal saline is recommended. Sodium bicarbonate may be cautiously added to the fluids to correct acidosis.

In oliguric or anuric animals, therapy to promote increased urine volume is often recommended if the animal is well hydrated and urine production is <0.5 mL/kg/hr.

This approach has been questioned because urine flow may increase without corresponding increases in renal blood flow and GFR. Administration of excess fluid to an animal in the maintenance phase of oliguric renal failure may result in life-threatening pulmonary and cerebral edema. Nonetheless, efforts to increase renal blood flow and GFR may enhance urine production and do have a role in the management of these animals.

For this therapy, urine production must be quantitatively monitored closely via an indwelling urethral catheter. Monitoring central venous pressure is advised to prevent overhydration. A sequential approach generally includes an initial slight overhydration by administration of a test dosage of 50 mL/kg of polyionic solution IV. If this fails to yield adequate urine flow within 3 hr, further measures include osmotic diuresis (10% or 20% mannitol or dextrose, 0.5-1 g/kg, IV, as a slow bolus over 15-30 min, alternated with infusion of lactated Ringer's solution, 30 mL/kg, IV, over 30 min).

Subsequent measures generally include furosemide (2 mg/kg, IV, which can be doubled and then tripled at 2-hr intervals if urine production does not increase above the target of 0.5 mL/kg/hr). However, furosemide may worsen the severity of acute renal failure caused by aminoglycosides.

Finally, renal vasodilators (dopamine diluted in 5% dextrose, IV, to provide 1-5 g/kg/min) plus furosemide (2 mg/kg, IV) may be tried for 2 hr. Dopamine may lead to ventricular arrhythmias and its use as a renal vasodilator has been questioned, particularly in cats.

High doses of dopamine may cause renal vasoconstriction. If attempts to restore urine flow fail, aggressive measures should be discontinued to avoid overhydration. Daily fluid therapy based on maintenance and rehydration needs is continued until renal function and clinical condition improve. Feeding tube placement greatly facilitates patient management at this stage and should be implemented for any animal with marked renal azotemia (serum creatinine >10 mg/dL after rehydration).

A second therapeutic option, rather than the aggressive measures discussed above, is to proceed directly to fluid therapy with polyionic solutions while waiting for renal regeneration. Again, feeding tube placement for parenteral nutrition should be implemented in anorectic animals with marked azotemia. Peritoneal dialysis, hemodialysis, or euthanasia may be necessary if none of the above measures restores urine production.

Glomerular Disease

Glomerular disease is a well-recognised cause of chronic (but not acute) kidney disease in dogs, and is also occasionally observed in cats. Animals with primary glomerular disease as a cause of chronic kidney disease may have somewhat different clinical and laboratory abnormalities than those with primary tubulointerstitial disease. Damage to the glomerular basement membrane results in albuminuria, which may lead to hypoalbuminemia. Animals may then exhibit signs related to hypoalbuminemia (eg, peripheral edema, hypercoagulability with thrombosis, hypercholesterolemia) instead of or in addition to uremia.

Secondary glomerulopathies, observed as sequelae of systemic or glomerular hypertension in animals with Stage III or IV chronic kidney disease, are common. Although the overall prevalence of a primary glomerulopathy as an inciting cause is not known, it is apparently more common in dogs than cats.

Immune-mediated glomerulonephropathy is characterized by deposition or in situ formation of immune complexes in the glomerular capillary wall, which then incite inflammatory changes. In one study of dogs, the mean age of presentation for glomerulonephritis was 4-8 yr; 55% were males, and there was no breed predilection. Immune-mediated glomerulonephritis has been associated with neoplasia, rickettsial diseases, systemic lupus erythematosus (SLE), heartworm disease, pyometra, chronic septicemia, and adenovirus infection, but it is usually idiopathic. Though multifactorial in origin, the glomerular disease associated with hyperadrenocorticism and diabetes mellitus in dogs is rarely attributable to immune complex formation. In one study of cats with glomerulonephritis, the mean age at presentation was 3-4 yr; 75% were males, and there was no breed predisposition. Primary glomerular disease in cats is most frequently associated with chronic infection by feline leukemia virus (FeLV), feline immunodeficiency virus (FIV), or feline infectious peritonitis (FIP) virus but has also been reported in association with neoplasia and systemic inflammatory diseases. The relatively young age and predilection for males reflects the high prevalence of FeLV infection as a cause in reported feline cases.

Familial glomerulopathies as a primary cause of chronic kidney disease have been reported in several breeds of dogs, including Bernese Mountain Dogs, English Cocker Spaniels, Doberman Pinschers, Greyhounds, Lhasa Apsos, Poodles, Rottweilers, Samoyeds, Shih Tzus, and Soft-coated Wheaten Terriers. These are not immune complex diseases, although some are characterized by proteinuria and associated clinical abnormalities that resemble those caused by immune-mediated glomerulonephropathy.

Amyloid is the name given to any of several chemically inert fibrillar protein subunits that can be deposited in tissue and interfere with normal organ function. All of these proteins are deposited in a â-pleated sheet conformation, which results in the unique appearance and chemical properties of amyloid. Most cases of amyloidosis in dogs and cats, including familial amyloidosis in Shar-Peis and Abyssinian cats, are reactive, or secondary, amyloidosis.

In this form of the disease, amyloid A protein is deposited in various tissues after serum levels increase as a result of chronic inflammation. When the kidneys are affected, amyloid deposition in the nonfamilial forms in dogs usually occurs in the glomerulus.

However, in Shar-Peis, at least 25% of Abyssinian cats, and in many domestic cats with the nonfamilial form of this disease, amyloid is found primarily in the medullary interstitium where it interferes with the renal concentrating mechanism and is more likely to produce nonproteinuric chronic kidney disease than protein-losing glomerular amyloid deposition. Glomerular amyloidosis usually leads to marked proteinuria. The nonfamilial form of amyloidosis usually affects middle-aged to older dogs and cats. Beagles, Collies, and Walker Hounds are reported to be at increased risk. Animals with the familial form of the disease are usually diagnosed at a younger age.

Clinical Findings: Glomerulopathy often leads to proteinuria (primarily albuminuria) and can produce hypoproteinemia, ascites, dyspnea (due to pleural effusion or pulmonary edema), and/or peripheral edema, which may be referred to as the nephrotic syndrome. Protein wasting can produce preferential loss of lean body mass that may be apparent on careful physical examination. Severe or chronic glomerular disease is a cause of chronic kidney disease; most dogs and many cats with glomerular disease eventually develop Stage III or Stage IV disease. Systemic hypertension may be more prevalent in proteinuric chronic kidney disease and may observed at any stage.

Proteinuria may result in loss of antithrombin III through the glomerular basement membrane, leading to a hypercoagulable state in dogs. Proteinuria also contributes to mild thrombocytosis and platelet hypersensitivity, which contribute to coagulation abnormalities in affected dogs, generally when plasma albumin levels are d"1.0 g/dL. Severe dyspnea secondary to pulmonary thromboembolism or other sequelae of thrombotic disease may be seen in dogs with glomerulonephritis or amyloidosis. It is unclear whether a hypercoagulable state also exists in proteinuric cats, because clinical signs from hypercoagulability have not been reported in cats.

Diagnosis: The serum urea nitrogen, creatinine, and phosphorus concentrations are usually increased, although the degree varies with the stage of chronic kidney disease at the time of diagnosis. Marked proteinuria with edema may be observed in the presence or absence of azotemia. Physical findings are usually nonspecific except that ascites, pleural effusion, and/or peripheral, pitting, nonpainful, subcutaneous edema, are evident in some animals (75% of cats and 15% of dogs). Although uncommon, urine specific gravity may be inappropriately high for the degree of renal dysfunction. Proteinuria is associated with all forms of glomerular disease, but it must be quantitated to determine whether the protein loss is significant. The urine protein to creatinine ratio is determined in a random urine sample to quantify urinary protein loss; a value >0.5 indicates proteinuria but does not define its origin (glomerular, tubular, or lower tract origin). If the sediment examination eliminates inflammatory urinary tract disease and hemorrhage as the source of proteinuria, then the degree of increase may help distinguish tubular proteinuria (typical ratio value of 0.5-2.5), glomerulonephritis (typical ratio value of 0.5-15), and glomerular amyloidosis (typical ratio value of 0.5-40). However, substantial overlap exists in these ranges, and the ratio will tend to be low in the initial stages of a glomerulopathy, increase in severity as the disease progresses, and then decline terminally as GFR falls to very low levels in late Stage IV disease.

Renal biopsy is often required to determine the type of glomerular disease. Membranous glomerulonephritis is reported most frequently in cats; there is a roughly equal distribution of histologic findings in dogs, with glomerular amyloidosis and membranous, proliferative, and membranoproliferative glomerulonephritis all represented. The degree of proteinuria does not always correlate with the severity of the histologic lesions or the degree of azotemia. Systemic hypertension develops in an unusually large proportion of animals with protein-losing glomerulonephritis; therefore, blood pressure should be determined in all animals with evidence of glomerular disease.

A careful search should be made for an inciting disease process. Abdominal and thoracic radiographs, ultrasonography, and specialized serologic tests can rule out various inflammatory, infectious, and neoplastic diseases. In dogs with glomerulonephritis, this includes tests for SLE (eg, antinuclear antibody titer and LE prep) and appropriate antigen or antibody screening tests for other infectious agents and heartworm disease; in cats, tests for infection with FeLV, FIV, FIP, SLE, and heartworm disease should be included.

Treatment: There are 6 basic principles to therapy in glomerulonephropathies: 1) If a cause of immune-complex disease can be identified, it should be treated. 2) Manifestations of the nephrotic syndrome, if present, should be managed with dietary salt restriction and judicious use of diuretics. 3) Antithrombotics (eg, aspirin) should be considered for hypoalbuminemic (plasma albumin <1.0 g/dL) animals as well as those with low serum levels of antithrombin III (<30% of normal). In dogs with marked proteinuria and serum albumin <2 g/dL, low-dose aspirin therapy is appropriate, unless melena is present or gastric ulceration is suspected. However, aspirin is bound to plasma proteins and is eliminated via the kidneys, so the dosage may need to be adjusted. 4) Because proteinuria may promote interstitial fibrosis, treatment to limit glomerular loss of protein is warranted and may include dietary protein restriction and administration of an ACE inhibitor. 5) Efforts to reduce the magnitude and consequences of glomerular immune complex deposition should be considered, especially in animals with biopsy-confirmed glomerular inflammation and no known primary antigenic stimulus. Immunosuppressive drugs (eg, azathioprine, cyclophosphamide, cyclosporine) can be used in dogs with glomerulonephritis, although results are variable. For amyloidosis, dimethylsulfoxide and colchicine have been tried, but without consistent results. These anti-inflammatory drugs should be administered only on a trial basis with owner consent. Corticosteroids seem to be beneficial only in mild glomerulopathy; they may worsen proteinuria in other glomerulopathies and should be avoided in animals with amyloidosis, as they are reported to enhance amyloid deposition. 6) Manifestations of chronic kidney disease will be observed in accordance with the stage of disease. Appropriate therapy has been discussed elsewhere.

Prognosis: Although one study found that mean survival time of dogs with glomerulonephritis was 87 days, the prognosis with early diagnosis and appropriate therapy is much better. In a recent study of dogs with glomerulonephritis, those receiving a placebo medication survived beyond the entire 6-mo duration of the study. The prognosis for animals with amyloidosis is guarded but variable, with reported mean survival times ranging from 49 days to 20 mo.

Renal Tubular Acidosis

The form of metabolic acidosis that occurs in Stages II-IV of acute and chronic kidney disease, referred to as uremic acidosis, is due to reduced urine-acidifying ability of diseased kidneys. In uremic acidosis, although the ability of some individual tubular cells to reabsorb bicarbonate and/or secrete hydrogen ions may be normal, there is generally far less total cell mass present. Acid accumulates if the animal is under metabolic or dietary acid pressure, which is common in carnivores and is particularly problematic in cats, which are often fed acidifying maintenance diets.

Rare renal tubular defects in dogs and cats may result in hyperchloremic metabolic acidosis, referred to as renal tubular acidosis. Two types of renal tubular acidosis have been described in dogs and one in cats. In Type I (distal), the ability of the distal tubule to secrete hydrogen ions against a concentration gradient is defective; in Type II (proximal), the ability to reabsorb bicarbonate in the proximal tubule is reduced. Type I has been reported in both species; Type II has also been described in dogs in conjunction with other proximal tubular defects in acquired (gentamicin nephrotoxicosis and an idiopathic form) and heritable (Fanconi syndrome, *see Fanconi Syndrome*) forms.

Type I renal tubular acidosis has been associated with demineralization of the skeleton (due to buffering of excess hydrogen ions) and nephrolithiasis (due to hypercalciuria from bone resorption) in dogs. Diagnosis is based on the presence of hyperchloremic metabolic acidosis with a urinary pH that is inappropriately high for the degree of systemic acidosis in the absence of bacterial urease modification of urine. Failure to produce acid urine after oral ammonium chloride loading is diagnostic; however, this test is contraindicated in animals that are already severely acidotic. Type II renal tubular acidosis is diagnosed by demonstrating increased urinary fractional excretion of bicarbonate when plasma bicarbonate levels are normal or decreased; this test is not practicable in the clinical setting and diagnosis is presumptively based on history, signalment, and clinical pathology findings.

Therapy consists of oral administration of an alkalinizing agent sufficient to maintain normal blood pH (1 mEq bicarbonate equivalent/kg/day for Type I and 1-6 mEq bicarbonate equivalent/kg/day for Type II, PO). Therapy is more problematic in dogs with Type II renal tubular acidosis, because supplemental bicarbonate is readily lost in the urine.

Fanconi Syndrome

Fanconi syndrome is a generalized proximal tubular reabsorptive defect resulting in excessive loss of many solutes in the urine. It has been reported as an acquired condition in dogs (gentamicin nephrotoxicosis and an idiopathic form) and in a heritable form in a variety of breeds (most notably Basenjis), in which it develops gradually in adults of both sexes. There is excessive urinary loss of glucose, sodium, potassium, phosphorus, uric acid, bicarbonate, and amino acids. Blood glucose concentrations are normal. Serum electrolytes are normal early in the disease, but hypophosphatemia, hypokalemia, and metabolic acidosis are seen in the later stages.

Clinical signs include polydipsia, polyuria, and weight loss. Signs of uremia may be present if the animal is in Stage III chronic kidney disease. Diagnosis is based on documentation of increased urinary fractional excretion of glucose, sodium, potassium, phosphorus, and bicarbonate in the presence of normal plasma concentrations.

Differential diagnoses include simple renal glucosuria and chronic kidney disease from other causes. The microscopic renal changes in the heritable form are not remarkable in the early stages but progress to nonspecific findings characteristic of chronic kidney disease.

A genetic marker has been developed. A treatment regimen to reverse the tubular defect has not been described. The histologic appearance of the acquired forms of Fanconi syndrome vary, depending on the cause.

Oral supplementation of sodium chloride, potassium, phosphate, and bicarbonate is indicated if the corresponding serum concentration is low. Dogs with acute or chronic kidney disease should be treated symptomatically as appropriate. The heritable disease is slowly progressive despite therapy and usually results in death from uremia.

Renal Glucosuria

This is usually a congenital defect in proximal tubular handling of glucose that results in glucosuria despite normal blood glucose concentration. Affected animals may be asymptomatic, have polydipsia and polyuria, or have recurrent urinary tract infections due to bacterial colonization in the presence of glucose. Diagnosis is made by demonstrating persistent glucosuria despite a normal blood glucose concentration and by identifying no other renal reabsorptive abnormalities. This disease is so uncommonly recognised that little is known about its biologic behaviour. The general consensus is that it is not progressive and does not require treatment.

Neoplasms of the Kidney

Neoplasms of the kidney are uncommon and represent ~0.5-1.7% of all neoplasms in dogs. Benign neoplasms are uncommon, usually incidental findings at necropsy, and generally of little clinical significance. Adenomas, lipomas, fibromas, and papillomas have been reported.

Primary malignant renal neoplasms (except nephroblastomas) are most common in middle-aged to older animals. No breed predilection has been found, except for heritable predilection for the development of bilateral, multifocal cystoadenocarcinomas in German Shepherds, generally between 5-11 yr of age. The most common primary malignant renal neoplasm is carcinoma, which originates from the renal tubular epithelium. Usually, it is unilateral, located at one pole of the kidney, and well demarcated. Size varies from microscopic to several times that of the normal kidney, and colour may be yellow, white, or gray. Renal carcinomas metastasize early to various organs; the opposite kidney, lungs, liver, and adrenals are involved most commonly.

Nephroblastomas (embryonal nephroma, Wilms' tumor) arise from vestigial embryonic tissue. They are seen in young animals and, in dogs, are most commonly diagnosed at <1 yr of age. There is no breed predilection. Males are affected twice as commonly as females. Nephroblastomas are usually unilateral but are occasionally bilateral. They can grow to immense proportions; it is not uncommon to have virtually the entire abdomen occupied by tumor. Metastasis occurs to regional lymph nodes, liver, and lungs.

Transitional cell carcinomas arise from transitional epithelium of the renal pelvis, ureter, bladder, or urethra. Other primary malignant renal neoplasms are uncommon and include hemangiosarcomas, fibrosarcomas, leiomyosarcomas, and squamous cell carcinomas.

The kidneys are a common site of metastatic or multicentric neoplasms. Metastatic lesions may be unilateral or bilateral. Lymphosarcoma is the most common multicentric tumor involving the kidneys. Up to 50% of dogs and cats with lymphosarcoma have renal lesions and, in some cases, only the kidneys or kidneys and brain are affected. Renal involvement is usually multifocal or diffuse, interstitial, and bilateral, and results in large, irregular kidneys. Lymphosarcoma in cats frequently is associated with infection by feline leukemia virus.

Clinical Findings: Signs are nonspecific and may include weight loss, anorexia, depression, and fever. Bilateral neoplasms may uncommonly destroy sufficient renal tissue to cause chronic kidney disease and associated signs of uremia. Astute owners may notice "lumps" in their animal's abdomen or abdominal enlargement. Persistent hematuria, usually microscopic, may occur. Rarely, renal tumors may produce excessive erythropoietin, which results in erythrocythemia (*Polycythemia: Introduction*).

Diagnosis: History and clinical signs may indicate a mass in the area of the kidneys or renomegaly, which can be confirmed by ultrasonography or radiography, although an excretory urogram or renal arteriogram may be required. Radiographs of the thorax may reveal metastatic disease. Neoplastic cells occasionally can be found in the urine sediment. Percutaneous needle aspiration and cytologic examination may be sufficient for the diagnosis of lymphosarcoma in cats and dogs, particularly when there is diffuse involvement or with ultrasonographic guidance when multifocal disease occurs. Histologic examination of tissue obtained by needle biopsy or surgical wedge biopsy is often necessary to determine the type of tumor.

Treatment: Treatment of all renal neoplasms except lymphosarcoma involves surgical removal; unilateral nephrectomy is usually required. Lymphosarcoma is best managed by combination chemotherapy. Chemotherapy is generally ineffective against renal tumors other than lymphosarcoma.

Neoplasms of the Lower Urinary Tract

Neoplasms of the ureters, bladder, and urethra are uncommon in dogs and rare in cats. The low incidence in cats may be due to a difference in tryptophan metabolism that results in low urinary concentrations of carcinogenic tryptophan metabolites. The mean age of affected dogs and cats is 9 yr. In the lower urinary tract, primary neoplasms are more likely to be malignant than benign. Papillomas, leiomyomas, fibromas, neurofibromas, hemangiomas, rhabdomyomas, and myxomas are found infrequently.

Among primary malignant neoplasms of the lower urinary tract, transitional cell carcinomas are diagnosed most frequently in both species. Squamous cell carcinomas, adenocarcinomas, fibrosarcomas, leiomyosarcomas, rhabdomyosarcomas, hemangiosarcomas, and osteosarcomas also are found. Transitional cell carcinomas may be solitary or multiple papillary-like projections from the mucosa or may develop as a diffuse infiltration of the ureter, bladder, prostate, and/or urethra. They are highly invasive and metastasize frequently, most commonly to the regional lymph nodes and lungs. Ureteral and bladder neoplasms can cause chronic obstruction to urine flow with secondary hydronephrosis. Urethral tumors are more likely to cause acute obstructive uropathy. Intractable secondary bacterial urinary tract infections are commonly associated with neoplasms of the bladder and urethra.

Clinical Findings: Hematuria, dysuria, stranguria, and pollakiuria are the most common signs. Animals with ureteral obstruction and unilateral hydronephrosis may show signs of abdominal pain and have a palpable, enlarged kidney. Signs of uremia may be apparent in animals with bilateral ureteral obstruction and hydronephrosis or with urethral obstruction. The bladder wall may be thickened, and a cord-like urethra or urethral mass(es) may be palpable rectally.

Diagnosis: History and clinical signs are highly suggestive of lower urinary tract disease in animals with tumors of the bladder or urethra. Urinalysis frequently reveals hematuria, and there may be evidence of secondary infection. Chronic, uncomplicated urinary tract infections must be differentiated from those associated with neoplasms. Neoplastic cells may be found in the sediment, particularly with transitional cell carcinomas. A cystourethrogram, retrograde urethrogram, or ultrasonography is generally necessary to determine the location and extent of the tumor. Biopsy of the tumor is required for definitive diagnosis.

Treatment: Excision of the tumor, if possible, is the most beneficial therapy. Transitional cell carcinomas are frequently located at the trigone of the bladder or in the urethra and may necessitate radical reconstructive surgery of the lower urinary tract. Prognosis is poor for these animals, even with surgery, because recurrence and metastasis occur rapidly. Chemotherapy with cisplatin or piroxicam may prolong the life of affected animals.

Disorders of Micturition

Disorders of micturition result from a dysfunction in the storage or voiding of urine and may be neurogenic or non-neurogenic in origin. Urinary incontinence is the failure of voluntarily control micturition, with constant or intermittent unconscious passage of urine. Incontinent animals may leave a pool of urine where they have been lying or may dribble urine while walking. The coat around the vulva or prepuce may be wet, and perivulvar or peripreputial dermatitis can result from urine scalding.

Failure of urine storage is characterized by inappropriate leakage of urine due to failure of bladder relaxation, urethral incompetence, anatomic defects, or overflow of stored urine. Urge incontinence is seen with detrusor irritability, usually associated with cystitis.

The most common non-neurogenic incontinence is attributed to deficiency of sex hormones in neutered animals, particularly female dogs, and is referred to as hormonal-responsive urethral incompetence. Idiopathic urethral sphincter incompetence also is seen. Urinary incontinence associated with anatomic defects may be detected in animals at an early age. For example, an animal with a unilateral congenital ectopic ureter may void normally but "dribbl" urine intermittently, whereas animals with bilateral ectopic ureters are less likely to void normally. Paradoxical urinary incontinence may develop when there is a partial obstruction of the urethra leading to bladder distention and overflow incontinence.

Failure of normal voiding is characterized by frequent attempts to urinate with stranguria, and passage of only small amounts of urine. Inability to urinate can be due to mechanical obstruction of the urethra by calculi, neoplasms, or strictures; detrusor atony from overdistention of the bladder; or neurologic disease. Animals with abnormalities of the voiding phase may develop overflow incontinence due to dribbling of urine associated with bladder overdistention.

Neurologic causes of micturition disorders can be categorized as upper (UMN) or lower motor neuron (LMN) lesions. Lesions in the sacral spinal cord, pelvic nerve, and detrusor atony lead to LMN signs, which are often characterized by a distended, easily expressed bladder. Dysautonomia in cats is a multisystemic disease characterized by widespread disruption of autonomic system functions, including urinary incontinence of LMN origin. Damage to the thoracolumbar spinal cord or disease of the cerebrum, cerebellum, or brain stem can lead to UMN signs, which are characterized by a distended bladder that is difficult to express. Another neurologic cause of inability to urinate is functional obstruction (detrusor-sphincter reflex dyssynergia), which occurs when there is incoordination of the normal micturition reflex; this is believed to result from overdischarge of sympathetic nerve impulses to the urethral sphincter, resulting in a failure of urethral relaxation during detrusor contraction. Animals with neurogenic incontinence may leak urine (LMN) and/or develop overflow incontinence due to dribbling of urine associated with bladder overdistension (any neurogenic cause).

Diagnosis: Clinical signs are usually suggestive of a micturition disorder. The history should include age of onset, sexual status of the animal, age at neutering, current medication, and history of previous urinary tract disorders. A thorough physical and neurologic examination is indicated, and the act of voiding should be observed, including estimation of initial and final bladder volume.

Animals with LMN lesions or an atonic bladder have a large, distended bladder that can be expressed with minimal pressure. Animals with mechanical or functional obstruction or with spinal lesions causing UMN also have a large distended bladder, but urine cannot be readily expressed. Caution must be exercised when attempting to express urine from these animals to avoid rupturing the bladder. Plain or contrast radiography, cystoscopy, or ultrasonography are necessary to determine the type and location of mechanical obstruction.

Animals with functional obstruction (reflex dyssynergia) generally exhibit pollakiuria with interrupted urine stream, distended urinary bladder, no identifiable structural cause of obstruction, and overflow incontinence, and generally have an abnormal neurologic examination. A catheter can easily be passed into the bladder in animals with functional obstruction but will not pass in animals with mechanical obstruction.

Treatment: Accurate diagnosis or localisation of the lesion is essential for appropriate pharmacologic management. Animals with hormonal incontinence were formerly treated with the appropriate sex hormone—diethylstilbestrol in females and testosterone in males. The dose should be adjusted to the minimum required to maintain continence. Diethylstilbestrol may be unavailable or difficult to obtain. Alternatively, an α-adrenergic agonist drug (eg, phenylpropanolamine, 2-4 mg/kg/day in divided doses) can be given to animals with urethral incompetence. Urge incontinence (detrusor instability) is treated with anticholinergic drugs such as oxybutin chloride (0.5 mg/kg, PO, sid) or propantheline (dogs <20 kg, 7.5 mg/day; dogs >20 kg, 15 mg/day; cats, 7.5 mg every 72 hr). Cholinergic drugs such as bethanechol are used in animals with detrusor atony. Functional obstruction is treated with sympatholytic drugs (eg, phenoxybenzamine, 2.5-10 mg, sid-tid); cholinergic drugs may also be necessary.

Complete mechanical obstruction of the urethra is a medical emergency and should be relieved by catheterization and retropulsion of the obstructing material into the bladder or by surgery. Animals with detrusor atony from overdistention but without neurologic lesions benefit from decompression of the bladder by placement of an indwelling urinary catheter for 3-7 days. This may be done continuously or intermittently. Those with neurogenic atony, which usually does not respond to medical management, may require manual expression of the bladder or catheterization several times daily.

Canine Urolithiasis

The most common canine uroliths are magnesium ammonium phosphate, calcium oxalate, or urate; less common uroliths include cystine, silica, calcium phosphate, and xanthine.

Struvite Stones: The most common urinary stones in dogs are composed of struvite. The mineral composition is mostly struvite ($MgNH_4PO_4 \cdot 6H_2O$), but frequently, small amounts of carbonate-apatite and ammonium urate are present. In most cases, struvite uroliths form in association with urinary tract infections with urease-producing Staphylococcus or Proteus spp . Unlike in cats, in which they are frequent, sterile struvite uroliths rarely form in dogs. They have been detected in a family of English Cocker Spaniels, suggesting a genetic predisposition.

Medical management involves dissolution and prevention of stone formation. In both instances, the aim of treatment is to reduce the concentrations of NH4+, Mg^{2+}, and PO4-3 in urine. For dissolution, urine should be extremely undersaturated for struvite; for prevention, the degree of struvite saturation should be sufficiently low to make crystallization unlikely. The choice between surgery, lithotripsy, and medical treatment may not be easy. Owner compliance, the animal's acceptance of the diet, availability of lithotripsy, practice philosophy, and knowledge of the indications and contraindications are necessary to make a decision. If stone dissolution is prolonged or fails, it may be more costly than surgical treatment. Surgical removal of uroliths is often incomplete, with small, hidden uroliths often inadvertently left in the urinary tract serving as a nidus for recurrence.

Before beginning stone dissolution by medical therapy, a physical examination, CBC, serum chemistry profile, urinalysis, urine culture and sensitivity, abdominal radiographs to document stone size, and blood pressure measurement (if possible) should be performed. Contraindications to stone dissolution include heart failure, edema, ascites, pleural effusion, hypertension, hepatic failure, renal failure, and hypoalbuminemia. Renal failure is not always a contraindication for dissolution of struvite nephroliths, however.

Dissolution Protocol: While the use of urinary acidification to reduce urine pH <6 and other individualized dietary maneuvers may prove effective, a few commercially available diets that are generally nutritionally balanced promote struvite stone dissolution. Dogs fed these rations generally have reduced intake of protein, phosphate, and magnesium and a high intake of sodium. This results in osmotic diuresis, reduced daily urea output, and enhanced urine volume. The low urinary urea concentration is one of the most important features of such diets and also reduces ammonia production by the action of urease-producing bacteria. No other food, including treats, should be fed, and adequate fresh water should be available at all times.

Urease-producing urinary tract infections must be treated. The choice of antibacterial should be based on sensitivity testing when possible. Most Staphylococcus and Proteus infections are sensitive to levels of amoxicillin or ampicillin achieved in the urine of normal dogs.

A urease inhibitor can be given but is not usually necessary. Concurrent treatment with a urease inhibitor such as acetohydroxamic acid enhances the rate of struvite stone dissolution, particularly when antibiotic resistance precludes effective antibacterial sterilization of the urine. A reasonably safe dose of acetohydroxamic acid appears to be 12.5 mg/kg, PO, bid. A reversible, mild hemolytic anemia has been seen in dogs given higher doses.

After ~4 wk of treatment, a physical examination, serum chemistry profile, urinalysis, and abdominal radiographs or ultrasonography should be repeated. The stone dissolution protocol should be discontinued if severe side effects develop, although a mild degree of hypoalbuminemia is to be expected and can be tolerated. With good compliance, the following results can be anticipated: urine pH <6.5; urine specific gravity <1.025; serum urea <10 mg/dL. The radiographic stone size should be compared with the size on previous radiographs. Routine testing should be repeated every 4 wk until 4 wk after the stone is no longer visible radiographically; this generally takes 8-12 wk but may take up to 20 wk. Stones that fail to reduce in size after 8 wk of treatment are probably not composed of struvite and should be treated another way, although failure could also result from poor treatment compliance. Renal stones tend to dissolve more slowly than bladder stones.

The recurrence rate after surgical treatment of struvite uroliths has been reported to be ~20-25%, with most recurrences within 1 yr. When surgery is performed to remove multiple small struvite calculi, removing all stone material is often difficult. In such cases, a 4-wk dissolution protocol starting at the time of suture removal aids in preventing recurrence due to residual crystalline material. Once the urinary tract is free of stones, prevention strategies are much more likely to be successful.

Prevention Protocol: The key to prevention of recurrence in animals with a struvite stone associated with infection is achieving and maintaining sterile urine. Routine testing of urine pH by the owner is important. If fresh urine is alkaline, a urinalysis and culture should be done, and the dog treated appropriately if an infection is present.

Once stone dissolution is completed, a prevention program can be considered. The aim is to prevent urinary tract infections with urease-producing microbes. The concentration of major struvite solutes in urine should also be reduced. A commercially available diet may be fed to lower urinary phosphate and magnesium and to maintain an acidic urine. Urease-producing infections should be eliminated, after which owners should regularly check the pH of the first voided urine in the morning after an overnight fast; in most dogs on a normal diet, the urine will be acidic. Checking urine pH weekly is sufficient.

Calcium Oxalate Stones: Calcium oxalate uroliths have been increasing in frequency in dogs. While they may develop in any breed, Miniature Schnauzers, Lhasa Apsos, Yorkshire Terriers, Bichon Frise, Shih Tzus, and Miniature Poodles may be predisposed. Most affected dogs are 2-10 yr old. Hypercalciuria leading to calcium oxalate stone formation can result from increased renal clearance of calcium due to excessive intestinal absorption of calcium (absorptive hypercalciuria), to impaired renal conservation of calcium (renal leak hypercalciuria), or to excessive skeletal mobilization of calcium (resorptive hypercalciuria).

Absorptive hypercalciuria is characterized by increased urine calcium excretion, normal serum calcium concentration, and normal or low serum parathormone concentration. Because absorptive hypercalciuria depends on dietary calcium, the amount of calcium excreted in the urine during fasting is normal or significantly reduced when compared with nonfasting levels. Renal leak hypercalciuria has been recognised in dogs less frequently than absorptive hypercalciuria. In dogs, renal leak hypercalciuria is characterized by normal serum calcium concentration, increased urine calcium excretion, and increased serum parathormone concentration. During fasting, these dogs do not show a decline in urinary calcium loss. The underlying cause of renal leak hypercalciuria in dogs is not known.

Resorptive hypercalciuria is characterized by excessive filtration and excretion of calcium in urine as a result of hypercalcemia. Hypercalcemic disorders have been associated only infrequently with calcium oxalate uroliths in dogs.

Routine laboratory determinations should include serum calcium, phosphate, total CO_2, and chloride to eliminate the possibility of hyperparathyroidism and renal tubular acidosis. Dissolution of calcium oxalate stones by medical means has not been established at present. Treatment requires surgical removal or lithotripsy followed by preventive strategies.

Prevention Protocol: Recurrence is a major problem with calcium oxalate uroliths. An "ideal" diet is considered to be low oxalate, low protein, and low sodium, and would maintain urine pH at 6.5-7.5 and urine specific gravity <1.020. A few commercially available canned foods achieve these goals and may minimize the risk of recurrence.

Potassium citrate may be added as needed to assure the urine pH is within the desired range; water may be used to provide appropriate reduction in urine concentration. If these urine conditions are achieved and calcium oxalate crystals are still observed in warm, fresh urine, then vitamin B_6 and/or thiazide diuretics can be considered (although of unproven efficacy). Effectiveness of therapy should be reevaluated at 1- to 4-mo intervals by urinalysis. Chlorothiazide diuretics may also be of value.

Urate Stones: Ammonium urate stones are most common in Dalmatians and in dogs with congenital portosystemic vascular shunts. The formation of ammonium urate calculi depends on the urine concentrations of urate and ammonium and on other poorly understood factors. Dalmatians fail to convert most of their metabolic urate to allantoin and thus excrete the bulk of nucleic acid metabolites as relatively insoluble urate. The biologic mechanism responsible for decreased hepatic conversion of urate to allantoin lies not in reduced uricase activity, but in reduced hepatic transport of urate; the rate of urate hepatic transport is about 3 times faster in breeds other than Dalmatians. The net result is only 30-40% of urate is converted to allantoin in Dalmatians compared with ~90% in other breeds. Feline Urolithiasis and Feline Lower Urinary Tract Disease (FLUTD).

(Feline Urologic Syndrome)

Hematuria, pollakiuria, and stranguria are the characteristic clinical signs of FLUTD in cats. Although the specific underlying etiology of this common disease may not be identified, 2 major disease categories have been suggested based on the presence or absence of mineral precipitates; this discussion is limited to feline urolithiasis.

Feline urolithiasis is a common disease that is seen with equal frequency in both sexes. Until recently, it was thought that most uroliths in cats were small and resembled sand or were gelatinous plugs that differed from typical uroliths in that they contained a greater amount of organic matrix, giving them a toothpaste-like consistency. Matrix-crystalline plugs are most commonly found within the urethra near the urethral orifice and are primarily responsible for urethral obstruction. Recently, prevalence of urolithiasis with grossly observable stones composed primarily of calcium oxalate has increased in cats. The most common feline uroliths are calcium oxalate, magnesium ammonium phosphate, and urate.

Urolithiasis is usually suspected based on clinical signs of hematuria, dysuria, or urethral obstruction. Urinalysis, urine culture, radiography, and ultrasonography may be required to differentiate uroliths from urinary tract infection or neoplasia. Radiography, cystoscopy, or ultrasonography are critically important to detect uroliths because only ~10% of feline urocystoliths can be detected by abdominal palpation. Uroliths with a diametre >3 mm are usually radiodense; however, because smaller uroliths are common, double contrast radiography may be required for detection. Radiographic evidence of uroliths is seen in ~20% of cats with hematuria or dysuria. The usual clinical approach to grossly observable urocystoliths is surgical removal or lithotripsy where available, followed by dietary therapy instituted as a preventive measure. For sterile struvite uroliths, medical dissolution is the preferred treatment.

Calcium Oxalate Stones: Calcium oxalate uroliths are the most common feline uroliths and the most common nephrolith, although their underlying cause is unknown. Common management schemes that involve feeding urine-acidifying diets with reduced magnesium, have reduced the incidence of feline struvite urolithiasis. Magnesium has been reported to be an inhibitor of calcium oxalate formation in rats and humans; thus, the reduced magnesium concentration in feline urine may partially explain the increase in calcium oxalate stones in cats.

Medical protocols that promote calcium oxalate dissolution are not known; therefore, surgery and lithotripsy are the primary means for removal (small bladder stones may be eliminated by voiding urohydropulsion). However, some calcium oxalate uroliths, especially those in the kidneys, may not cause clinical signs for months to years. Because of the unavoidable destruction of nephrons during nephrotomy, this procedure is not recommended unless it can be established that the stones are a cause of clinically significant disease. Recurrence remains problematic. A variety of diets has been formulated to restrict the formation of calcium oxalate uroliths and should be considered appropriate for maintenance in cats with nephroliths and following the removal of urocystoliths. Eliminating any associated urinary tract infections, avoiding mineral and vitamin C and D supplementation, and encouraging water consumption are critical.

Struvite Stones: Three distinct types of struvite uroliths are recognised in cats: amorphous urethral plugs with a large quantity of matrix, sterile struvite uroliths (which form perhaps as a result of certain dietary ingredients), and struvite uroliths that form as a sequela of urinary tract infection with urease-producing bacteria. Struvite uroliths induced by infection are less common than sterile struvite uroliths. An additional type of struvite urolith in cats consists of a sterile struvite nidus that predisposes to urinary tract infection with urease-producing bacteria and subsequent formation of infected struvite laminations around the sterile nidus.

Treatment of sterile struvite urolithiasis focuses on reducing the urine pH to ≤ 6.0 and on reducing the urine magnesium concentration by feeding magnesium-restricted diets. Reducing urine pH and magnesium concentration is best accomplished by feeding a commercially available prescription diet formulated for this purpose. Generally, neither sodium chloride nor urine acidifiers should be given concurrently with these diets because they are already supplemented with sodium chloride and formulated to produce aciduria. In addition, these diets should not be fed to cats that are acidemic, have azotemia of any cause, or have cardiac dysfunction or hypertension. Urolith size and crystalluria should be monitored every 4 wk by radiographs or ultrasonography and urinalysis, respectively. Struvite crystals should not form if therapy has been effective in producing urine that is undersaturated with magnesium, ammonium, and phosphate. Because small uroliths may not be detected radiographically, the calculolytic diet should be continued for ≥4 wk after radiographic documentation of urolith dissolution. If treatment does not induce complete dissolution of uroliths, it is likely that either the wrong mineral component was identified, the nucleus of the urolith is composed of a different mineral than the outer portion of the urolith, or the owner is not complying with therapeutic recommendations.

Other Feline Stones: Ammonium urate, uric acid, calcium phosphate, and cystine uroliths are less common in cats, but ammonium urate and uric acid account for ~6% of feline uroliths. Although a renal tubular reabsorptive defect and portovascular anomalies have been incriminated as causes in a few cases, the cause of most urate uroliths in cats has not been established. Nonetheless, formation of highly acidic and concentrated urine associated with consumption of diets high in purine precursors (especially liver) appears to be a risk factor.

Medical protocols that consistently promote dissolution of ammonium urate uroliths in cats have not been developed, and surgery remains the most common method of removal. For small stones, voiding urohydropulsion may be effective. Prevention should include feeding a diet low in purine precursors and promoting formation of less acidic urine that is not highly concentrated. Although allopurinol may reduce the formation of urate in cats, studies of the efficacy and potential toxicity of allopurinol in cats are required before meaningful guidelines can be established.

Chapter 7

Behavioural Medicine Introduction

An animal's "behaviour" is the product of its genetic composition, the environment in which the animal functions, and the animal's experience (ie, what it has learned given its previous genetic × environment interaction). While this section focuses primarily on abnormal behaviour of domestic animals, the extent to which an animal's behaviour is abnormal is defined by its deviation from "normal." For each group of domestic animals, normal social and group behaviour is outlined and followed by a listing of the common behavioural disorders and treatment approaches.

In behavioural medicine, diagnoses are not diseases; correlation is not causality. Behavioural conditions for which there is putative etiologic and pathophysiologic heterogeneity (multifactorial disorders) are complex (*Table: Levels of "Causality" to Consider in Behavioural Diagnosis*).

Phenotypic (functional, phenomenologic) diagnoses are open to various mechanistic bases of all subsequent levels. Some of these more reductionistic levels can be tested using treatment (eg, specific pharmacologic agents), but few phenotypic diagnoses can be specifically tested using behaviour modification. Most of the behavioural diagnoses for farm animals are descriptive and relatively nonspecific. Behavioural diagnoses for dogs and cats have been more fully developed and are discussed in the context of the "necessary and sufficient" conditions (or criteria) for diagnosis. The use of "necessary and sufficient" conditions, using the terms as they are used in logical and mathematical applications, is a refinement over descriptive definitions. These conditions act as qualitative, and potentially quantitative, exclusion criteria, allowing for uniform and unambiguous assessment of aberrant, abnormal, and undesirable behaviours.

A necessary condition is one that must be present for the listed diagnosis to be made. A sufficient condition is one that can stand alone to singularly identify the condition. Sufficiency is an outcome of knowledge: as more becomes known about the genetics, molecular response, neurochemistry, and neuroanatomy of any condition and its behavioural correlates, a sufficient condition can be defined more succinctly and accurately. Definition of necessary and sufficient conditions is not synonymous with a compendium of signs associated with the behaviour. The number of signs present and their intensity may be a gauge for the severity of the condition, or act as a flag when there can be variable, nonoverlapping presentations of the same condition.

Principles of Behavioural Diagnosis and Treatment

Many "health" problems faced by pet dogs and cats are associated with behavioural pathologies or unmet behavioural expectations. A good behavioural history is required before making any behavioural diagnosis. History taking should include the following items: 1) sex, breed, and age of animal (breed predispositions); 2) age at onset of condition or complaint; 3) duration of condition or complaint; 4) description of actual behaviour; 5) frequency of condition or behaviour (hourly, daily, weekly, monthly); 6) duration of average bout (seconds, minutes, hours); 7) range of duration of bouts; 8) any changes in pattern, frequency, intensity, and duration of bouts; 9) any corrective measures tried and the response (possibly none); 10) any activities that stop the behaviour (eg, animal collapses); 11) 24-hr schedule of animal and owner, as well as any day-to-day variability; 12) animal's familial history; 13) anything else that the owner thinks is relevant.

Modern veterinary care should include routine screening questions about specific behavioural complaints (eg, "Any inappropriate or undesirable chewing, any growling, any odd behaviours?") in addition to routine questions that alert veterinarians to potential somatic medical problems. This accomplishes two goals. First, it initiates a dialog with the clients about behaviour and lets clients know that behaviour is central to good veterinary care. Clients will then feel comfortable asking their veterinarian about behavioural issues. Such dialog represents the best chance for learning of a client's behavioural concerns before these concerns threaten the pet's life. Second, it establishes a baseline of the pet's behaviours. Such a behavioural profile will identify "normal" for that pet and provide a context in which to evaluate behavioural change or client complaints about behaviour. This is exactly what is done by recommending routine laboratory evaluation for healthy pets. Length of dysfunction—whether the dysfunction involves a "medical" or a "behavioural" complaint—can affect prognosis, and the extent to which this is true in behavioural medicine is profound.

Basic questionnaires on canine behaviour can be easily completed at each visit to encourage routine assessment. Questionnaires should be standardized so that no topic is left uncovered for any patient, and should provide the veterinarian with background data about the dog's history and husbandry. Such data are particularly important if the dog has a behavioural condition that may be genetic in origin or if the veterinarian has not had the dog as a patient since puppyhood. Additional questionnaires can focus on specific behaviours (eg, problems with elimination, interactions with humans or other animals, etc). These questionnaires give clients the vocabulary and opportunity to discuss their pet's behaviours with their veterinarian in an efficient, consistent, and meaningful way. If the veterinarian suspects a problem, but feels that more data are needed, the clients can complete the questionnaires about specific behaviours again in a month or two. When the answers are compared, any trends will become clear and early intervention is then possible. For veterinarians who do not wish to formulate their own questionnaires, there are many published examples that can be incorporated into daily practice. When used continuously from the outset of the relationship with a particular pet, these tools will allow the veterinarian to intervene before many behaviour problems become complex.

Veterinarians should also assess how the clients have "trained' their dog and how they have tried to alter the dog's behaviours. The answers may indicate either deliberate or inadvertent abuse. In the USA, the Association of Pet Dog

Trainers and American Humane have published guidelines for appropriate and humane training and behaviour modification. Without questioning the client about their training experiences, the veterinarian cannot discuss less desirable techniques and explain why replacing them with modern and humane techniques is so important. For clients who are stuck in an abuse cycle, the veterinarian may be able to direct them to help that they otherwise would not have received had the vet not known how the dog was "disciplined."

Because behavioural diagnoses cannot be made on the basis of a one-time event, having the client complete a questionnaire at each visit can clarify the pattern of the animal's behaviour. The veterinarian can then ask if the pattern of nonspecific signs (eg, barking, growling, lunging, etc) meets specified diagnostic criteria (eg, fear aggression, protective aggression, etc). The veterinarian and the client must use the same definitions for the same nonspecific signs, and they both must accurately recognise and describe individual behaviours and behavioural sequences that are a concern. Videotapes of patient behaviours can ensure that such communication occurs. Questionnaires rely on client reports and because of this are more subjective. However, when combined with videotapes, the veterinarian can use questionnaires to assess whether the behaviours meet certain diagnostic criteria and how accurately the client can recognise the affiliated patterns. Client understanding and compliance are critical if patients with behavioural disorders are to improve. Only when clients can recognise the behaviours leading to or associated with the problematic ones can they avoid or prevent the provocative situation. By showing the client the problematic behaviour on videotape and then working with him or her to substitute a more desirable response, the veterinarian is able to preserve the human-animal bond and help treat the condition.

Principles of Behaviour Modification and Treatment

The most commonly used behavioural techniques include habituation, extinction, desensitization, counterconditioning, and shaping. Flooding is often talked about but seldom used because it has the potential to make most animals worse. While it is claimed that punishment is frequently used, with varying degrees of success, few people correctly employ punishment. For punishment to occur, the aversive stimulus (eg, screaming at the dog, startling the cat with a loud noise, etc) must occur sufficiently close to the onset of the behaviour that the probability of the behaviour occurring in the future is lessened. Most aversive stimuli are inappropriate in context, duration, or time of application and are more about the client's anger than about changing the behaviour.

Most of the humane, passive, or positive techniques involved in behaviour modification are not hard to learn and are equally successfully employed as preventive techniques. The following is a short review of the basic principles involved in the techniques and their associated strategies.

Habituation: Habituation is an elementary form of learning that involves no rewards. It is merely the cessation or decrease in a response to a stimulus that results from repeated or prolonged exposure to that stimulus. The stimulus can be positive, neutral, or negative. For example, horses placed in a pasture bordering a road may at first run away when traffic passes, but eventually learn to ignore it. As would be expected, stimuli associated with potentially adverse consequences are more difficult to extinguish with habituation than other stimuli. In prey species, responses to sounds associated with predators should be difficult to habituate because they have been selected for and generally are adaptive; the predator does not have to be present very often for the response to be rewarded. Furthermore, if such responses are even occasionally rewarded, the habituation response will be inhibited. In such circumstances, prolonged exposure to the stimulus may be associated with hypervigilance, exhaustion, and increased anxiety. In fact, this is one explanation for the feedback between anxiety and environmental events, even in situations when the anxiety is pathologic and potentially maladaptive.

Spontaneous Recovery: This phenomenon is associated with habituation. If there is an extended interval between the time the animal last experienced a stimulus to which it had habituated and re-exposure to the stimulus, the animal may again react. Habituation usually occurs more rapidly following spontaneous recovery if no overt fearful associations are involved.

Dishabituation

Dishabituation is the reinstatement of a habituated response as a result of exposure to a stimulus that provokes a response similar to the original. The classic examples of this involve mildly fearful responses—if habituation had just occurred to a certain hand gesture, and another movement occurred that was also worrisome for the animal, the animal could dishabituate to the hand gesture. Rehabituation is the rule unless the event is compounded and made more fearful, or the animal's reaction is extreme (suggesting something innate about the animal's response, not the event itself).

Conditioning: Conditioning refers to associations between stimuli and responses. Classical conditioning does not require a reward structure to make these associations, while operant or instrumental conditioning uses a reward structure. In operant conditioning, learning is fastest if the positive reinforcer occurs immediately (within 0.5 sec).

Delayed and intermittent reinforcements slow the acquisition of the response but work well to reinforce its maintenance. In addition to timing (quantity), value (quality) is also important—the more an animal values a reinforcer, the more quickly and reliably it will acquire the response. Hence, a food treat that dogs do not usually get (eg, cheese, boiled chicken, etc) will be better than their standard kibble in teaching them a new behaviour. It is important to realise that not all dogs value food above all else—some prefer interactive play or petting.

Reinforcement

Reinforcement is the application of a stimulus or an event that increases the probability that a certain behaviour or class of behaviours will be repeated. A positive reinforcer is a stimulus or an event that occurs after a response that leads to an increase in the response in the future. A negative reinforcer is an aversive event or stimulus that increases the frequency of a behaviour, but does so through escape or avoidance. Because people tend to use negative reinforcers in a way consistent with the potential for abuse, they should be avoided by those who feel less than absolutely confident in their timing and control.

Negative reinforcement is *not* to be confused with punishment. Punishment is the application of an aversive or negative stimulus after a response, which leads to a decrease in the frequency of the response. Negative reinforcement is the removal of an aversive stimulus that then leads to an increase in a response.

Second-order reinforcers are signals that can be used at a distance to convey that the reward or the valuable stimulus is coming. Commonly used second-order reinforcers are words ("Good girl!"), hand signals, and clickers or whistles.

By carefully pairing these with the reward with which the response to the command has already been paired, second-order reinforcers can elicit the same response as the reward would (at least temporarily—suddenly switching from a first-order reward to only a second-order one should not be done without at least intermittent pairing of the first- and second-order rewards).

"Positive" training and "clicker" training have recently become fashionable. It is possible to do an excellent job at positive training without using any secondary reinforcers. Clicker training requires frequent practice and excellent timing. In situations involving problem behaviours, the animal must be confused as seldom as possible.

The incorrect use of clickers may hinder, rather than expedite, a behaviour modification program. However, the correct use of clickers is an excellent way to immediately "mark" desirable responses or to associate a positive emotional response with the stimulus. A competent trainer and clear and accurate instructions are therefore needed.

Stimulus and Response Generalization

This occurs when an operantly or classically conditioned response is provoked not only by the object or event that originally provoked it, but by similar objects or events. A common example of stimulus response generalization in dogs is to people in uniforms: if a delivery person or metre-reader initially scared the dog or provoked a protective response, this response may then be generalized to others in uniform although the circumstances might not be the same. The more similar the original and subsequent stimuli are, the more similar the responses will be. Stimulus and response generalization may be associated with the development of profoundly anxious or fearful and phobic responses, and understanding this may be key to diminishing the worrisome behaviour.

Extinction: A response that ceases when reinforcement/reward is stopped is called extinction. A classic example of extinction of a response involves the dog that jumps up on people for attention.

If people pet the dog, the behaviour continues; if they stop at once and forever, the dog will eventually extinguish its response because the reward is no longer there. However, any form of intermittent reinforcement—even occasional petting of the dog in response to its jumping—will enhance the continuation of the response.

The more valuable the original reinforcer, the longer the reinforcement has been continuing, and the more uncertainty there is about whether the response has been truly removed (ie, presence or absence of intermittent reinforcement), the greater the resistance to extinction.

Resistance to extinction can also occur even without reinforcement, if the reward was good enough and it is tightly coupled with the behaviour. Because there is often an association between eliciting the reward and the intensity or rapidity of the performance of the behaviour, the intensity or frequency of the behaviour one is attempting to extinguish usually increases at the beginning of an extinction process. It is critical that clients *not* give in. Giving in will only make extinction more difficult because the animal has learned that although the client's threshold has increased, the animal can override it.

Overlearning: Overlearning is the repeated evocation and expression of an already learned response. It is a phenomenon that is frequently employed in training for specific events, but may be underused in preventing fearful responses in dogs. Overlearning accomplishes 3 things: it delays forgetting, it increases the resistance to extinction, and it increases the probability that the response will become a "knee-jerk" one, or response of first choice, when the circumstances are similar. This last aspect can be extremely useful in teaching an animal to overcome a fear or anxiety.

Shaping: This learning technique works well for animals that do not know what response is desired by the trainer. Shaping works through gradual approximations and allows the animal to be rewarded initially for any behaviour that resembles the desired behaviour. For instance, when teaching a puppy to sit, following a slight squat with a food reward will enhance the probability that squatting will be repeated. This squatting behaviour is then rewarded only when it becomes more exaggerated, and finally, when it becomes a true sit.

Avoidance: Avoidance is essential until clients can seek qualified help, particularly in the case of aggression. With treatment it may be possible to desensitize the dog to circumstances in which aggressive behaviour is exhibited, but avoidance is key in minimizing danger. Clients may be concerned that avoidance means that the dog will now have control, ie, that they are giving in to the dog. This is not what is happening; rather, the dog is not being given the chance to exert control in the manner to which it is accustomed. Every time a dog becomes aggressive, it learns that aggression may help it cope with the situation, thus reinforcing the problem. Even if the event is eventually aborted by an outside force, they learn the experience of exhibiting aggression.

Desensitization: Desensitization is a decrement in response that is produced by gradual exposure to a stimulus that elicits the response. For example, if a puppy has become fearful of or stimulated by the doorbell, use of a tape recording of the doorbell could help stop the undesired response. If the tape is played very softly at first and then only gradually increased in volume at increments designed to elicit no response, the puppy may become desensitized to the doorbell.

In counterconditioning, negative or undesirable behaviour is extinguished or controlled by teaching the animal to do another behaviour (preferably favourable and fun) that competitively interferes with the execution of the undesirable behaviour. This is best coupled with desensitization. In the doorbell example, the puppy will learn faster if it is first taught to sit, stay, and relax in exchange for a treat. The puppy must be absolutely quiet and calm, and convey by the look in its eyes, body posture, and facial expressions that it would do anything for its owner. Once this behaviour is learned, the desensitization component is added by playing the tape recording at gradually increasing volume. Performing the adoration act for a food reward is incompatible with or competitively exclusive of barking. If at any point the puppy starts to act anxious or to not attend to the client, the tape recording should be lowered in volume until it can relax again. Relaxing is the key—the sitting and staying is merely a facilitator for the relaxation. There is no point in having the dog sit and stay if it is clearly distressed. Relaxation is the first step to changing the behaviour.

Counterconditioning coupled with desensitization is an extremely time-consuming technique. The exercises must be constantly repeated so that the response lessens until there is none, and all the patient's communicatory signals must be considered. Clients who are least successful with this technique want both quicker fixes and less work. However, moving too quickly provokes anxiety and sabotages any behaviour modification program.

Flooding: Flooding involves prolonged exposure at a level that provokes the response so that the animal eventually gives up. This is exactly the opposite of the approach taken in desensitization. It is far more stressful than any of the other therapy strategies and, used inappropriately, could damage the animal. The most common side effect is enhanced fear. This technique should be used only by those with extensive experience and as a last resort.

Aversive Conditioning/Punishment: This strategy involves the presentation of an aversive stimulus in response to an inappropriate or undesirable behaviour; the stimulus is intended to abort the behaviour and to decrease the probability of it occurring in the future (the correct definition of punishment). To be most successful, the stimulus designed to abort the behaviour must occur as early as possible but certainly within the first 30-60 sec of the onset of the behavioural sequence, and it must be consistent and appropriate. The critical factors in punishment include timing, consistency, appropriate intensity, and the presence of a conditioned response (ie, when the undesirable behaviour ends there must be some favourable stimulus or reward, even if it is just praise or a pat). This is the most frequently ignored part of therapy for people whose pets have behavioural problems. People often resort to physical punishment as the correction method of choice, but punishment does not need to be physical. Furthermore, "good" punishment is just as hard work as appropriately executed counterconditioning and desensitization. Punishment is never an "easy out" and has a high probability of failure unless the client understands that its focus is to decrease the probability of future inappropriate events.

Principles of Pharmacologic Treatment

Facile drug use, particularly in the absence of a diagnosis, is not a component of rational treatment and should be avoided. Drug treatment for almost any behavioural condition is most useful when combined with behaviour modification. Prior to incorporating behavioural pharmacology into any treatment program, practitioners should have a reasonable diagnosis or list of diagnoses, an appreciation for the putative mechanism of action of the available drugs, and a clear understanding of potential side effects. In addition, they should have some idea of how the drug will specifically alter the behaviour in question. This is critical because it will not only help clients to watch for adverse effects and improvements, but can also help confirm or reject the original diagnosis. Without these guidelines, behavioural drugs may not be given long enough or at a sufficient dosage to attain the desired effect, clients will be unable to participate in the evaluation process, and there will be no objective behavioural criteria with which to assess improvement.

It is important to teach clients to be observant and recognise specific signs of potential adverse reactions. Such reactions can be minimized by performing a premedication CBC, urinalysis, and serum biochemistry profile and by taking a complete behavioural and medical history.

Baseline ECGs are recommended for patients with a history of arrhythmia, heart disease, or prior drug reactions; that are on more than one medication; or that may undergo anesthesia or sedation. Liver dyscrasias and cardiac arrhythmias may not rule out the use of a drug, but knowing that they exist can serve as a guide to dosage and anticipated side effects. Because clients may be distressed after a behavioural consultation, a written reminder of situations for which they should be alert may be helpful. It should also be kept in mind that with few exceptions (eg, clomipramine for separation anxiety in dogs, selegiline for cognitive dysfunction in dogs), the use of the majority of medications prescribed for behavioural problems in pets is extra-label.

Most medications used to treat behavioural problems are tricyclic antidepressants or selective serotonin reuptake inhibitors. Prolonged treatment may be necessary for some pets to prevent relapse, but with good physical and laboratory monitoring there are few associated risks. *See Table: Drugs that May Be Useful in the Treatment of Canine Behavioural Diagnoses* and *Table: Drugs that May Be Useful in the Treatment of Feline Behavioural Diagnoses* for recommended dosages for canine and feline behavioural drugs. There have been few well-designed, prospective clinical trials of medication use for behavioural problems in animals, so it should be kept in mind that many of these dosages are based on extrapolation from human use and clinical experience with pets.

Normal Social Behaviour and Behavioural Problems of Domestic Animals

Horses Social Behaviour

Domestic horses are social animals. In feral situations, they live in a harem group or band with one to several stallions, multiple mares, and those mares' offspring. One stallion (the highest-ranking or "dominant" animal) is primarily responsible for most of the breeding. In many species, rank is associated with age or some ability to survive and thrive in challenged environments. Old age can be a gauge of the latter. High-ranking males are the first to secure access to a receptive female and the first to displace a female from another band. In the absence of conception, horses cycle every 21 days, except when seasonally anovulatory (fall and winter). Within a harem group, the highest-ranking individual is usually, but not always, a stallion. This high-ranking stallion will force foals to leave the group once they are ~2 yr old, as they begin to become sexually and socially mature.

Snapping (tooth clapping or champing) is a facial expression given by young horses to adults, particularly stallions. It peaks in frequency at 2 mo of age, after which it decreases; it may function to decrease aggression from adults, but is also compatible with displaced nursing behaviour. This is not the same behaviour as smacking, which is an aggressive threat in which the ears are laid back and the mouth is open with lips smacking, but the lips are not retracted. Social maturity is not attained until 5 yr of age. Most fillies and all colts leave the natal herd at about this age. Fillies that remain in their natal group may have decreased reproductive success. Young stallions form bachelor herds, and the highest-ranking stallion within this group is usually the next one to acquire a mate. Fillies can join a bachelor herd but are often incorporated into other bands. Stallions are rarely solitary; when this occurs, the stallions appear to be old or infirm.

While hierarchical rank in males is evaluated primarily on the basis of access to females, hierarchical rank in females is determined by effect on group behaviour and activity (ie, seeking out resources such as water holes). Horse groups are largely structured by females, and females make the decision about whether to leave or to stay within a harem.

Such decisions are usually based not on specific stallions or their characteristics, but on the female's assessment of food resources. High-ranking females can successfully interfere with the nursing of foals by lower-ranking females. Mares have preferred associates, are preferentially groomed, and will groom certain individuals. This pattern is typical of many social animals in that rank is conferred largely by the deference of other animals—not by the results of outright combat. Hierarchical relationships within groups also depend on the age and sex distribution of the group. The more members of the herd, and the more within each age and sex group, the less likely it is for a linear dominance hierarchy to exist. Relationships within most horse bands are triangular and complex.

Hierarchical rank depends on multiple factors and probably their interaction, eg, age or length of residence in the social group, sex (although probably less important than age), size, and inheritance (rank of the mother). These factors are important to consider when addressing problems that may arise in stabled horses. Hierarchical social effects also exist between herds. Multi-stallion herds are dominant over single-stallion bands, possibly because lower-ranking stallions within a herd conduct most of the fighting that occurs between groups.

Herds that are currently occupying an area or using a resource (eg, a water hole) tend to retain it. Groups, as well as individuals within them, follow specific patterns of fecal marking.

Many behavioural problems are associated with confinement. Under free-ranging circumstances, horses will wander and spend >60% of their day foraging. The remainder of their time is spent standing, lying down, or engaging in another activity. This same pattern is the preferred one under barn conditions; even with free choice of grain, horses will choose to eat many small meals a day. Horses also use free-ranging locomotion as part of their play development. Until ~3 mo of age, most play is solitary. Interactive play peaks at 3-4 mo of age. There are sex differences in play; colts play more than fillies and play different games than do fillies. Colt games focus more on fighting and mounting, while filly games focus more on running and mutual grooming. Fillies will groom both colts and fillies; colts tend to groom only fillies, which has been interpreted as practice for later courtship behaviour.

Recent data on the role of play in carnivores suggests such behaviours may be best interpreted as learning how to make and recover from social mistakes. The ability to make a mistake successfully may be more important than previously appreciated. The social experience of play is important for normal social interaction in adult life.

Behavioural Problems

Aggression to People or Savagery: The most common correlates of aggression to people are sexual behaviour, dominance-associated/impulse dyscontrol aggression (abnormal and out-of-context) and fear. Understanding which of these is occurring will greatly aid in treatment. Fear can be induced by the behavioural environment (eg, physical abuse or harsh treatment) or by the physical environment (eg, night blindness associated with confinement in a dark stall followed by introduction to pasture with other horses). Savage horses that are exhibiting dominance-associated/impulse dyscontrol aggression behaviour toward people have been considered too dangerous to keep. There have been cases of horses killing people in such circumstances. The extent to which early intervention can help modulate these behaviours is unknown.

Treatment involves counterconditioning and desensitization, using rewards for nonaggressive approaches. Rewards could be frequent feedings of highly desirable foods (eg, molasses, apples, vanilla, watermelon), attention, caretaking (epimeletic) behaviours such as grooming, or exercise. The purpose of the frequent feedings is to mimic the natural grazing situation and to associate that and the food reward with the person's presence. All aggressive animals should probably be neutered because there appears to be a genetic basis (albeit poorly understood) for most aggressions, and removal of hormones is associated with less reactive behaviours. Progestins have been recommended as a substitute for castration or ovariohys-terectomy but have many side effects that involve multiple organ systems and render the reproductive option moot.

More forceful interventions include techniques designed to increase the equine perception of vulnerability and may include hobbling, the use of paralytic agents (succinylcholine), and controlling access and frequency of light. Because of the danger involved, people have been less willing to try neuropharmacologic intervention, instead resorting to euthanasia. If recognised early, treatment with selective serotonin reuptake inhibitors (eg, fluoxetine) may be successful when combined with behaviour modification.

Horses like to turn on lights and can be rewarded with the ability to do so. Horses are prey species and are wary of dogs and other predators; learning to associate light with people, especially if coupled with positive reinforcement, may help.

Aggression to Horses: Aggression to other horses is usually associated with sex, secondary to a fear as described above, or idiosyncratic. Horses have preferred grooming and grazing partners; the extent to which these preferences may be a factor in aggression to other horses is unknown. Treatment can include castration, the use of progestins, and desensitization and counterconditioning that require that the horses are fed by the handler only when in each others' presence. This can be done gradually by introducing horses across one or two fences so that they do not injure each other. Two fences are optimal because they reduce the possibility that the horses could strike each other with their feet. Shock has also been used to treat aggression to horses, based on the principle that fleeing will be rendered undesirable, while concomitantly rendering attack punitive. In cases of profound fear or anxiety, shock will usually either worsen the aggression or render other aspects of the horse's behaviour undesirable. Horses are a prey species and have a heightened avoidance system. Accordingly, shock may produce a cessation of the undesirable behaviour but also render the horse less interactive, more wary, and more fearful in general. Animal welfare concerns should be a rational component of any cogent behavioural treatment.

Wood-Chewing: Wood-chewing may be a residual behaviour associated with the equid pattern of browsing. Under free-ranging circumstances, horses will graze 12-14 hr/day. Most wood-chewing occurs in the winter, and it appears to be seen more often in horses that are fed pelleted diets. If horses receive <1 kg of hay/100 kg body wt, wood-chewing can become extreme. It is important to address the primary problem (ie, learn why the horse is engaging in this behaviour), rather than merely trying to prevent it, which can make the horse even more secretive.

Treatment involves increasing both roughage (hay, sawdust, etc) and exercise through work or increased pasture time. Because of the social factors involved in grazing under free-ranging conditions, animals who chew wood may have less easily recognised, but still extant, social needs that are unmet.

Coprophagia

Coprophagia is a normal behaviour in foals that may play a role in B-vitamin supplementation and influence the intestinal flora. It is most common in the first month of life, after which it usually declines. When it is seen in adults, it is usually associated with low roughage, low protein, or a dietary deficiency. In these cases, the primary dietary problem must be addressed; treatment always involves increasing the amount of roughage in the diet and may involve increasing the amount of protein.

Pica: In horses, pica is usually manifest by ingestion of sand or gravel and can result in colonic impaction. In profound circumstances, this may be a ritualistic behaviour. Early intervention is important and involves providing the horse with alternative substances that are acceptable (eg, increasing hay). Texture may be important, and the addition of roughage and salt blocks may have a role. In small animals, such behaviours appear to have familial associations, but comparable data are lacking for horses.

Anorexia: Horses form close affiliative attachments with other horses, and anorexia can be associated with changes in these relationships. The most common situation involves separation anxiety in the absence of a preferred equine companion. Addressing the underlying social problem through social facilitation is critical, and treatment with anxiolytic drugs that may also stimulate appetite (eg, benzodiazepines such as diazepam) can help.

Foals usually feed when the mare feeds. During the first month, foals graze only 5 min/hr, but this increases to 45 min/hr by 6 mo of age. Accordingly, weaning methods may be important to prevent anorexia in young horses. Aggressive mares may attack foals that try to share food. Barriers should be erected that safely permit normal development and feeding patterns. Foals may not eat the same plant or same plant part as the mare, and the parts they choose may be based on the height of the plant. Management should address this problem. Creep feeders should be placed near the mare so that the foal does not have to choose between food and contact with its dam. Foals on pasture and those that are nursing do not drink water, but the mares need access to good, clean water.

Obesity: Obesity can be the result of decreased exercise, increased palatable food, and under-stimulation (horses that eat in the absence of other activities). To avoid hyperlipemia, food should not be abruptly removed from obese horses. Reducing intake (by feeding the horse decreased amounts) while increasing exercise is preferable. Horses fed rations that are calorically diluted will compensate by eating more if fed ad lib.

Stall Walking or Circling: Confined, stabled horses can spend >25% of their time in nondirected motor activity within their stall. They may become exhausted or tangled in their bedding; in warm climates, they may become overheated. Classic stall walking or circling is usually in response to separation from another horse or to claustrophobia; it is usually rapid and accompanied by vocalization. Clients should watch for nonspecific signs of anxiety (eg, pacing, startling, changes in typical ingestive and elimination behaviours, changes in vocalization, etc) when stablemates or housing conditions change. The less appreciated form of stall walking involves stereotypic behaviour. In this case, the motor activity itself becomes a manifestation of an obsessive-compulsive disorder; it is not accompanied by vocalization. Treatment should address the primary problem, including increasing exercise; providing social company (which need not be a horse); allowing the horse to see other horses; providing thick, clean bedding; feeding frequently (or at least twice per day); providing more open stalls and better access to outside views; and antianxiety or anti-obsessive-compulsive medication. Stall toys are unlikely to fix the problem unless the horse is young and frisky and played with the toys before the problem became apparent.

Weaving: Weaving occurs when a horse that stall walks is tied or prohibited from walking because of restricted space. Horses prohibited from performing other locomotor movements weave. Treatment includes untying the horse, providing a larger stall, turning the horse out onto pasture, and the other treatments recommended for stall walking.

Pawing: Pawing is a potentially injurious behaviour because it can change the surface of the floor and can cause wear to the horses' hooves. It is a normal, anticipatory behaviour and can occur when horses on winter pasture are forced to dig for feed. When horses are confined and fed highly palatable foods, pawing can occur more frequently and more intensely than it would otherwise. Pawing also may be associated with signalling that accompanies escape behaviour. The underlying problem should be identified to determine treatment, which should not be directed solely at the nonspecific behaviour of pawing. Specific treatments are as for stall walking. The pawing should not be rewarded, which is what inadvertently happens when horses paw in anticipation of feeding. The food should be presented to the horse only when the horse is not pawing, or the horse should be brought to the food.

Kicking: Kicking damages horses' legs and stalls. It is often an aggressive behaviour that appears when another horse is nearby or when the horse perceives that another horse is nearby. Kicking can also occur in anticipation of food or environmental stimulation (as does pawing). It may occur when the horse cannot achieve its goals (eg, exercise, mating opportunities, monitoring the outside world, etc). All nonspecific kicking is not the same; the underlying basis for the kicking should be determined and treated. Treatment is as for stall walking. If aggression is involved, it may require rearranging the social grouping in the barn. Horses can find their own compatible neighbours and can be permitted to choose their own stalls. Hand-feeding the horse can be one way to implement counterconditioning, ie, the horse is fed only when calm and quiet.

Cribbing

Cribbing (windsucking, crib biting) is a distinct behaviour, different from wood-chewing, that involves grasping a horizontal surface with the incisors and flexing the neck without swallowing air. In extreme cases, the horse may do this 3,000 times/day. The activity makes a strange, nonflatulent sound. Cribbing is most easily diagnosed by noting the missing U-shaped pieces from the available fencing. Horses that crib have worn teeth and develop thick neck muscles. Cribbers tend to have lower levels of endogenous opiates, and cribbing is postulated to stimulate opiate release. Accordingly, treatment with exogenous opiate blockers (eg, naloxone, nalmefene) may help because it blocks a self-perpetuating loop. Some sweet (and palatable) feeds may also release endogenous opiates and worsen cribbing through positive feedback. Therefore, treatment may involve increasing roughage in the diet, changing companions, and providing greater access to more varied environments (eg, pasture). Unless the horse is very thin or afflicted by flatulent colic, it may be easiest to do nothing.

The assertion that horses learn to crib from other horses has never been substantiated. Cribbing may be more closely related to the group conditions and any resultant anxiety. Cribbing straps prevent the behaviour (in theory) by placing pressure on the horse, causing pain when the neck is flexed. Highly motivated horses will crib despite the straps; in such cases, the cribbing may be more a manifestation of an obsessive-compulsive disorder, and treatment with an antiobsessive-compulsive drug may be useful. Experimentally, treatment with narcotic antagonists has reduced cribbing, but these may not be practical for longterm use. Surgical treatments that have been recommended but are often unsuccessful include ventral accessory neurectomy and myotomy. It may be preferable to address the social, physical (eg, duration and form of exercise), and welfare needs of the horse prior to resorting to surgery. If the horse is harming itself when cribbing, a cribbing muzzle may be useful.

Self-Mutilation: This may be due to an underlying medical problem (eg, a dermatologic or GI condition involving colic and parasitemia). The progression of the problem should help differentiate a medical problem from one that is primarily behavioural. In horses, most self-mutilation involves biting of the limbs, chest, or flanks. Self-mutilation can appear in sexually frustrated (usually male) or socially incompatible horses, or as a manifestation of an obsessive-compulsive disorder. Treatment should involve correction of the underlying condition. Self-mutilation associated with sexual frustration can be addressed by castration, pasturing with a mare, removing all mares (or horses that induce the behaviour, if the problem is primarily social) from the environment, increasing exercise, increasing roughage and decreasing grain, and treatment with progestins or opiate blockers. In the case of an obsessive-compulsive disorder, treatment should involve behavioural and environmental modification and antianxiety or anti-obsessive-compulsive medication.

Foal Rejection

Foal rejection is seen in 3 main forms: mares that will accept the foal but will not let it suckle, mares that are fearful of the foal and run away, and mares that exhibit stallion-like behaviour and attempt to kick and bite the foal. Mares may paw at foals to stimulate them to rise from recumbency. This behaviour must be differentiated from rejection. Mares can kill their foals if they are experiencing a nutritional stress, and this can be a normal, although uncommon behaviour.

The first step in treatment is to protect the foal. If the mare will accept the foal but not let it suckle, the mare should be helped for several nursings until she learns that suckling is pleasurable. Holding her in such a way that she cannot injure the foal may involve either cross-ties or partial barriers through which she can see and smell the foal but that prohibit her from reaching for it. The mare should be examined for mastitis in case she is refusing to suckle because of a painful udder. Pressure resulting from infrequent nursings can be treated using warm water baths and soaks, light massage using a hose, and milking the mare. Foals can suckle up to every 5 min for the first few days of their life, so access to the nipple is important. This nursing and contact form the basis for an ongoing maternal-foal bond. Mares that are afraid of their foals should be treated in the same manner, but the addition of relaxation cues (including darker, quieter stalls and food treats) and mild tranquilizers may help. Dogs have been used to evoke maternal "herding" behaviour by stimulating the mare to protect the foal from a potential threat. Mares that attempt to injure their foals must be restrained using stocks or bars. At the same time, the mare can be counterconditioned (preferably prior to foaling) using a stanchion and positive reward. Olfactory and hormonal cues may be important. Noses of mares and foals can be rubbed with fetal membranes, or immediate postpartum cervical stimulation can be practiced. Both of these may stimulate mares to lick, which is important in the first phase of attachment. Mares that lick exuberantly in the first hour may be willing to adopt an orphaned foal. After the first hour postpartum, licking behaviour decreases and is replaced by nickering between the foal and mare. These are characteristic behaviours that can be monitored in the course of normal development of the mare-foal bond. Tranquilization can be helpful, if relatively mild uncertainty and anxiety are involved.

Poor Libido: Stallions experience poor libido if they are overused for breeding, have experienced inhibition through the use of antimasturbation devices, are used out of season, or are injured while breeding. Experience is paramount with stallions, and all of these etiologies support the role of bad experiences; owners who want to restrict show or performance horses from masturbating should be so informed. Masturbation is a normal equine behaviour and there is no truth to the myth that masturbation depletes semen value—horses that masturbate rarely ejaculate. Although measurement of testosterone levels may be worthwhile, it is usually uninformative because few horses are truly testosterone-deficient. Stallions that have poor libido should be rested if overused. Letting such stallions watch other stallions mate may have a beneficial effect on their libido.

Providing them with a variety of teaser mares, mating partners (the Coolidge effect, ie, an increase in mating attempts following introduction of a new partner), and other stallions can also stimulate their interest. Pasturing with a mare in estrus may help. Using an artificial vagina to desensitize a stallion that has been injured can be useful. Treatment with diazepam (to address anxiety) and oxytocin, testosterone, or gonadotropin-releasing hormone (to address the hormonal basis of erection, intromission, and ejaculation) can help. Stallions that will intromit, but not ejaculate, may benefit from hormone-based treatments.

Aggression When Breeding: Stallions that are aggressive when used for breeding are often overused or used out of season. These stallions can benefit from the use of an artificial vagina out of season so that they learn that the experience is pleasurable. Stallions can develop preferences for mating and may not be compatible with the chosen mare; changing the mare may help.

If stallions were stabled with mares when they were colts, they may have some social inhibition for mating, and forced mating can result in aggression. The social role is also emphasized by the finding that there is more breeding/hr if bachelor stallions are present. Physical devices (eg, hobbles) or pharmacologic intervention (eg, succinylcholine) have been used to control stallions and to induce learned helplessness. Treating the primary aggression is preferred.

Nymphomania

Nymphomaniac mares "wink" (show clitoris), squat, and urinate frequently. Urine scalding is a real, secondary problem. Mating behaviours and those involved in solicitation are not considered abnormal if they occur every 21 days when the mares cycle. Treatments usually focus on the underlying physiologic correlates of the behaviours. Nympho-maniac mares should be checked for granulosa cell tumors. Treatment has involved the use of progestins and ovariohy-sterectomy. If behaviour problems persist after ovariohysterectomy, the use of dexamethasone will suppress adrenal androgens.

Psychic Estrus: Mares with psychic estrus show estrous behaviour without any of the physiologic correlates of heat. Treatment is as for nymphomania.

Silent Estrus: Mares exhibiting silent estrus show all of the physiologic correlates of heat without any of the behavioural signs. Tape-recorded sounds of a stallion soliciting mares and breeding them can help, as can the presence of stallion odor. The presence of a known stallion with whom the mare has a good social relationship can help. It may be necessary to permanently or temporarily wean the last foal.

Intraspecific Mounting: Intraspecific mounting is usually mare-mare. Males seldom mount other males unless they bite them, in which case aggression is the primary problem. Mares that mount other mares should be checked for granulosa cell tumors. This can be a normal behaviour in some estrous or pregnant mares.

Geldings that Act Like Stallions: Geldings that act like stallions will mount mares, attack foals, fight with other males, and self-mutilate. Some of these geldings are "proud cut" and have residual epididymis. Retained testes may also be implicated. Geldings that still have testosterone may have larger manes, tails, and forelocks than other geldings in their cohort. These geldings can destabilize other social relationships. The behaviour of the geldings can encompass the entire range of mating-associated behaviours, including herding, courting (piaf), and flehmen responses. Treatment involves protecting the rest of the group (ie, removing the mares and foals) and using progestins or cyproheptadine, which may block release of adrenocorticotropic hormone from the pituitary gland, or the newer selective serotonin reuptake inhibitors, which address the increased reactivity at a central level.

Bibliography

Adams, H. Richard: *Veterinary pharmacology and therapeutics*, Wiley-Blackwell, NY, 2011.

Aspinall, Victoria; Cappello, Melanie; Bowden, Sally; Jeffery, Andrea,: *Introduction to Veterinary Anatomy and Physiology Textbook*, Elsevier Health Sciences, 2019.

Baker, Rebecca, and Lumsden, John H.: *Colour Atlas of Cytology of the Dog and Cat,* Mosby, St. Louis, MO, 2010.

Boden, Edward; West, Geoffrey Philip.: *Black's Veterinary dictionary*, Rowman & Littlefield, 2008.

Bryant, Susan: *Anesthesia for Veterinary Technicians*, John Wiley and Sons, NY, 2018.

Campbell, Terry W.: *Avian Hematology and Cytology,* Iowa State University Press, IA, 2015.

Cannon, Martha; Hijfte, Myra Forster-van (2006), *Feline medicine: a practical guide for veterinary nurses and technicians*, Elsevier Health Sciences, 2017.

Capen, Charles C.: *Pathobiology of the Aging Dog*. Iowa State University Press, Ames, IA, 2011.

Cowell, Rick L., and Tyler, Ronald D.: *Diagnostic Cytology and Hematology of the Horse,* Mosby, St. Louis, MO, 2021.

Feldman, Bernard F.: *Schalm's Veterinary Hematology,* Lippincott Williams & Wilkins, Philadelphia, PA, 2000.

Goldschmidt, Michael H., and Shofer, Francis: *Skin Tumors of the Dog and Cat,* Butterworth-Heinemann, Woburn, MA, 2004.

Gopinath, C.: *Atlas of Experimental Toxicological Pathology,* MTP Press, Lancaster, UK, 2009.

Griner, Lynn A.: *Pathology of Zoo Animals: A Review of Necropsies Conducted Over a Fourteen-Year Period at the San Diego Zoo,* Zoological Society of San Diego, San Diego, CA, 2013.

Jones, Thomas Carlyle: *Veterinary Pathology,* Williams & Wilkins, Baltimore, MD, 2017.

Latimer, Kenneth S.: *Duncan and Prasse's Veterinary Laboratory Medicine: Clinical Pathology,* Iowa State University Press, Ames, IA, 2013.

Maronpot, Robert: *Pathology of the Mouse,* Cache River Press, Vienna, IL, 2019.

McEntee, Kenneth: *Reproductive Pathology of Domestic Mammals,* Academic Press, San Diego, CA, 2010.

McGavin, M. Donald: *Thomson's Special Veterinary Pathology,* Mosby, St. Louis, MO, 2011.

Percy, Dean H., and Barthold, Stephen W.: *Pathology of Laboratory Rodents and Rabbits,* Iowa State University Press, Ames, IA, 2011.

Raskin, Rose E., and Meyer, Denny J.: *Atlas of Canine and Feline Cytology,* W. B. Saunders, Philadelphia, PA, 2011.

Roberts, Ronald J.: *Fish Pathology,* W. B. Saunders, New York, 2019.

Slauson, David O., and Cooper, Barry J.: *Mechanisms of Disease: A Textbook of Comparative General Pathology,* Mosby, St. Louis, MO, 2020.

Stockham, Steven L., and Scott, Michael A.: *Fundamentals of Veterinary Clinical Pathology,* Iowa State Press, Ames, IA, 2020.

Summers, Brian A.: *Veterinary Neuropathology,* Mosby, St. Louis, MO, 2015.

Ward, Jerrold Michael: *Pathology of Genetically Engineered Mice,* Iowa State University Press, Ames, IA, 2010.

Wynn, Susan G., and Marsden, Steve: *Manual of Natural Veterinary Medicine: Science and Tradition,* Mosby, St. Louis, MO, 2013.

Index

❑❑❑